Challenges in Inflammatory Bowel Disease

Guest Editors

MIGUEL REGUEIRO, MD
ARTHUR M. BARRIE III, MD

MEDICAL CLINICS OF NORTH AMERICA

www.medical.theclinics.com

January 2010 • Volume 94 • Number 1

SAUNDERS an imprint of ELSEVIER, Inc.

W.B. SAUNDERS COMPANY
A Division of Elsevier Inc.

1600 John F. Kennedy Boulevard • Suite 1800 • Philadelphia, Pennsylvania 19103-2899

http://www.theclinics.com

MEDICAL CLINICS OF NORTH AMERICA Volume 94, Number 1
January 2010 ISSN 0025-7125, ISBN-13: 978-1-4377-1834-8

Editor: Rachel Glover
Developmental Editor: Donald Mumford

Medical Clinics of North America (ISSN 0025-7125) is published bimonthly by Elsevier Inc., 360 Park Avenue South, New York, NY 10010-1710. Months of issue are January, March, May, July, September, and November. Periodicals postage paid at New York, NY, and additional mailing offices. Subscription prices are USD 204 per year for US individuals, USD 361 per year for US institutions, USD 105 per year for US students, USD 259 per year for Canadian individuals, USD 469 per year for Canadian institutions, USD 165 per year for Canadian students, USD 314 per year for international individuals, USD 469 per year for international institutions and USD 165 per year for international students. To receive student/resident rate, orders must be accompanied by name of affiliated institution, date of term, and the *signature* of program/residency coordinator on institution letterhead. Orders will be billed at individual rate until proof of status is received. Foreign air speed delivery is included in all *Clinics* subscription prices. All prices are subject to change without notice. **POSTMASTER:** Send address changes to *Medical Clinics of North America*, Elsevier Health Sciences Division, Subscription Customer Service, 3251 Riverport Lane, Maryland Heights, MO 63043. **Customer Service: Telephone: 1-800-654-2452** (U.S. and Canada); **1-314-447-8871** (outside U.S. and Canada). **Fax: 1-314-447-8029. E-mail: journalscustomerservice-usa@elsevier.com** (for print support); **journalsonlinesupport-usa@ elsevier.com** (for online support).

Reprints. For copies of 100 or more of articles in this publication, please contact the Commercial Reprints Department, Elsevier Inc., 360 Park Avenue South, New York, NY 10010-1710. Tel.: 212-633-3812; Fax: 212-462-1935; E-mail: reprints@elsevier.com.

Medical Clinics of North America is also published in Spanish by McGraw-Hill Interamericana Editores S. A., P.O. Box 5-237, 06500 Mexico, D.F., Mexico.

Medical Clinics of North America is covered in *MEDLINE/PubMed (Index Medicus), Current Contents, ASCA, Excerpta Medica, Science Citation Index,* and *ISI/BIOMED.*

Printed in the United States of America.

GOAL STATEMENT

The goal of *Medical Clinics of North America* is to keep practicing physicians up to date with current clinical practice by providing timely articles reviewing the state of the art in patient care.

ACCREDITATION

The *Medical Clinics of North America* is planned and implemented in accordance with the Essential Areas and Policies of the Accreditation Council for Continuing Medical Education (ACCME) through the joint sponsorship of the University of Virginia School of Medicine and Elsevier. The University of Virginia School of Medicine is accredited by the ACCME to provide continuing medical education for physicians.

The University of Virginia School of Medicine designates this educational activity for a maximum of 15 *AMA PRA Category 1 Credits*™ for each issue, 90 credits per year. Physicians should only claim credit commensurate with the extent of their participation in the activity.

The American Medical Association has determined that physicians not licensed in the US who participate in this CME activity are eligible for a maximum of 15 *AMA PRA Category 1 Credits*™ for each issue, 90 credits per year.

Credit can be earned by reading the text material, taking the CME examination online at http://www.theclinics.com/home/cme, and completing the evaluation. After taking the test, you will be required to review any and all incorrect answers. Following completion of the test and evaluation, your credit will be awarded and you may print your certificate.

FACULTY DISCLOSURE/CONFLICT OF INTEREST

The University of Virginia School of Medicine, as an ACCME accredited provider, endorses and strives to comply with the Accreditation Council for Continuing Medical Education (ACCME) Standards of Commercial Support, Commonwealth of Virginia statutes, University of Virginia policies and procedures, and associated federal and private regulations and guidelines on the need for disclosure and monitoring of proprietary and financial interests that may affect the scientific integrity and balance of content delivered in continuing medical education activities under our auspices.

The University of Virginia School of Medicine requires that all CME activities accredited through this institution be developed independently and be scientifically rigorous, balanced and objective in the presentation/discussion of its content, theories and practices.

All authors/editors participating in an accredited CME activity are expected to disclose to the readers relevant financial relationships with commercial entities occurring within the past 12 months (such as grants or research support, employee, consultant, stock holder, member of speakers bureau, etc.). The University of Virginia School of Medicine will employ appropriate mechanisms to resolve potential conflicts of interest to maintain the standards of fair and balanced education to the reader. Questions about specific strategies can be directed to the Office of Continuing Medical Education, University of Virginia School of Medicine, Charlottesville, Virginia.

The faculty and staff of the University of Virginia Office of Continuing Medical Education have no financial affiliations to disclose.

The authors/editors listed below have identified no professional or financial affiliations for themselves or their spouse/partner:

Waqqas Afif, MD; Ashwin N. Ananthakrishnan, MD, MPH; Arthur M. Barrie III, MD, PhD (Guest Editor); Meenakshi Bewtra, MD, MPH; Su Min Cho, MBBS; Sung W. Cho, MBBS, MSc; Rachel Glover (Acquisitions Editor); Mazen Issa, MD; Bard E. Maltz, MD; Miguel Regueiro, MD (Guest Editor); Cary G. Sauer, MD, MSc; Andrew Wolf, MD (Test Author); Hao Wu, MB; and Timothy L. Zisman, MD, MPH.

The authors/editors listed below identified the following professional or financial affiliations for themselves or their spouse/partner:

David G. Binion, MD serves on the advisory board for Abbott Laboratories, Centocor, and UCB Pharma, and is an industry funded research/investigator for Centocor.

Shane M. Devlin, MD is on the Speakers' Bureau for Schering-Plough, Abbott, UCB, Proctor and Gamble, and Shire, and is an industry funded research/investigator and consultant for Schering-Plough.

Subra Kugathasan, MD is an industry funded research/investigator and is on the advisory committee/board for UCB and Centocor.

James D. Lewis, MD, MSCE receives research support from Takeda and Shire, and expects research support from Centocor; and is a consultant for Astra Zeneca, GlaxoSmithKline, and Millenium.

Edward V. Loftus, Jr., MD is an industry funded research/investigator for Abbott, UCB, Schering-Plough, Otsuka, and ActoGeniX, and is a consultant for Abbott, UCB, Centocor, Procter & Gamble, and Shire.

Uma Mahadevan, MD is on the Advisory Committee/Board for P+G, Centocor, UCB, Abbott, Elan, and Shire.

Remo Panaccione, MD is a consultant for Astra Zeneca, Ferring, Abbott Laboratories, Schering-Plough, Shire, Centocor and Elan Pharmaceuticals; is on the Speakers' Bureau for Astra Zeneca, Abbott Laboratories, Byk Solvay, Jansen, Schering-Plough and Centocor; is on the Advisory Board for Ferring, Abbott Laboratories, Schering-Plough, Shire and Elan Pharmaceuticals; has received educational grants from Ferring, Axcan and Schering-Plough; has received research grants from Abbott Laboratories, Schering-Plough, Centocor and Millenium Pharmaceuticals; and has received occasional honoraria from Axcan, Shire and Jansen.

David T. Rubin, MD receives grant support from Procter and Gamble Pharmaceuticals, Salix Pharmaceuticals, Prometheus Pharmaceuticals, Abbott Immunology, and Elan Pharmaceuticals; serves as a consultant for Salix Pharmaceuticals, Abbott Immunology, UCB Pharma, Shire, Millenium Pharma, Centocor, Elan Pharmaceuticals, and Genentech; and, is Co-Founder of Cornerstones Health, Inc. (non-profit medical education company).

David A. Schwartz, MD is a consultant for P&G, Abbott, UCB, Centocor, Cellerix, Shire and Axcan; and receives grant support from Abbott, UCB, and P&G.

Bo Shen, MD has a research grant from Salix, and has honorarium and a research grant from Ocera.

Disclosure of Discussion of Non-FDA Approved Uses for Pharmaceutical Products and/or Medical Devices.

The University of Virginia School of Medicine, as an ACCME provider, requires that all faculty presenters identify and disclose any off-label uses for pharmaceutical and medical device products. The University of Virginia School of Medicine recommends that each physician fully review all the available data on new products or procedures prior to clinical use.

TO ENROLL

To enroll in the Medical Clinics of North America Continuing Medical Education program, call customer service at 1-800-654-2452 or visit us online at http://www.theclinics.com/home/cme. The CME program is available to subscribers for an additional fee of USD 205.

FORTHCOMING ISSUES

March 2010
Chest Pain
Guy D. Eslick, PhD, MMedSc and
Michael Yelland, MBBS, PhD,
Guest Editors

May 2010
Sleep Medicine
Christian Guilleminault, MD,
Guest Editor

July 2010
Drug Hypersensitivity
Werner J. Pichler, MD,
Guest Editor

RECENT ISSUES

November 2009
**Cutaneous Manifestations of Internal
Diseases**
Neil S. Sadick, MD, *Guest Editor*

September 2009
Preoperative Medical Consultation
Lee A. Fleisher, MD and
Stanley H. Rosenbaum, MD,
Guest Editors

July 2009
Care of the Cirrhotic Patient
David A. Sass, MD, *Guest Editor*

RELATED INTEREST

Gastroenterology Clinics of North America, June 2009 (Volume 38, Issue 2)
Peptic Ulcer Disease
F.K.L. Chan, MD, *Guest Editor*

THE CLINICS ARE NOW AVAILABLE ONLINE!

Access your subscription at:
www.theclinics.com

Contributors

GUEST EDITORS

MIGUEL REGUEIRO, MD
Associate Professor, Department of Medicine; Associate Chief for Education;
Co-Director, Inflammatory Bowel Disease Center; Head, IBD Clinical Program; Director,
Gastroenterology Fellowship Program, University of Pittsburgh School of Medicine,
Pittsburgh, Pennsylvania

ARTHUR M. BARRIE III, MD, PhD
Assistant Professor of Medicine, University of Pittsburgh School of Medicine, Pittsburgh,
Pennsylvania

AUTHORS

WAQQAS AFIF, MD
Instructor of Medicine, Division of Gastroenterology and Hepatology, Mayo Clinic,
Rochester, Minnesota

ASHWIN N. ANANTHAKRISHNAN, MD, MPH
Fellow, Division of Gastroenterology and Hepatology, Medical College of Wisconsin,
Milwaukee, Wisconsin

MEENAKSHI BEWTRA, MD, MPH
Instructor, Division of Gastroenterology, Department of Medicine, University
of Pennsylvania, Philadelphia, Pennsylvania

DAVID G. BINION, MD
Co-Director, Inflammatory Bowel Disease Center; Director, Translational Inflammatory
Bowel Disease Research, UPMC IBD Center; Visiting Professor of Medicine,
Division of Gastroenterology, Hepatology and Nutrition, University of Pittsburgh
School of Medicine, Pittsburgh, Pennsylvania

SU MIN CHO, MBBS
Fellow in Gastroenterology, Hepatology and Nutrition, University of Pittsburgh Medical
Center, Pittsburgh, Pennsylvania

SUNG W. CHO, MBBS, MSc
Department of General Surgery, University of Pittsburgh Medical Center, Pittsburgh,
Pennsylvania

SHANE M. DEVLIN, MD
Clinical Assistant Professor, Inflammatory Bowel Disease Clinic, Division
of Gastroenterology, Department of Medicine, University of Calgary, Calgary, Alberta,
Canada

MAZEN ISSA, MD
Assistant Professor of Medicine, Division of Gastroenterology and Hepatology, Medical College of Wisconsin, Milwaukee, Wisconsin

SUBRA KUGATHASAN, MD
Professor of Pediatrics and Human Genetics, Emory University School of Medicine; Division of Pediatric Gastroenterology, Emory Children's Center, Atlanta, Georgia

JAMES D. LEWIS, MD, MSCE
Associate Professor of Medicine, Division of Gastroenterology; Center for Clinical Epidemiology and Biostatistics, University of Pennsylvania, Philadelphia, Pennsylvania

EDWARD V. LOFTUS Jr, MD
Professor of Medicine, Division of Gastroenterology and Hepatology, Mayo Clinic, Rochester, Minnesota

UMA MAHADEVAN, MD
Associate Professor of Medicine and Director of Clinical Research, Center for Colitis and Crohn's Disease, University of California, San Francisco, San Francisco, California

BRAD E. MALTZ, MD
Gastroenterology Fellow, Vanderbilt University; The Vanderbilt Clinic, Nashville, Tennessee

REMO PANACCIONE, MD
Associate Professor, Director, Inflammatory Bowel Disease Clinic, Division of Gastroenterology, Department of Medicine, University of Calgary, Calgary, Alberta, Canada

MIGUEL REGUEIRO, MD
Associate Professor, Department of Medicine; Associate Chief for Education; Co-Director, Inflammatory Bowel Disease Center; Head, IBD Clinical Program; Director, Gastroenterology Fellowship Program, University of Pittsburgh School of Medicine, Pittsburgh, Pennsylvania

DAVID T. RUBIN, MD
Assistant Professor of Medicine, Inflammatory Bowel Disease Center, University of Chicago Medical Center, Chicago, Illinois

CARY G. SAUER, MD, MSc
Assistant Professor, Department of Pediatrics, Division of Pediatric Gastroenterology, Emory University School of Medicine; and Emory Children's Center, Atlanta, Georgia

DAVID A. SCHWARTZ, MD
Associate Professor of Medicine; Director, IBD Center, Division of Gastroenterology, Vanderbilt University Medical Center, Nashville, Tennessee

BO SHEN, MD
Digestive Disease Institute, Cleveland Clinic, Cleveland, Ohio

HAO WU, MB
Department of Gastroenterology, Zhongshan Hospital, Fudan University, Shanghai, China

TIMOTHY L. ZISMAN, MD, MPH
Assistant Professor of Medicine, Division of Gastroenterology, University of Washington Medical Center, Seattle, Washington

Contents

Crohn disease (CD) and ulcerative colitis (UC) comprise a group of inflammatory disorders of the gastrointestinal tract that can vary in severity of disease, anatomic extent of inflammation, presence and nature of extraintestinal manifestations, and response to therapeutic approaches. There have been attempts to classify CD based on the location and behavior of disease. Advances in understanding of genetic susceptibility to inflammatory bowel disease (IBD) suggest that CD and UC may represent a continuum of overlapping disorders. This has led to an attempt to classify IBD on clinical, molecular, and serologic grounds. Differences in clinical, genetic, and immunologic profiles may require more targeted, refined treatment approaches to help clinicians make decisions regarding recently introduced biologic agents. This article provides an overview of the current approaches to therapy for CD and UC and focuses on the evidence supporting the rationale for changing paradigms in the management of IBD, including mucosal healing as an end point and earlier use of immunosuppressive and biologic agents, particularly in CD (so-called top-down therapy).

Fistulas manifest frequently in Crohn disease and can result in significant morbidity and often lead to the need for surgical intervention. Historically, it has been more difficult to obtain complete fistula closure in patients with perianal Crohn disease. Anti-tumor necrosis factor-alpha agents and the use of more accurate imaging modalities such as magnetic resonance imaging and rectal endoscopic ultrasound have enhanced the ability to manage fistulizing Crohn disease. A combined medical and surgical approach usually presents the best option for most patients.

Inflammatory bowel disease (IBD) includes Crohn disease and ulcerative colitis, and is often diagnosed in late childhood and early adulthood. What determines the age of onset remains unexplained. Early onset may represent the "pure" form of the disease process and hence may hold secrets of the initiating events of IBD pathogenesis. Clinical scientists continue to focus on pediatric IBD because it may shed light on the cause and prevention of this lifelong disease. Over the last decade, data in pediatric IBD studies have demonstrated many similarities and differences between pediatric and adult onset, which continue to add pieces to an increasingly complex IBD puzzle. The mechanism responsible for these similarities and differences remains unanswered. This article discusses clinically relevant epidemiology and treatment aspects of pediatric IBD, with special focus on similarities and differences in pediatric and adult IBD. Evidence-based treatment algorithms, with special focus on pediatric studies and care for children, are also highlighted.

This review covers important questions that arise for physicians caring for women with inflammatory bowel disease. Fertility, pregnancy outcomes and the safety of medications in pregnancy and lactation are discussed.

Restorative proctocolectomy with ileal pouch-anal anastomosis has become the surgical treatment of choice for most patients with ulcerative colitis who require surgery. Although the surgical procedure offers a cure in some patients, postoperative inflammatory and noninflammatory complications are common. Pouchitis is the most common long-term complication of the procedure. Pouchitis represents a spectrum of disease processes with heterogeneous risk factors, clinical phenotypes, natural history, and prognosis. Accurate diagnosis and classification are important for proper treatment and prognosis.

This article describes the cancer risks of commonly used inflammatory bowel disease (IBD) medications, with an emphasis on hematologic malignancy risks. The increasing use of immunosuppressant therapies in the treatment of IBD has raised this question to an even greater importance. Studies evaluating these medications are complicated due to varying disease severity and concomitant use of other immunosuppressant medication. The potential risks of all therapies must be weighed against the benefits these therapies can offer these patients.

Over the last decade, the medical treatment of inflammatory bowel disease (IBD) has been revolutionized, with increasing use of both immunomodulatory and biologic medications. Corticosteroids have increasingly been associated with an elevated risk of serious and opportunistic infections, both independently and in combination with immunomodulator and biologic agents. There are limited data on the infectious risk of immunomodulators. It is unclear if anti-tumor necrosis factor agents increase overall infectious risk in patients with IBD, but the available literature has demonstrated an increased risk of opportunistic infections, particularly in terms of tuberculosis and histoplasmosis. Combination therapy likely increases the risk of opportunistic infections in patients with IBD but this has not yet been conclusively proved.

Preface

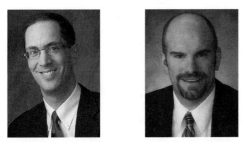

Miguel Regueiro, MD   Arthur M. Barrie III, MD, PhD
Guest Editors

We are honored to serve as the editors for this issue of *Medical Clinics of North America* titled "Challenges in Inflammatory Bowel Disease." The authors comprise a distinguished group of physician scientists and clinicians who are leaders in the field of inflammatory bowel disease (IBD). In this issue, they share their insights and expertise into how they manage challenging IBD presentations. We believe this issue provides an invaluable consulting reference for all health care providers.

This issue covers a wide range of IBD topics. Drs. Remo Panaccione and Shane Devlin report on how to treat IBD patients in this evolving era of biologic agents. Drs. David Schwartz and Brad Maltz describe the standard of care for the vexing problem of fistulizing disease. Drs. Subra Kugathasan and Cary Sauer highlight the unique aspects of pediatric IBD. Dr. Uma Mahadevan explains the management of pregnant IBD patients. Drs. Bo Shen and Hao Wu illustrate the biologic and clinical ramifications of an ileal pouch-anal anastomosis. Drs. James Lewis and Meena Bewtra report on how we should proceed with IBD therapy given the controversial malignancy risk. Similarly, Drs. Edward Loftus and Waqqas Afif detail the infectious risks of various IBD medications. Drs. Ashwin Ananthakrishnan and Mazen Issa, along with our colleague, Dr. David Binion, share their insight into the *Clostridium difficile* epidemic in IBD patients, and Drs. David Rubin and Timothy Zisman describe the exciting developments in novel diagnostic and prognostic tools for IBD. Lastly, we describe our own experiences with postoperative management of IBD, including the use of tumor necrosis factor alpha inhibitors.

We are confident that readers of this issue will significantly benefit from the authors' contributions. We are extremely appreciative of the authors' hard work and sacrifice of

This article originally appeared in *Gastroenterology Clinics of North America* Volume 38 Issue 4.

Med Clin N Am 94 (2010) xiii–xiv
doi:10.1016/j.mcna.2009.10.004
0025-7125/09/$ – see front matter © 2010 Elsevier Inc. All rights reserved.

time. We truly enjoyed working with all of them and commend them on their efforts. We are also very thankful for the guidance and assistance of Kerry Holland, senior editor, and her staff.

Miguel Regueiro, MD
University of Pittsburgh School of Medicine UPMC-PUH
Mezzanine Level, C-Wing
200 Lothrop Street
Pittsburgh, PA 15213, USA

Arthur M. Barrie III, MD, PhD
University of Pittsburgh School of Medicine
Pittsburgh, PA, USA

E-mail addresses:
mdr7@pitt.edu (M. Regueiro)
amb145@pitt.edu (A.M. Barrie)

Evolving Inflammatory Bowel Disease Treatment Paradigms: Top-Down Versus Step-Up

Shane M. Devlin, MD, Remo Panaccione, MD*

KEYWORDS

- Inflammatory bowel disease • Crohn disease
- Ulcerative colitis • Management • Anti-TNF • Biologic
- Therapy • Top-down

Crohn disease (CD) and ulcerative colitis (UC) comprise a group of inflammatory disorders of the gastrointestinal (GI) tract that can vary significantly in many aspects, including severity of disease, anatomic extent of inflammation, the presence and nature of extraintestinal manifestations, and response to therapeutic approaches.[1–5] This clinical heterogeneity has led to attempts at classifying CD based on the location and behavior of disease.[6] More recently, advances in understanding of genetic susceptibility to inflammatory bowel disease (IBD) suggest that CD and UC may represent a continuum of overlapping disorders,[7,8] which has led to an attempt to better classify IBD on clinical, molecular, and serologic grounds.[9] Beyond classification, differences in clinical, genetic, and immunologic profiles may require more targeted, refined treatment approaches based on more than disease location and severity. These approaches may help clinicians who make decisions in the rapidly evolving area of recently introduced biologic agents.

This article provides an overview of the current approaches to therapy for CD and UC. An in-depth review is beyond the scope of this article and can best be accomplished by referring to published guidelines.[1,4,5,10] This article focuses on the evidence supporting the rationale for changing paradigms in the management of IBD, including mucosal healing as an end point and earlier use of immunosuppressive and biologic agents, particularly in CD (so-called top-down therapy).[11] This review does not focus on the current controversy regarding concomitant immunosuppressive therapy versus

This article originally appeared in *Gastroenterology Clinics of North America* Volume 38 Issue 4.
Division of Gastroenterology, Inflammatory Bowel Disease Clinic, Department of Medicine, University of Calgary, 3280 Hospital Dr NW, Calgary, Alberta, Canada T2N 4N1
* Corresponding author.
E-mail address: rpanacci@ucalgary.ca (R. Panaccione).

Med Clin N Am 94 (2010) 1–18
doi:10.1016/j.mcna.2009.08.017
0025-7125/09/$ – see front matter © 2010 Elsevier Inc. All rights reserved.

medical.theclinics.com

monotherapy with the use of biologic agents. Although the majority of the proposed approaches outlined are based on the interpretation of evidence, some are reflective of the authors' opinion and may diverge from published guidelines.

THE CHALLENGE OF CHOOSING THE APPROPRIATE THERAPY FOR THE NEWLY DIAGNOSED PATIENT WITH CD

The therapeutic approach to the patient with newly diagnosed CD is confounded by the clinical heterogeneity of the disease. The approach should differ based on the clinical presentation of the new patient. Patients presenting at diagnosis with a complicated disease phenotype, such as internal penetrating disease or perianal CD, are different from patients presenting with mild diarrhea and an ileocolonoscopy demonstrating scattered and superficial colonic aphthae. In considering initial therapeutic options, the clinician must consider the evidence that may point to differences in the history of an individual patient with CD.

CD is a chronic relapsing disease characterized by periods of apparent remission and obvious disease activity. Population-based data from Denmark have demonstrated that within a year of diagnosis more than 50% of patients are in remission, about one-third have highly active disease, and 15% have only mild disease.[12] A Markov model of a population-based inception cohort from Olmsted County, Minnesota, suggested a patient with CD would spend 24% of the time in medical remission on no medical therapy, 27% of the time being treated with mesalamine only, 41% of the time in postoperative remission, and only 7% of the time in a state requiring therapy with corticosteroids or immunosuppressants.[13] However, as discussed later in this article, the meaning of clinical or postoperative remission in the context of these studies and whether it is truly reflective of remission as it pertains to mucosal healing must be considered. Similar to the heterogeneity of clinical presentation, the natural history of CD is equally diverse and the ideal is to have tools to aid in the prediction of a severe disease course versus a more indolent type of disease so that a more aggressive therapeutic approach can be instituted earlier instead of a more graduated approach.

Several tools are available to the clinician that may aid in predicting a more aggressive course of disease in patients with CD. These include clinical, endoscopic, serologic, and genetic variables (a more expansive review is available in the article by Rubin in this issue). The most useful tools for clinicians are simple-to-use clinical predictors that can easily be applied in practice. Clinical parameters, largely derived from retrospective studies, that predict a more aggressive disease course include a younger age of disease onset, active smoking, extensive small bowel disease, deep colonic ulcers, perianal disease, and an initial need for corticosteroids.[14–18] Other clinical factors that should be considered are extensive upper GI tract disease or disease of an undesirable location that would require extensive, complicated surgery. More recently, two commercially available panels of antibodies to microbial antigens have been associated with complicated small bowel disease behavior in adult and pediatric CD in cross-sectional and prospective studies.[19–24] These panels include antibodies directed at several microbial antigens including oligomannan (anti-*Saccharomyces cerevisiae* or ASCA), *Escherichia coli* outer membrane porin C (anti-OmpC), flagellin (anti-CBir1), antilaminaribioside (ALCA), antimannobioside (AMCA), antichitobioside (ACCA), antichitin (anti-C), and antilaminarin (anti-L).[21,25–30] The clinical utility of these panels is an area of ongoing interest, but their greatest potential may lie in their predictive capacity (for a more detailed review see the article by Rubin in this issue).

THE CURRENT APPROACH TO MANAGING CD

Traditionally the goals of therapy have been to eliminate all symptoms related to a patient's CD. More recently, other goals have been advocated such as improving a patient's quality of life and reducing hospitalization, surgery, and mucosal healing. The means to achieve these goals may differ depending on the clinical presentation and presence or absence of extraintestinal manifestations of a patient's CD.

The standard therapies available to a clinician include 5-aminosalicylates, sulfasalazine, antimicrobial therapy, corticosteroids, immunosuppressive agents, and monoclonal antibodies (MAbs). The only commercially available MAbs include the three antitumor necrosis factor (TNF) antibodies, infliximab, adalimumab, and certolizumab pegol, and natalizumab, an MAb directed against the α4-integrin.[31–35] Therapy for CD should be thought of as acute or induction therapy, followed by maintenance therapy.

Induction therapy for patients with mild-to-moderate CD has traditionally consisted of 5-aminosalicylates or sulfasalazine or antimicrobial agents such as ciprofloxacin and metronidazole.[36–46] However, the evidence is clear that, with the possible exception of patients with mild colonic disease, these agents are ineffective and their routine use is not recommended.[5,41,46,47] Induction therapy with corticosteroids, however, is a highly effective strategy. Population-based studies demonstrate that after 30 days prednisone results in remission in 48% to 58% of patients, response in 26% to 32%, and lack of response in 16% to 20%.[48,49] Similar results were observed in a comparable cohort from the United Kingdom.[50] However, prolonged response occurs in only 32% to 44% and corticosteroid dependence occurs in 28% to 36%.[45,46] For patients with mild disease the systemic side effects of prednisone often do not warrant its use.[51] For patients who have mild-to-moderate CD that is limited to the ileum and right colon, controlled-release oral budesonide is a good option at a dose of 9 mg/d, which has been shown to be more effective than placebo or mesalamine at inducing response and remission and causes fewer corticosteroid side effects than systemic glucocorticoids.[52–55] Immunosuppressive agents such as azathioprine (AZA), 6-mercaptopurine (6-MP) and methotrexate (MTX) have been studied for induction of active moderate-to-severe corticosteroid-dependent CD.[56,57] In a meta-analysis examining the use of AZA/6-MP, the odds ratio for response for active CD was 3.09; 16 weeks of parenteral MTX at a dose of 25 mg weekly led to remission in 39% of patients. However, neither agent is rapidly acting and they generally require concomitant corticosteroids for induction therapy. The only other therapeutic option associated with a rapid induction of response and remission is the anti-TNFα agents. Infliximab, adalimumab, and certolizumab pegol induction therapy is associated with response rates of approximately 40% to 80% at 4 to 12 weeks in patients for whom other standard therapies have failed.[33,58–60] Natalizumab was associated with sustained response and remission from weeks 4 to 8 in patients with an elevated C-reactive protein (CRP) in 48% and 26% of patients, respectively.[35]

Induction therapy serves to downregulate acutely the adaptive immune response that drives gut inflammation in CD. However, the underlying genetic and environmental predisposition remains unchanged, and hence maintenance therapy is generally required. Although the theoretical Markov model cited earlier in this article estimated that patients with CD would spend only 7% of their time in a disease state requiring immunosuppressive therapy or corticosteroids, this is in contrast to studies of actual patients. The data on short- and long-term response to corticosteroids found that a long-term response occurs in only 32% to 44% of patients and corticosteroid dependence occurs in 28% to 36%.[48,49] Data from a clinical trial comparing the use of infliximab induction with AZA versus a more traditional approach of induction with corticosteroids followed by the addition of AZA on relapse (the top-down trial) found that at 52 weeks, 65% of patients had relapsed after corticosteroids and were eventually treated with AZA.[11] Therefore, the majority of patients with CD, particularly those treated with corticosteroid induction, require maintenance therapy. Fewer therapeutic agents are available for maintenance therapy than for induction therapy. Only the immunosuppressive agents (AZA, 6-MP, and MTX) and biologic agents have documented efficacy in the maintenance of response and remission in CD.[31–33,56,61–63]

Many clinicians still commonly apply a stepwise approach to the management of mild CD, using induction therapy with agents with limited systemic toxicity (eg, antimicrobials, mesalamine, or budesonide for ileal-right colonic disease) followed by maintenance therapy with an immunosuppressive agent after 1 or 2 episodes of symptomatic relapse,[64] particularly in patients who lack obvious clinical predictors of severe disease. In patients with moderate-to-severe CD, most clinicians would use systemic corticosteroids for induction therapy with the addition of an immunosuppressive agent concomitant with induction corticosteroids or after one symptomatic relapse.[64] In recent years, the use of immunosuppressive therapy has increased significantly.[65] Biologic agents have traditionally been used only after failure of or intolerance to immunosuppressive therapy. In general, this escalating approach is referred to as "step-up therapy."

THE NATURAL HISTORY OF UC

UC has a heterogeneous course. Disease activity is generally described as mild, moderate, or severe, based on the number of bowel movements, presence and degree of rectal bleeding, and presence or absence of other systemic features.[1] Work from Denmark followed 1161 UC patients for 25 years and studied changes in disease activity.[66] This study found a rate of colectomy of 24% after 10 years of disease activity. Between the third and seventh year after diagnosis, 18% of patients had active disease on a yearly basis, 25% had persistent remission, and 57% had intermittent relapses. The only features that were found to be predictive of active disease course were the disease activity in the preceding years, the number of years with disease relapses, and the presence of systemic symptoms. A study from the same group, studying part of the same cohort, found that the disease location is not static.[67] Patients with proctosigmoiditis at diagnosis had a 53% likelihood of proximal extension within 25 years and, conversely, 75% of patients with pancolonic involvement developed less extensive overt disease during the same period. Discrepant from this study is a more recent Norwegian study of a 10-year follow-up of an inception cohort of UC patients, which found that proximal extension of distal disease occurred in only 20% of patients.[68] However, consistent with the Danish cohort, 83% of patients had a relapsing course and approximately one-half of patients were relapse free during the previous 5 years. The presence of pancolonic disease with an elevated erythrocyte sedimentation rate (ESR) was predictive of a higher likelihood of colectomy (which occurred in 9.8% of patients at 10 years). These studies show that UC is a heterogeneous disease in terms of location, extent, change over time, and disease course. Ability to predict disease course in UC is not so well developed as in CD.

THE CURRENT APPROACH TO MANAGING UC

The goals of therapy in UC are the same as those cited for CD. The therapies available to a clinician are identical to those that are available for CD, with a few key exceptions.

The anti-TNF agents adalimumab and certolizumab pegol and the anti-α; 4-integrin natalizumab are not currently indicated for UC. Antimicrobial agents lack efficacy in UC and their use is not advocated.[69,70] Cyclosporine has proven efficacy in acute, severe UC.[71,72] Similarly, therapy should be thought of as induction and maintenance therapy.[4]

Induction therapy for mild-to-moderate UC generally consists of 5-aminosalicylate therapy (sulfasalazine or mesalamine), which, unlike CD, is a highly effective strategy.[4,73,74] Approximately 40% to 80% of patients will respond within 4 weeks to orally administered 5-aminosalicylates.[4,73,74] Many of the symptoms of UC, such as urgency and tenesmus, arise from rectal inflammation. The optimal approach to therapy, regardless of the extent of disease, is combined oral and rectal aminosalicy-lates.[75,76] For those patients who do not initially respond to 5-aminosalicylates or who have more severe symptoms, corticosteroids are an effective induction therapy. Population-based data from Olmsted County, Minnesota have demonstrated that at 30 days, 54% of patients achieve complete remission, 30% achieve partial remission, and 16% fail to respond.[49] At 1 year, 49% maintain response, 22% are corticosteroid dependent, and 29% go on to require colectomy. Therefore, the requirement for a course of corticosteroids in UC can also be seen as a bad prognostic indicator. As in CD, the use of 6-MP/AZA in UC requires a significant time of onset; these are not good inductive agents and usually require concomitant use of corticosteroids. The role of these agents is less clear than in CD because there is considerable hetero-geneity in study design. A recent meta-analysis evaluated the use of 6-MP/AZA for induction of remission in UC and, using a pooled analysis of 4 studies that met inclu-sion criteria, found an odds ratio of 1.59 favoring 6-MP/AZA, but the confidence interval was not significant (0.59–4.29).[77] This pooled analysis of 4 studies included a total of only 89 patients, reflecting the small nature of many of the studies evaluating these agents in UC. The only other agent with well-documented efficacy in inducing remission in UC is infliximab. In the active ulcerative colitis trial (ACT) 1 and ACT 2 trials for moderate-to-severe UC, the use of 5 mg/kg of infliximab induction therapy was associated with a 67% response rate and a 36% remission rate at 8 weeks in patients who had active disease despite standard therapies (aminosalicylates, corticosteroids, or 6-MP/AZA).[78] Maintenance of response and remission can be achieved in UC with 5-aminosalicylates, 6-MP/AZA, and infliximab.[4,78,79] Similar to induction studies, the PEGylated antibody Fragment Evaluation in Crohn Diseases Safety and Efficacy (PRECiSE) role and efficacy of 6-MP/AZA is unclear, although a recent meta-analysis including 4 studies and 232 patients found a significant odds ratio favoring 6-MP/AZA over control. A clinical trial evaluating AZA versus infliximab versus combination therapy with both agents in patients naive to these therapies for induction and main-tenance of UC is ongoing and may clarify the role of these agents in UC.

WHICH IS THE BETTER WAY TO DETERMINE RESPONSE TO THERAPY IN IBD: SYMPTOMS OR ENDOSCOPIC ASSESSMENT?

In clinical practice, the assessment of disease activity in UC and CD has traditionally been accomplished by assessing clinical symptoms such as the presence or absence of blood, the number of stools per day, and the presence or absence of evidence of systemic toxicity. In addition, other means such as elevation in the ESR or CRP can be useful.[80,81] More recently, fecal markers such as fecal calprotectin have shown significant promise.[82] In clinical trials, investigators rely on activity indices that are highly symptom based, such as the Crohn Disease Activity Index (CDAI) or Harvey-Bradshaw Index (HBI) in CD, and the Mayo score, among others, for UC.[83–85]

Patients with IBD often have symptoms that are not related to inflammatory lesions of the GI tract. Symptoms can have many causes, including medication side effects, choleretic diarrhea after ileal resection in CD, and postsurgical diarrhea. Many patients with IBD will develop a syndrome of postinflammatory irritable bowel that is not reflective of demonstrable inflammation at a mucosal level, which may explain the high placebo response rates that have been seen in some clinical trials evaluating the use of biologic agents for CD.[34,60] Subsequent stratification of patients by more objective evidence of inflammation, such as elevated CRP, has demonstrated efficacy among patients with active inflammation versus lack of efficacy in those who probably lack significant inflammation.[35,60] With the more recent practice of incorporating mucosal assessment into clinical trial protocols, this efficacy can be demonstrated even more clearly. In the Study of Biologic and Immunomodulator Naive Patients in Crohn Disease (the SONIC study), evaluating AZA, infliximab monotherapy, and infliximab in combination with AZA for patients with active CD who were naive to both classes of medications, there was strong evidence for the superiority of infliximab alone or in combination with AZA in patients with mucosal lesions at baseline, but no difference in efficacy in patients who lacked mucosal lesions at baseline but still qualified based on CDAI.[86] CDAI has been shown to lack correlation to the presence and degree of endoscopic lesions in CD.[80] This demonstrates that relying on clinical symptoms alone when making key therapeutic decision is fraught with difficulty and represents an error-prone approach to management.

The disconnect between mucosal lesions and symptoms is illustrated by studies of postoperative recurrence of CD. Within a year after intestinal resection, at least 70% of patients have recurrent disease endoscopically, yet clinical recurrence occurs in only one-third by 3 years, implying that endoscopic lesions and symptoms may not correlate.[87–90] A recent study, presented in abstract form, demonstrated that determination of the clinical impression of disease activity had a sensitivity and specificity of only 56.4% and 80.9%, respectively when compared with colonoscopy as the gold standard.[91] In clinical trials of mesalamine and infliximab for UC, endoscopic healing has been demonstrated to exceed the proportion of patients meeting criteria for clinical improvement or remission, emphasizing that noninflammatory processes can drive symptoms in IBD.[78,92] This led to attempts at developing disease activity indices that are more comprehensive and take into account not only clinical symptoms but also noninvasive markers of inflammation such as fecal lactoferrin.[93]

THE VALUE OF MUCOSAL HEALING AS AN END POINT IN IBD

The notion that mucosal assessment is a more representative means of assessing disease activity is important, but more important is the relevance of achieving such an end point. Healing of mucosal ulceration should be a superior strategy to achieving clinical remission or improvement alone in the presence of persistent mucosal lesions. However, until recently, there was not much evidence to support such an intuitive assertion.

Data from a large Norwegian population-based cohort of incident UC and CD patients provides insight into the value of achieving mucosal healing.[94] Of 740 patients in the cohort, baseline and repeat endoscopic assessment was available in 495. In UC patients, the presence of mucosal healing 1 year after diagnosis was significantly associated with a reduced need for colectomy at 5 years. In patients with CD, the presence of mucosal healing at 1 year was associated with reduced subsequent need for corticosteroids. In addition, there was a numerical, but not a statistical, reduction in the need for surgery. Mucosal healing at 1 year in CD was associated with mucosal healing at 5 years. This incident cohort spanned 1990 to 1994, before the advent of biologic agents, and signifies that the achievement of mucosal healing by any means is valuable and is not reflective only of the effect of biologic agents.

There are important data about the advantages of achieving mucosal healing in the specific context of biologic agents. Data from the ACCENT-I (A Crohn Disease Clinical Trial Evaluating Infliximab in a New Long-term Treatment Regimen) trial for infliximab demonstrated that patients on infliximab who achieved mucosal healing tended toward lower rates of hospitalization.[95] More recent longitudinal data from a large cohort of CD patients in Leuven demonstrates that the presence of mucosal healing during therapy with infliximab was strongly associated with a lower risk of major abdominal surgery.[96]

Data should be examined with respect to the ability of the available therapeutic agents in terms of inducing mucosal healing, as this is likely to be better reflective of their true efficacy.

In IBD, mucosal healing data are available for corticosteroids, AZA/6-MP, MTX, infliximab, certolizumab pegol, and adalimumab.

Mucosal healing data for corticosteroids are limited and the definition of mucosal healing in older studies is markedly less rigorous than by current defined endoscopic scoring systems. In CD and UC, the use of corticosteroids has not been associated with significant degrees of mucosal healing.[97,98] A more recent study using a more contemporary definition of mucosal healing compared AZA with budesonide for patients with ileal or ileocolonic CD and budesonide was associated with complete or near-complete mucosal healing in only 24% of patients.[99]

Until recently, there were limited data regarding mucosal healing with the use of mesalamine in UC. However, with the recent development of Multi-Matrix System (MMX) mesalamine, there are mucosal healing data from trials in UC.[73,74] At 8 weeks, approximately 35% to 40% of patients on 2.4 to 4.8 g/d of MMX mesalamine achieved mucosal healing in 2 pivotal trials of this agent. There are no mucosal healing data for mesalamine in CD.

Data for AZA/6-MP come from two lines of evidence: postoperative prevention studies and a recent prospective randomized controlled trial for active CD.[86,100,101] Postoperative prevention studies have been inconsistent and largely disappointing. An open-label randomized trial of 2 mg/kg/d of AZA versus 3 g/d of mesalamine failed to demonstrate a difference in clinical recurrence at 24 months, but there was no endoscopic component to this study.[100] A later study evaluating 50 mg/d of 6-MP versus mesalamine and placebo demonstrated a lower endoscopic recurrence rate with 6-MP compared with placebo, but the endoscopic recurrence rate at 24 months with 6-MP was still 43%.[101] The best and most informative data regarding the efficacy of AZA in induction of mucosal healing come from the SONIC trial mentioned earlier in this article that evaluated AZA versus infliximab versus infliximab in combination with AZA in patients with active CD, naive to infliximab and AZA, requiring corticosteroids to control symptoms.[86] As discussed later in this article, the rate of mucosal healing at 26 weeks was only 16.5% with AZA. There are no mucosal healing data for AZA in UC, although a study similar in design to the SONIC trial is ongoing.

There are few data regarding mucosal healing with the use of MTX. One small pilot study in patients with CD and UC and a second small study published only in abstract form suggested some ability to induce healing of mucosal lesions but more data are needed.[102,103]

The data for mucosal healing in CD with infliximab are discussed in detail later in this article. Recently, data have been published in abstract form regarding mucosal healing in CD with certolizumab pegol and adalimumab.[104,105] In a prospective trial

135 patients were randomized to either adalimumab induction therapy (160 mg/80 mg) followed by 40 mg every other week, or induction alone followed by placebo for 52 weeks. Adalimumab induction and maintenance were associated with complete mucosal healing at 52 weeks in 24.2% versus 0% in patients induced but not maintained on adalimumab. In an open-label study, patients were treated with 400 mg of certolizumab pegol at 0, 2, and 4 weeks and then every 4 weeks up to week 54. Endoscopic remission as defined by the Crohn Disease Endoscopic Index of Severity was noted by week 10 in 55.1% of patients, but complete mucosal healing (a more stringent end point used in the infliximab and adalimumab data) occurred in only 6.1% of patients. In UC, infliximab, 5 mg/kg induction and maintenance were associated with an approximately 45% to 50% rate of mucosal healing at week 30 in the ACT 1 and ACT 2 trials evaluating this agent for induction and maintenance of moderate to severe UC (defined as an endoscopy subcore of 0 or 1).[78] There are currently no mucosal healing data for adalimumab or certolizumab pegol in UC and neither agent is currently indicated for this disease. Studies with adalimumab are ongoing.

WHAT IS THE RATIONALE FOR TOP-DOWN THERAPY IN CD?

There is mounting evidence that a strategy of earlier use of more potent immunosuppressive therapies may be the optimal approach to therapy in properly selected patients. The key to understanding this lies in the natural history of CD, particularly that of small bowel disease and those patients who require corticosteroids. In a retrospective study of more than 2000 patients with CD, the long-term evolution of disease behavior was investigated.[106] Patients progress in a stepwise fashion from inflammatory lesions (likely most amenable to therapy) toward irreversible structural disease such as strictures and penetrating disease. Antiinflammatory therapy presents a limited opportunity for treatment. A direct analogy can be made with inflammatory joint disease, in which irreversible structural damage occurs early and rapidly and may not necessarily be related to symptoms. Rheumatologists have used immunosuppressive therapy early in the course of rheumatoid arthritis and more recent data suggest that the early introduction of anti-TNF agents not only slows or halts progression of structural damage but may also allow the eventual withdrawal of immunosuppressive therapy.[107,108]

Although the historical standard in terms of a treatment approach to treating UC and CD has been a stepwise process as described earlier in this article, this uniform approach has failings that put patients with a high likelihood of progressive disease at risk. There is a process by which biologic agents, specifically TNFα; antagonists, are used as the initial induction therapy, and this therapeutic paradigm has been referred to as a top-down strategy. There is compelling evidence to substantiate this approach.

The first example of top-down therapy may have been a randomized, placebo-controlled trial of 6-MP and prednisone in pediatric patients with newly diagnosed CD published by Markowitz and colleagues.[109] Patients were randomized within 8 weeks of diagnosis to 6-MP 1.5 mg/kg/d plus a tapering course of prednisone versus placebo and prednisone. Maintenance therapy with 6-MP or placebo was continued for 18 months. Remission was achieved in 89% of patients overall, but in patients maintained with 6-MP, the 18-month relapse rate was only 9% versus 47% in those maintained with placebo ($P = .007$). Those patients treated with 6-MP were exposed to a lower cumulative dose of corticosteroids. Although in the current paradigm initial use of an immunosuppressive agent such as 6-MP would not be considered top-down, that study represented at the time a departure from traditional practice.

The next evidence comes from retrospective analyses of large randomized controlled trials of the anti-TNF agents adalimumab and certolizumab pegol. In the Crohn Trial of the Fully Human Antibody Adalimumab for Remission Maintenance (the CHARM trial), which evaluated maintenance of response and remission to adalimumab, the week-26 rate of maintenance of remission with adalimumab 40 mg every other week was 56% in patients with a disease duration less than 2 years, 35% in those with a disease duration of 2 to 5 years, and 37% in those with disease longer than 5 years.[110] In the PRECiSE 2 study evaluating maintenance of response and remission with certolizumab pegol in CD, 62% of patients maintained response at week 26.[63] However, in those with an elevated CRP and a disease duration of less than 2 years, the maintenance of response was 90% ($P = .02$), suggesting that early use of an anti-TNF agent was more successful.[111] Although comparing clinical trials of differing designs and with different patient populations should be discouraged, some insight can be drawn from a comparison of the ACCENT-I trial evaluating induction and maintenance of response and remission with infliximab for adult CD and the Randomized, Multicenter, Open-Label Study to Evaluate the Safety and Efficacy of Anti-TNFα; Chimeric Monoclonal Antibody in Pediatric Subjects with Moderate to Severe Crohn Disease (REACH) trial evaluating infliximab in pediatric patients.[31,112] The median disease duration in ACCENT-I was approximately 8 years, whereas in REACH it was approximately 2 years. The week 10 and 54 response rates in REACH were 88.4% and 63.5% versus 70% and 43%, respectively for the same time points in ACCENT-I.

The most compelling data in support of the top-down strategy come from prospective studies of patients with newly diagnosed CD naive to all therapy apart from mesalamine or antibiotics (the top-down trial), and in relatively newly diagnosed CD naive to biologic agents and immunosuppressive therapy (SONIC) and patients who have undergone ileocecal resection for CD.[11,86,113]

In a randomized control trial of patients with newly diagnosed CD who were naive to corticosteroids, immunomodulators, and anti-TNFα; agents, treatment was initiated as a top-down approach with infliximab 5 mg/kg at weeks 0, 2, and 6, and AZA 2.5 mg/kg/d with infliximab being delivered subsequently on an episodic, as-needed schedule or as a more traditional step-up approach with corticosteroids followed by the initiation of AZA on relapse or in cases of corticosteroid dependence, only then to be followed by infliximab in cases of ongoing disease activity.[11] The primary end point was clinical remission without corticosteroids and without surgery at weeks 26 and 52. At weeks 26 and 52, 60% and 62%, respectively of patients treated with early infliximab met this end point versus 36% and 42%, respectively in the step-up group. The trial demonstrated that active CD could be treated without using corticosteroids. At 104 weeks, there was no longer a difference between the two groups in terms of clinical remission. However, in patients treated with early infliximab, the rate of mucosal healing at 104 weeks was 71% versus only 30% in patients treated in a conventional step-up manner. The achievement of mucosal healing at 2 years was a strong predictor of remission from steroids, absence of subsequent relapse, or need for further anti-TNF therapy up to follow-up of 4 years, implying that early, aggressive therapy could have long-term benefits,[114] despite the trial design of episodic use of infliximab rather than regularly scheduled therapy, which is now advocated. The results might have been even more compelling had patients been on further maintenance therapy with infliximab, which is a subject in need of further study.

Although the SONIC trial is not strictly top-down, it provides similar insight into the advantage of earlier use of an anti-TNF agent. The median disease duration in the SONIC trial was just more than 2 years. Patients with active CD requiring corticosteroids were randomized to AZA 2.5 mg/kg/d, infliximab 5 mg/kg induction and maintenance, or the combination of both agents. The primary end point was remission from corticosteroids at week 26, but important secondary end points included mucosal healing at week 26 and pharmacokinetic data on infliximab levels and antibodies to infliximab. At 26 weeks, 30.6% of patients on AZA were in remission from corticosteroids compared with 44.4% with infliximab monotherapy and 56.8% for those on combination therapy with both agents. Mucosal healing at the same time was even more striking at 16.5% with AZA, 30.1% with infliximab monotherapy, and 43.9% with combination therapy.

The ultimate top-down therapy is to initiate treatment before the development of disease. Although this is impossible at present, a rough approximation of this model is the paradigm of prevention of surgically induced remission, before the development of recurrent mucosal disease. There is an insight into the benefit of anti-TNFα; therapy in this setting in the context of a small randomized controlled trial of 24 CD patients comparing postoperative infliximab induction and maintenance therapy to standard postoperative therapy. At 1 year, infliximab induction and maintenance were associated with a 9.1% rate of endoscopic recurrence versus 84.6% with placebo. Of the placebo-treated patients, 53.8% were on immunosuppressive therapy during the trial.

This evidence unequivocally demonstrates several key points. Intervention earlier in the course of disease with effective therapy is likely to be more successful. This type of early intervention may decrease the likelihood of disease progression to more aggressive phenotypes that require surgical intervention. Anti-TNF agents appear to be more successful in patients with shorter duration disease and, at least for infliximab, are markedly superior to AZA at inducing mucosal healing. Achieving early mucosal healing appears to have long-term benefits that may truly alter the natural history of a patient's CD. From a health economic perspective, a top-down approach was studied using administrative claims data, which have been presented in abstract form.[115] Rubin and colleagues studied the claims data for more than 3000 CD patients who were treated with biologic agents. A step-up approach was identified if the biologic agent followed other therapies and a top-down approach was identified if a biologic agent was initiated within 30 days of diagnosis of CD. Those patients treated with biologic agents earlier were noted to have a lower rate of CD-related surgery. Although the study did not investigate costs directly, this is likely to be a less expensive strategy.

IS THERE RATIONALE FOR TOP-DOWN THERAPY IN UC?

Unlike CD in which longer duration of disease is associated with a higher likelihood of irreversible structural damage, the same cannot be said of UC. One important long-term issue with UC is the development of dysplasia, for which the presence of unchecked inflammation is a key risk factor.[116] Theoretically, therefore, earlier use of an agent known to exert a potent biologic effect and lead to mucosal healing could have a long-term benefit. However, the best evidence for prevention of dysplasia currently exists for 5-aminosalicylates, and similar evidence is lacking for infliximab.[117] A subanalysis of the ACT 1 and ACT 2 trials failed to demonstrate any difference in response rates to infliximab with patients with disease duration of less than 3 years versus greater than 3 years.[118] Therefore, at present, there is little rationale for a top-down approach to managing UC. There will be patients who will have an accelerating disease course and would likely benefit from earlier intervention, but the current tools do not allow reliable advance identification of these patients. Further study is needed in this area of of IBD management.

THE FUTURE APPROACH TO THE MANAGEMENT OF IBD

The future management approach to IBD will be based on accurate and detailed phenotype and risk assessment at diagnosis based on clinical, serologic and genetic profiling. Those patients with a global risk that puts them at higher likelihood of rapidly progressive disease and the development of disabling complications should be treated with the most effective therapy as early as possible (currently anti-TNFα; agents). Similar arguments can be made to use a top-down approach with anti-TNFα; agents in CD patients with disease of an undesirable time span or location. It still remains a point of debate whether a biologic agent needs to be combined with AZA initially, although this has clearly been demonstrated to be superior in efficacy in the SONIC trial. Conversely, patients with a lower risk profile can be managed with a more traditional stepwise approach. Paramount to both treatment paradigms, however, is use of tools for the assessment of mucosal disease as the key measure of response, given the clear evidence that this is most reflective of disease activity and is most predictive of long-term success.

This approach is nearing realization in CD given the advances in understanding of genetics of this disorder, but more work is clearly needed in UC.

If a top-down approach is adopted by clinicians, several critically important questions remain. Does top-down therapy and successful induction of mucosal healing require an ongoing maintenance biologic or can it be withdrawn? Will this approach truly alter the natural history of CD in the long-term, or simply delay complications? Will this approach reduce the number of hospitalizations and operations universally? Will this approach be safe? Each answer leads to new questions but it is clear that the management of IBD in the 21st century will continue to evolve and unprecedented progress seems imminent.

REFERENCES

1. Kornbluth A, Sachar DB. Ulcerative colitis practice guidelines in adults. American College of Gastroenterology, Practice Parameters Committee. Am J Gastroenterol 1997;92:204–11.
2. Podolsky DK. Inflammatory bowel disease. N Engl J Med 2002;347:417–29.
3. Sands BE. From symptom to diagnosis: clinical distinctions among various forms of intestinal inflammation. Gastroenterology 2004;126:1518–32.
4. Kornbluth A, Sachar DB. Ulcerative colitis practice guidelines in adults (update): American College of Gastroenterology, Practice Parameters Committee. Am J Gastroenterol 2004;99:1371–85.
5. Lichtenstein GR, Hanauer SB, Sandborn WJ. Management of Crohn's disease in adults. Am J Gastroenterol 2009;104:465–83 [quiz 464, 484].
6. Gasche C, Scholmerich J, Brynskov J, et al. A simple classification of Crohn's disease: report of the Working Party for the World Congresses of Gastroenterology, Vienna 1998. Inflamm Bowel Dis 2000;6:8–15.
7. Barrett JC, Hansoul S, Nicolae DL, et al. Genome-wide association defines more than 30 distinct susceptibility loci for Crohn's disease. Nat Genet 2008;40:955–62.

8. Anderson CA, Massey DC, Barrett JC, et al. Investigation of Crohn's disease risk loci in ulcerative colitis further defines their molecular relationship. Gastroenterology 2009;136:523–9, e3.

9. Silverberg MS, Satsangi J, Ahmad T, et al. Toward an integrated clinical, molecular and serological classification of inflammatory bowel disease: report of a Working Party of the 2005 Montreal World Congress of Gastroenterology. Can J Gastroenterol 2005;19(Suppl A):5–36.

10. Travis SP, Stange EF, Lemann M, et al. European evidence based consensus on the diagnosis and management of Crohn's disease: current management. Gut 2006;55(Suppl 1):i16–35.

11. D'Haens G, Baert F, van Assche G, et al. Early combined immunosuppression or conventional management in patients with newly diagnosed Crohn's disease: an open randomised trial. Lancet 2008;371:660–7.

12. Munkholm P, Langholz E, Davidsen M, et al. Disease activity courses in a regional cohort of Crohn's disease patients. Scand J Gastroenterol 1995;30: 699–706.

13. Silverstein MD, Loftus EV, Sandborn WJ, et al. Clinical course and costs of care for Crohn's disease: Markov model analysis of a population-based cohort. Gastroenterology 1999;117:49–57.

14. Allez M, Lemann M, Bonnet J, et al. Long term outcome of patients with active Crohn's disease exhibiting extensive and deep ulcerations at colonoscopy. Am J Gastroenterol 2002;97:947–53.

15. Cosnes J, Carbonnel F, Beaugerie L, et al. Effects of cigarette smoking on the long-term course of Crohn's disease. Gastroenterology 1996;110:424–31.

16. Cosnes J, Carbonnel F, Carrat F, et al. Effects of current and former cigarette smoking on the clinical course of Crohn's disease. Aliment Pharmacol Ther 1999;13:1403–11.

17. Lichtenstein GR, Olson A, Travers S, et al. Factors associated with the development of intestinal strictures or obstructions in patients with Crohn's disease. Am J Gastroenterol 2006;101:1030–8.

18. Franchimont DP, Louis E, Croes F, et al. Clinical pattern of corticosteroid dependent Crohn's disease. Eur J Gastroenterol Hepatol 1998;10:821–5.

19. Mow WS, Vasiliauskas EA, Lin YC, et al. Association of antibody responses to microbial antigens and complications of small bowel Crohn's disease. Gastroenterology 2004;126:414–24.

20. Arnott ID, Landers CJ, Nimmo EJ, et al. Sero-reactivity to microbial components in Crohn's disease is associated with disease severity and progression, but not NOD2/CARD15 genotype. Am J Gastroenterol 2004;99:2376–84.

21. Targan SR, Landers CJ, Yang H, et al. Antibodies to CBir1 flagellin define a unique response that is associated independently with complicated Crohn's disease. Gastroenterology 2005;128:2020–8.

22. Amre DK, Lu SE, Costea F, et al. Utility of serological markers in predicting the early occurrence of complications and surgery in pediatric Crohn's disease patients. Am J Gastroenterol 2006;101:645–52.

23. Dubinsky MC, Lin YC, Dutridge D, et al. Serum immune responses predict rapid disease progression among children with Crohn's disease: immune responses predict disease progression. Am J Gastroenterol 2006;101:360–7.

24. Rieder F, Wolf A, Schleder S, et al. The novel anti-Glycan antibodies anti-L and anti-C in conjunction with ALCA, ACCA, gASCA and AMCA predict early development of fistuae, stenoses and surgery in patients with Crohn's disease: a prospective analysis [abstract]. Gastroenterology 2008;134:A53.

25. Main J, McKenzie H, Yeaman GR, et al. Antibody to *Saccharomyces cerevisiae* (bakers' yeast) in Crohn's disease. BMJ 1988;297:1105–6.
26. Quinton JF, Sendid B, Reumaux D, et al. Anti-*Saccharomyces cerevisiae* mannan antibodies combined with antineutrophil cytoplasmic autoantibodies in inflammatory bowel disease: prevalence and diagnostic role. Gut 1998;42: 788–91.
27. Sutton CL, Kim J, Yamane A, et al. Identification of a novel bacterial sequence associated with Crohn's disease. Gastroenterology 2000;119:23–31.
28. Landers CJ, Cohavy O, Misra R, et al. Selected loss of tolerance evidenced by Crohn's disease-associated immune responses to auto- and microbial antigens. Gastroenterology 2002;123:689–99.
29. Ferrante M, Henckaerts L, Joossens M, et al. New serological markers in inflammatory bowel disease are associated with complicated disease behaviour. Gut 2007;56:1394–403.
30. Seow CH, Stempak JM, Xu W, et al. Novel anti-glycan antibodies related to inflammatory bowel disease diagnosis and phenotype. Am J Gastroenterol 2009;104:1426–34.
31. Hanauer SB, Feagan BG, Lichtenstein GR, et al. Maintenance infliximab for Crohn's disease: the ACCENT I randomised trial. Lancet 2002;359:1541–9.
32. Colombel JF, Sandborn WJ, Rutgeerts P, et al. Adalimumab for maintenance of clinical response and remission in patients with Crohn's disease: the CHARM trial. Gastroenterology 2007;132:52–65.
33. Sandborn WJ, Feagan BG, Stoinov S, et al. Certolizumab pegol for the treatment of Crohn's disease. N Engl J Med 2007;357:228–38.
34. Ghosh S, Goldin E, Gordon FH, et al. Natalizumab for active Crohn's disease. N Engl J Med 2003;348:24–32.
35. Targan SR, Feagan BG, Fedorak RN, et al. Natalizumab for the treatment of active Crohn's disease: results of the ENCORE Trial. Gastroenterology 2007; 132:1672–83.
36. Summers RW, Switz DM, Sessions JT Jr, et al. National Cooperative Crohn's Disease Study: results of drug treatment. Gastroenterology 1979;77:847–69.
37. Malchow H, Ewe K, Brandes JW, et al. European Cooperative Crohn's Disease Study (ECCDS): results of drug treatment. Gastroenterology 1984;86:249–66.
38. Prantera C, Cottone M, Pallone F, et al. Mesalamine in the treatment of mild to moderate active Crohn's ileitis: results of a randomized, multicenter trial. Gastroenterology 1999;116:521–6.
39. Tremaine WJ, Schroeder KW, Harrison JM, et al. A randomized, double-blind, placebo-controlled trial of the oral mesalamine (5-ASA) preparation, Asacol, in the treatment of symptomatic Crohn's colitis and ileocolitis. J Clin Gastroenterol 1994;19:278–82.
40. Singleton JW, Hanauer SB, Gitnick GL, et al. Mesalamine capsules for the treatment of active Crohn's disease: results of a 16-week trial. Pentasa Crohn's Disease Study Group. Gastroenterology 1993;104:1293–301.
41. Sutherland L, Singleton J, Sessions J, et al. Double blind, placebo controlled trial of metronidazole in Crohn's disease. Gut 1991;32:1071–5.
42. Ursing B, Alm T, Barany F, et al. A comparative study of metronidazole and sulfasalazine for active Crohn's disease: the cooperative Crohn's disease study in Sweden. II. Result. Gastroenterology 1982;83:550–62.
43. Ambrose NS, Allan RN, Keighley MR, et al. Antibiotic therapy for treatment in relapse of intestinal Crohn's disease. A prospective randomized study. Dis Colon Rectum 1985;28:81–5.

44. Colombel JF, Lemann M, Cassagnou M, et al. A controlled trial comparing ciprofloxacin with mesalazine for the treatment of active Crohn's disease. Groupe d'Etudes Thérapeutiques des Affections Inflammatoires Digestives (GETAID). Am J Gastroenterol 1999;94:674–8.

45. Arnold GL, Beaves MR, Pryjdun VO, et al. Preliminary study of ciprofloxacin in active Crohn's disease. Inflamm Bowel Dis 2002;8:10–5.

46. Steinhart AH, Feagan BG, Wong CJ, et al. Combined budesonide and antibiotic therapy for active Crohn's disease: a randomized controlled trial. Gastroenterology 2002;123:33–40.

47. Hanauer SB, Stromberg U. Oral Pentasa in the treatment of active Crohn's disease: a meta-analysis of double-blind, placebo-controlled trials. Clin Gastroenterol Hepatol 2004;2:379–88.

48. Munkholm P, Langholz E, Davidsen M, et al. Frequency of glucocorticoid resistance and dependency in Crohn's disease. Gut 1994;35:360–2.

49. Faubion WA Jr, Loftus EV Jr, Harmsen WS, et al. The natural history of corticosteroid therapy for inflammatory bowel disease: a population-based study. Gastroenterology 2001;121:255–60.

50. Ho GT, Chiam P, Drummond H, et al. The efficacy of corticosteroid therapy in inflammatory bowel disease: analysis of a 5-year UK inception cohort. Aliment Pharmacol Ther 2006;24:319–30.

51. Singleton JW, Law DH, Kelley ML Jr, et al. National Cooperative Crohn's Disease Study: adverse reactions to study drugs. Gastroenterology 1979;77:870–82.

52. Kane SV, Schoenfeld P, Sandborn WJ, et al. The effectiveness of budesonide therapy for Crohn's disease. Aliment Pharmacol Ther 2002;16:1509–17.

53. Otley A, Steinhart AH. Budesonide for induction of remission in Crohn's disease. Cochrane Database Syst Rev 2005;(4):CD000296.

54. Thomsen OO, Cortot A, Jewell D, et al. A comparison of budesonide and mesalamine for active Crohn's disease. International Budesonide-Mesalamine Study Group. N Engl J Med 1998;339:370–4.

55. Rutgeerts P, Lofberg R, Malchow H, et al. A comparison of budesonide with prednisolone for active Crohn's disease. N Engl J Med 1994;331:842–5.

56. Pearson DC, May GR, Fick GH, et al. Azathioprine and 6-mercaptopurine in Crohn disease. A meta-analysis. Ann Intern Med 1995;123:132–42.

57. Feagan BG, Rochon J, Fedorak RN, et al. Methotrexate for the treatment of Crohn's disease. The North American Crohn's Study Group Investigators. N Engl J Med 1995;332:292–7.

58. Targan SR, Hanauer SB, van Deventer SJ, et al. A short-term study of chimeric monoclonal antibody cA2 to tumor necrosis factor alpha for Crohn's disease. Crohn's Disease cA2 Study Group. N Engl J Med 1997;337:1029–35.

59. Hanauer SB, Sandborn WJ, Rutgeerts P, et al. Human anti-tumor necrosis factor monoclonal antibody (adalimumab) in Crohn's disease: the CLASSIC-I trial. Gastroenterology 2006;130:323–33 [quiz 591].

60. Schreiber S, Rutgeerts P, Fedorak RN, et al. A randomized, placebo-controlled trial of certolizumab pegol (CDP870) for treatment of Crohn's disease. Gastroenterology 2005;129:807–18.

61. Feagan BG, Fedorak RN, Irvine EJ, et al. A comparison of methotrexate with placebo for the maintenance of remission in Crohn's disease. North American Crohn's Study Group Investigators. N Engl J Med 2000;342:1627–32.

62. Sandborn WJ, Hanauer SB, Rutgeerts P, et al. Adalimumab for maintenance treatment of Crohn's disease: results of the CLASSIC II trial. Gut 2007;56: 1232–9.

63. Schreiber S, Khaliq-Kareemi M, Lawrance IC, et al. Maintenance therapy with certolizumab pegol for Crohn's disease. N Engl J Med 2007;357:239–50.

64. Vermeire S, van Assche G, Rutgeerts P. Review article: altering the natural history of Crohn's disease–evidence for and against current therapies. Aliment Pharmacol Ther 2007;25:3–12.

65. Cosnes J, Nion-Larmurier I, Beaugerie L, et al. Impact of the increasing use of immunosuppressants in Crohn's disease on the need for intestinal surgery. Gut 2005;54:237–41.

66. Langholz E, Munkholm P, Davidsen M, et al. Course of ulcerative colitis: analysis of changes in disease activity over years. Gastroenterology 1994;107:3–11.

67. Langholz E, Munkholm P, Davidsen M, et al. Changes in extent of ulcerative colitis: a study on the course and prognostic factors. Scand J Gastroenterol 1996;31:260–6.

68. Solberg IC, Lygren I, Jahnsen J, et al. Clinical course during the first 10 years of ulcerative colitis: results from a population-based inception cohort (IBSEN study). Scand J Gastroenterol 2009;44:431–40.

69. Dickinson RJ, O'Connor HJ, Pinder I, et al. Double blind controlled trial of oral vancomycin as adjunctive treatment in acute exacerbations of idiopathic colitis. Gut 1985;26:1380–4.

70. Rubin DT, Kornblunth A. Role of antibiotics in the management of inflammatory bowel disease: a review. Rev Gastroenterol Disord 2005;5(Suppl 3):S10–5.

71. Lichtiger S, Present DH, Kornbluth A, et al. Cyclosporine in severe ulcerative colitis refractory to steroid therapy. N Engl J Med 1994;330:1841–5.

72. Van Assche G, D'Haens G, Noman M, et al. Randomized, double-blind comparison of 4 mg/kg versus 2 mg/kg intravenous cyclosporine in severe ulcerative colitis. Gastroenterology 2003;125:1025–31.

73. Lichtenstein GR, Kamm MA, Boddu P, et al. Effect of once- or twice-daily MMX mesalamine (SPD476) for the induction of remission of mild to moderately active ulcerative colitis. Clin Gastroenterol Hepatol 2007;5:95–102.

74. Kamm MA, Sandborn WJ, Gassull M, et al. Once-daily, high-concentration MMX mesalamine in active ulcerative colitis. Gastroenterology 2007;132:66–75 [quiz 432–3].

75. Safdi M, DeMicco M, Sninsky C, et al. A double-blind comparison of oral versus rectal mesalamine versus combination therapy in the treatment of distal ulcerative colitis. Am J Gastroenterol 1997;92:1867–71.

76. Marteau P, Probert CS, Lindgren S, et al. Combined oral and enema treatment with Pentasa (mesalazine) is superior to oral therapy alone in patients with extensive mild/moderate active ulcerative colitis: a randomised, double blind, placebo controlled study. Gut 2005;54:960–5.

77. Gisbert JP, Linares PM, McNicholl AG, et al. Meta-analysis: efficacy of azathioprine and mercaptopurine in ulcerative colitis. Aliment Pharmacol Ther 2009;30:126–37.

78. Rutgeerts P, Sandborn WJ, Feagan BG, et al. Infliximab for induction and maintenance therapy for ulcerative colitis. N Engl J Med 2005;353:2462–76.

79. Timmer A, McDonald JWD, MacDonald JK. Azathioprine and 6-mercaptopurine for maintenance of remission in ulcerative colitis. Cochrane Database Syst Rev 2007:CD000478.

80. Jones J, Loftus EV Jr, Panaccione R, et al. Relationships between disease activity and serum and fecal biomarkers in patients with Crohn's disease. Clin Gastroenterol Hepatol 2008;6:1218–24.

81. Vermeire S, Van Assche G, Rutgeerts P. Laboratory markers in IBD: useful, magic, or unnecessary toys? Gut 2006;55:426–31.

82. Langhorst J, Elsenbruch S, Koelzer J, et al. Noninvasive markers in the assessment of intestinal inflammation in inflammatory bowel diseases: performance of fecal lactoferrin, calprotectin, and PMN-elastase, CRP, and clinical indices. Am J Gastroenterol 2008;103:162–9.

83. Best WR, Becktel JM, Singleton JW, et al. Development of a Crohn's disease activity index. National Cooperative Crohn's Disease Study. Gastroenterology 1976;70:439–44.

84. Harvey RF, Bradshaw JM. A simple index of Crohn's-disease activity. Lancet 1980;1:514.

85. Schroeder KW, Tremaine WJ, Ilstrup DM. Coated oral 5-aminosalicylic acid therapy for mildly to moderately active ulcerative colitis. A randomized study. N Engl J Med 1987;317:1625–9.

86. Sandborn WJ, Rutgeerts PM, Reinisch WM. Sonic: a randomized double-blind, controlled trial comparing infliximab and infliximab plus immunomodulators and biologic therapy [abstract]. Am J Gastroenterol 2008;1117:S436.

87. Olaison G, Smedh K, Sjodahl R. Natural course of Crohn's disease after ileocolic resection: endoscopically visualised ileal ulcers preceding symptoms. Gut 1992;33:331–5.

88. Rutgeerts P, Geboes K, Vantrappen G, et al. Predictability of the postoperative course of Crohn's disease. Gastroenterology 1990;99:956–63.

89. Sachar DB. The problem of postoperative recurrence of Crohn's disease. Med Clin North Am 1990;74:183–8.

90. Regueiro M, Schraut WH, Kip K, et al. Silent Crohn's disease (CD): poor correlation between Crohn's Disease Activity Index (CDAI) and endoscopic activity scores one year after intestinal resection and ileocolonic anastamosis [abstract]. Gastroenterology 2009;136:A685.

91. Rodemann JF, Kip K, Binion DG, et al. Clinical assessment of ulcerative colitis activity correlates poorly with endoscopic disease activity [abstract]. Gastroenterology 2009;136:A668.

92. Hanauer SB. Dose-ranging study of mesalamine (PENTASA) enemas in the treatment of acute ulcerative proctosigmoiditis: results of a multicentered placebo-controlled trial. The U.S. PENTASA Enema Study Group. Inflamm Bowel Dis 1998;4:79–83.

93. Langhorst J, Boone JH, Rueffer A, et al. A new simple highly accurate quantitative disease activity index with improved correlation to endoscopy for assessing intestinal inflammation in IBD [abstract]. Gastroenterology 2009;136:A668.

94. Froslie KF, Jahnsen J, Moum BA, et al. Mucosal healing in inflammatory bowel disease: results from a Norwegian population-based cohort. Gastroenterology 2007;133:412–22.

95. Rutgeerts P, Diamond RH, Bala M, et al. Scheduled maintenance treatment with infliximab is superior to episodic treatment for the healing of mucosal ulceration associated with Crohn's disease. Gastrointest Endosc 2006;63:433–42 [quiz 464].

96. Schnitzler F, Fidder H, Ferrante M, et al. Mucosal healing predicts long-term outcome of maintenance therapy with infliximab in Crohn's disease. Inflamm Bowel Dis 2009 [Epub ahead of print].

97. Truelove SC, Witts LJ. Cortisone in ulcerative colitis: preliminary report on a therapeutic trial. Br Med J 1954;14:375–8.

98. Modigliani R, Mary JY, Simon JF, et al. Clinical, biological, and endoscopic picture of attacks of Crohn's disease. Evolution on prednisolone. Groupe d'Etude Thérapeutique des Affections Inflammatoires Digestives. Gastroenterology 1990;98:811–8.

99. Mantzaris GJ, Christidou A, Sfakianakis M, et al. Azathioprine is superior to budesonide in achieving and maintaining mucosal healing and histologic remission in steroid-dependent Crohn's disease. Inflamm Bowel Dis 2009;15:375–82.

100. Ardizzone S, Maconi G, Sampietro GM, et al. Azathioprine and mesalamine for prevention of relapse after conservative surgery for Crohn's disease. Gastroenterology 2004;127:730–40.

101. Hanauer SB, Korelitz BI, Rutgeerts P, et al. Postoperative maintenance of Crohn's disease remission with 6-mercaptopurine, mesalamine, or placebo: a 2-year trial. Gastroenterology 2004;127:723–9.

102. Kozarek RA, Patterson DJ, Gelfand MD, et al. Methotrexate induces clinical and histologic remission in patients with refractory inflammatory bowel disease. Ann Intern Med 1989;110:353–6.

103. Panaccione R. The use of methotrexate is associated with mucosal healing in Crohn's disease [abstract]. Gastroenterology 2005;128(Suppl):A49.

104. Rutgeerts P, D'Haens GR, Van Assche GA, et al. Healing in patients with moderate to severe ileocolonic Crohn's disease: first results of the EXTEND trial [abstract]. Gastroenterology 2009;136:A116.

105. Colombel J, Lemann M, Bouhnik Y, et al. Endoscopic mucosal improvement in patients with active Crohn's disease treated with certolizumab pegol: first results of the MUSIC clinical trial [abstract]. Inflamm Bowel Dis 2008;14:S25.

106. Cosnes J, Cattan S, Blain A, et al. Long-term evolution of disease behavior of Crohn's disease. Inflamm Bowel Dis 2002;8:244–50.

107. Goekoop-Ruiterman YP, de Vries-Bouwstra JK, Allaart CF, et al. Clinical and radiographic outcomes of four different treatment strategies in patients with early rheumatoid arthritis (the BeSt study): a randomized, controlled trial. Arthritis Rheum 2005;52:3381–90.

108. Breedveld FC, Weisman MH, Kavanaugh AF, et al. The PREMIER study: a multicenter, randomized, double-blind clinical trial of combination therapy with adalimumab plus methotrexate versus methotrexate alone or adalimumab alone in patients with early, aggressive rheumatoid arthritis who had not had previous methotrexate treatment. Arthritis Rheum 2006;54:26–37.

109. Markowitz J, Grancher K, Kohn N, et al. A multicenter trial of 6-mercaptopurine and prednisone in children with newly diagnosed Crohn's disease. Gastroenterology 2000;119:895–902.

110. Schreiber S, Reinisch W, Colombel JF, et al. Early Crohn's disease shows high levels of remission to therapy with adalimumab: sub-analysis of CHARM [abstract]. Gastroenterology 2007;132:A147.

111. Schreiber S, Hanauer SB, Lichtenstein GR, et al. Superior efficacy of certolizumab pegol in early Crohn's disease is independent of CRP status [abstract]. Gastroenterology 2007;132:T1298.

112. Hyams J, Crandall W, Kugathasan S, et al. Induction and maintenance infliximab therapy for the treatment of moderate-to-severe Crohn's disease in children. Gastroenterology 2007;132:863–73 [quiz 1165–6].

113. Regueiro M, Schraut W, Baidoo L, et al. Infliximab prevents Crohn's disease recurrence after ileal resection. Gastroenterology 2009;136:441–50, e1, [quiz 716].

114. Baert FJ, Moortgat L, Van Assche GA, et al. Mucosal healing predicts sustained clinical remission in early Crohn's disease. Gastroenterology 2008;134:W1133.

115. Rubin DT, Sederman R. Maintenance of response to biologic therapy in Crohn's disease is improved with "Early Use" v. "Step Up" treatment using health claims data [abstract]. Gastroenterology 2009;136:A735.

116. Rutter M, Saunders B, Wilkinson K, et al. Severity of inflammation is a risk factor for colorectal neoplasia in ulcerative colitis. Gastroenterology 2004;126:451–9.

117. Velayos FS, Terdiman JP, Walsh JM. Effect of 5-aminosalicylate use on colorectal cancer and dysplasia risk: a systematic review and metaanalysis of observational studies. Am J Gastroenterol 2005;100:1345–53.

118. Reinisch W, Sandborn WJ, Rutgeerts P, et al. Infliximab treatment for ulcerative colitis: comparable clinical response, clinical remission, mucosal healing in patients with disease duration <3 years Vs >3 years [abstract]. Gastroenterology 2008;134:A495.

Treatment of Fistulizing Inflammatory Bowel Disease

David A. Schwartz, MD[a],*, Brad E. Maltz, MD[b,c]

KEYWORDS

- Fistula • Inflammatory bowel disease • Crohn disease
- Biologic agents • Anti-TNF • Perianal • Abscess • Treatment

Crohn disease can manifest in many different ways including fibrostenotic (stricturing) or nonperforating, nonstricturing (inflammatory) disease or predominantly perforating (fistulizing) disease. Patients with fistulizing Crohn disease tend to have a more aggressive disease course. Fistulas can be either external (enterocutaneous or perianal) or internal, such as enteroenteral or enterocystic. The morbidity is increased greatly in those patients with fistulizing disease. Perianal disease and fistulas can lead to fecal incontinence, abscess formation, and anal strictures. External fistulas, including enterocutaneous and perianal fistulas, are associated with pain, abscesses, and drainage. In contrast, internal fistulas are frequently asymptomatic and therefore hard to diagnose. The treatment of fistulas depends on many factors, including location, severity, and previous surgical history.

Understanding of perianal disease continues to grow, and newer therapies such as antitumor necrosis factor anti-(TNF) agents have expanded therapeutic treatment options and changed the practitioner's goal of treatment for fistulas from reduction in fistula drainage to true closure or fibrosis of the fistula tract.

The estimated incidence of fistulas (enterocutaneous or perianal) in patients with Crohn disease is approximately 35%.[1] Approximately 21% of patients with Crohn will have perianal fistulas within 10 years of diagnosis. Before the introduction of biologic agents, most fistulas required surgical intervention, and the rate of fistula recurrence was estimated to be 34%.[1–3] Internal fistulas are often silent but perhaps just as common. In a study by Michelassi and colleagues, one third of all patients undergoing

This article originally appeared in *Gastroenterology Clinics of North America*, Volume 38, Issue 4.
[a] Division of Gastroenterology, Vanderbilt University Medical Center, Suite 514, 1211 21st Avenue, Nashville, TN 37232, USA
[b] Vanderbilt University, TN, USA
[c] 1600 The Vanderbilt Clinic, Nashville, TN 37232-5280, USA
* Corresponding author.
E-mail address: David.a.schwartz@vanderbilt.edu (D.A. Schwartz).

an operation for Crohn disease were found to have internal fistulas. Of those patients, 25 of 36 (69%) with enterovesicular fistula had symptoms of internal fistula such as pneumoturia or fecaluria. In the other 147 patients with internal fistulas, only 54% had accurate preoperative diagnostic evaluation (radiographic or endoscopic).[4]

UNDERSTANDING THE ANATOMY AND PATHOGENESIS

Current understanding shows that fistulas in Crohn disease develop secondary to multiple causes. Internal fistulas, or fistulas from the small bowel or colon to the adjacent bowel or organs, are likely secondary to transmural inflammation of the bowel wall. This inflammation then can penetrate into adjacent organs, tissue, or skin. These fistulas are more likely to occur at the site of a stricture and may represent a bypass tract. These types of fistulas are categorized by their location and the connection with contiguous organs such as enterovesicular fistulas or enteroenteric fistulas.[5] One proposed mechanism for perianal fistula formation is that fistulas begin as an ulcer within the anal canal. When feces are forced into this ulcer, they cause penetration of the lesion through the wall. This track then extends over time with increased pressure from the fecal stream.[6] Another hypothesis of fistula formation involves an abscess of one of the anal glands, which can be present within the intersphincteric space. This abscess then grows, and a fistula forms as a way to drain this area of the purulence under pressure. The fistula can extend through the external anal sphincter (trans-sphincteric fistula), track down to the skin (intersphincteric fistula), or track upward to become a suprasphincteric fistula. It is important to diagnose and categorize fistulas correctly, as correct categorization impacts which treatment modality will be most useful or successful in an individual patient.

In order to understand how best to treat fistulizing Crohn disease, one must have a thorough understanding of the anatomy of the anal canal (**Fig. 1**). The anal canal is formed by three layers:

The internal anal sphincter, which is made of smooth muscle of the rectum
The intersphincteric space
External anal sphincter, which is comprised of skeletal muscle arising from an extension of the puborectalis and levator ani muscles

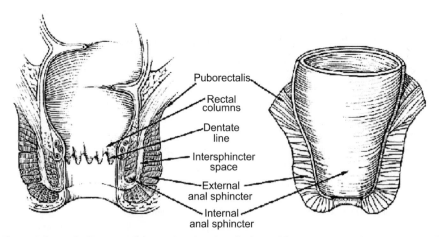

Fig. 1. Schematic diagram of the perianal region. (*Adapted from* Fry RD, Kodner IJ. Anorectal disorders. Clin Symp 1985;37:2–32; with permission.)

The dentate line is the midway point of the internal anal sphincter. It is the area that marks the interface of the columnar and transitional epithelium of the rectum from the squamous epithelium of the anus. Within this area, one finds the anal crypts with anal glands located at the bases of the crypts.

A careful physical examination and endoscopic examination must be performed prior to initiating treatment for the fistulizing disease, with special attention to location of the fistula in relation to the dentate line. Fistulas can be classified many different ways. The most anatomically precise method is the Parks classification.[5,7] This classification system uses the external sphincter as a central point of reference and includes five types of perianal fistulas: (1) intersphincteric, (2) trans-sphincteric, (3) suprasphincteric, (4) extrasphincteric, and (5) superficial. An intersphincteric fistula tracks between the internal anal sphincter (IAS) and the external anal sphincter (EAS) in the intersphincteric space. A trans-sphincteric fistula tracks from the intersphincteric space through the EAS. A suprasphincteric fistula leaves the intersphincteric space over the top of the puborectalis and penetrates the levator muscle before tracking down to the skin. An extrasphincteric fistula tracks outside of the EAS and penetrates the levator muscle into the rectum. Finally, a superficial fistula tracks below both the IAS and EAS complexes.

Although the Parks system is the most accurate method of describing fistula anatomy and helps clinicians communicate with the surgeons taking care of patients with perianal fistulas, there are several limitations to this system, including the fact that associated abscesses and connections to other structures such as the vagina or bladder are not part of this schema but are clinically important.

The other methods for classifying fistulas are to divide them into simple or complex fistulas. This was proposed in 2003 by American Gastroenterological Association Technical Review Panel as an alternative and more clinically relevant classification system for perianal fistula (**Fig. 2**).[8] Within this system, a simple fistula is superficial or begins low in the rectal canal, has a single opening on the skin, is not associated with an abscess, and does not connect to other structures such as the vagina or scrotum. A fistula is complex if it begins high in the canal, is associated with an abscess, has multiple openings, or connects to an adjacent structure. Another important distinction is to determine if the fistula is associated with obvious inflammation of the colonic mucosa. If so, this too would be considered complex. This classification is

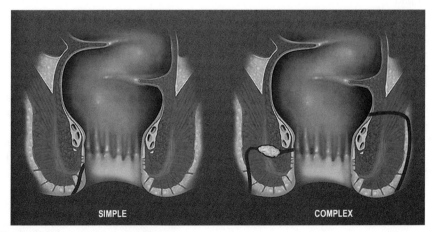

Fig. 2. Simple versus complex fistulas.

clinically relevant, because complex fistulas involve more of the sphincter complex, reducing the chance for fistula healing, and placing patients at increased risk for incontinence with aggressive surgical intervention.

DIAGNOSTIC MODALITIES FOR ASSESSING FISTULAS

Occult abscesses or fistulas are difficult but important to recognize. Missing occult lesions can result in recurrent fistulas or abscesses or convert a simple fistula into a complex fistulizing process.[9,10] Once the fistulizing process becomes complex, the chance for healing is reduced greatly.[9,11,12] In order to prevent the development of a complex fistula and increase the chance of closure, one must identify and optimize the medical and surgical treatment early at disease onset. The fistula must be defined fully so appropriate therapy can be started. The goal is to establish drainage of any abscess that may be present and control fistula healing to prevent abscess formation during treatment of fistulas. Ideally, this initial assessment could be done with a simple digital rectal exam (DRE), although because of the associated induration and scarring, the accuracy of this examination in defining fistula anatomy is reportedly low, 62% in one study.[13]

Because of the low accuracy of the DRE, imaging should be used as a means to provide a therapeutic roadmap to ensure that all potential areas are treated. The various imaging modalities that have been used to assess perianal fistulas include fistulography, computed tomography (CT), pelvic magnetic resonance imaging (MRI), and rectal endoscopic ultrasound (EUS).

FISTULOGRAPHY AND CT

Fistulography involves the placement of a small catheter into the cutaneous opening of a fistula tract and injection contrast under pressure. Fistulography can cause pain during the examination and the theoretical potential for dissemination of septic fistulous contents. Fistulography has a low overall accuracy for determining the tract of the fistula, ranging from 16% to 50%.[14–17]

CT has been used to assess perianal disease but is limited by poor spatial resolution in the pelvis. It is not commonly used, because its accuracy also is low, ranging from 24% to 60%.[18–22]

EUS MRI

The most accurate way to evaluate perianal Crohn fistulas is by MRI[23–26] or rectal EUS.[18,19,27–30] A prospective blinded study compared the accuracy of MRI, EUS, and examination under anesthesia (EUA) in 34 patients with suspected Crohn perianal fistulas.[28] In this study, all three methods demonstrated high accuracy when compared with the consensus gold standard (EUS, 91%; MRI, 87%; and EUA, 91%). The consensus gold standard was determined by the coinvestigators after reviewing all of the test results and the patients' history. When any of the imaging modalities were combined with EUA, the accuracy was 100% in these patients and was the most cost-effective approach. The role of MRI and EUS to monitor the fistula response to medical therapy is still being explored but may help guide treatment decisions in these patients.[31–33]

TREATMENT OPTIONS

After a fistula has been assessed properly and categorized as simple versus complex, the most appropriate treatment course can be determined. The decision between medical therapy and surgical therapy or a combination medical and surgical therapy is determined by the type of fistula and the degree of rectal inflammation present.

MEDICAL TREATMENT
Antibiotics

Multiple studies have been performed utilizing antibiotics for treating fistulizing Crohn disease, with only modest results. Most of these are open-label case series involving few patients.[34–36] Antibiotics are used for both their activity in perianal sepsis and for their anti-inflammatory properties. The most common antibiotics used are metronidazole at doses of 750 to 1000 mg/d or ciprofloxacin at 1000 to 1500 mg/d for up to 2 to 4 months. Adverse events commonly associated with metronidazole include metallic taste, glossitis, nausea, and a distal peripheral sensory neuropathy. Adverse events with ciprofloxacin occur less commonly but include headache, nausea, diarrhea, and rash.

Recently, a randomized, double-blinded, placebo-controlled trial was performed looking at ciprofloxacin and metronidazole for treating perianal fistulas in patients with Crohn disease.[37] Twenty-five patients were randomized to ciprofloxacin 500 mg (10 patients), metronidazole 500 mg (7 patients), or placebo (8 patients) twice daily for 10 weeks. Response (at least 50% reduction in the number of draining fistulas) at week 10 was seen in four patients (40%) treated with ciprofloxacin, one patient (14.3%) treated with metronidazole, and one patient (12.5%) with placebo ($P = .43$). One patient each from both the ciprofloxacin and placebo groups, and five (71.4%) treated with metronidazole dropped out of the study ($P<.02$). This small study suggested that remission and response occurred more often in patients treated with ciprofloxacin, but the differences were not significant.

Immunomodulators

There have been several trials of 6-mercaptopurine and azathioprine (AZA/6MP) for luminal Crohn disease where the treatment of perianal disease was a secondary endpoint.[38] A meta-analysis of these trials looked at fistula closure as a secondary endpoint for post hoc analysis. This analysis found that 22 of 42 (54%) of patients with perianal Crohn disease who received AZA/6MP responded versus only 6 of 29 (21%) patients who received placebo (odds ratio [OR] = 4.44) Caution should be taken, as the primary goal of these studies was to treat active inflammatory Crohn disease, and they were not designed primarily to look at the effect on perianal fistulas. In fact, only one of the studies stratified the patients for the presence of fistulas at randomization.

In a study by Dejaco and colleagues, antibiotics were used along with immuno-modulator therapy. The use of metronidazole or ciprofloxacin induced an early response (at least 50% reduction in the number of draining fistulas) at week 8, with fistula closure occurring in 25% of cases. In patients who received additional azathioprine therapy, the response was better (48% vs 15%) at week 20. Most of the patients in this study had simple fistulas, and only 9 of the 52 cases were classed as complex fistulas.[39]

Tacrolimus

Tacrolimus has been studied for perianal Crohn disease in a randomized placebo-controlled study.[6] Forty-eight patients with Crohn perianal fistulas were randomized to tacrolimus standard dose 0.2 mg/kg/d versus placebo for 10 weeks. In the tacrolimus group, 43% had fistula improvement (closure of at least 50% of fistulas for longer than 4 weeks) compared with 8% placebo patients (P = .004). Complete fistula closure, however, was only achieved in 10% of the patients who received tacrolimus. Fistula closure in the treatment group was not improved with concomitant immuno-suppressive therapy with AZA/6MP (38% closure with therapy vs 50% without). The number of adverse events was higher in the treatment group (5.2 vs 3.9, P = .009), including headache, insomnia, elevated creatinine, paresthesias, and tremor. The use of tacrolimus requires regular monitoring of renal function and drug levels, which limits its ease of use.

In the study by Gonzalez-Lama, tacrolimus was used to treat patients with fistulizing Crohn disease that was refractory to conventional therapy including infliximab. In this open-label study, patients received oral tacrolimus (0.05 mg/kg every 12 hours). Ten patients were included in the study (enterocutaneous fistula, three patients; perianal fistula, four patients; rectovaginal fistula, three patients) with 6 to 24 months of follow-up. Four patients (40%) achieved complete clinical responses. Five patients (50%) achieved partial responses (decrease in fistula drainage, size, discomfort) (P<.05).[40]

Cyclosporine

Studies with cyclosporine for fistulizing Crohn disease also have been performed. These are all uncontrolled small studies that showed improvement in fistula drainage, but most patients relapsed after transition to oral therapy or discontinuation of the drug.[41–43] The toxicity profile of cyclosporine may preclude use for fistulizing disease given safer, better-tolerated alternatives. Methotrexate also has been studied in an uncontrolled case series for treatment of perianal Crohn disease[44,45]; however, there currently are not enough data to support use of methotrexate for fistulizing disease.

TNF ANTAGONISTS

Prior to the introduction of anti-TNF antibodies, the goal of treatment was primarily control of symptoms in order to improve the patient's quality of life. Long-term reso-lution had not been demonstrated in a large group of patients. Now it is realistic to strive for complete fibrosis of the fistula when using biologic agents, especially in those patients with simple fistulas.

Several biologic therapies have been developed for treating Crohn disease—including adalimumab (a fully human immunoglobulin [Ig]G1 anti-TNF-alpha monoclonal antibody), infliximab (a chimeric monoclonal antibody to TNF-alpha), and certolizumab pegol (a humanized anti-TNF Fab' monoclonal antibody fragment linked to polyethylene glycol)—which antagonize TNF-alpha and have been shown to decrease clinical severity of disease.

There have been two double-blind placebo-controlled trials of an anti-TNF anti-body with a primary focus being on fistulizing Crohn disease. Both of these trials have been with infliximab.[7,8] The initial fistula trial with an anti-TNF-alpha agent looked at the short-term effect of infliximab on fistula drainage.[7] Ninety-four patients were randomized to treatment with infliximab 5 mg/kg, infliximab 10 mg/kg, or placebo. Patients were given an infusion at weeks 0, 2, and 6. The primary endpoint was a greater than or equal to 50% reduction from baseline in the number of draining fistulas. A fistula was considered to be draining if the examiner could express puru-lent material with gentle pressure on the fistula tract. Results showed a 68% response rate (achievement of the primary endpoint) in the 5 mg/kg infliximab treat-ment arm compared with only 26% in the placebo cohort; 55% of patients who received infliximab 5 mg/kg had complete cessation of drainage (ie, closure) of all fistulas. The fistulas, however, tended to become active again once infliximab was discontinued.

This study led to the ACCENT II (A Crohn Disease Clinical Trial Evaluating Infliximab in a New Long-term Treatment Regimen in Patients With Fistulizing Crohn Disease) trial,[8] which investigated whether cessation of fistula drainage could be preserved over the course of a year with infliximab maintenance therapy given every 8 weeks. Patients who had active fistulas and who responded to the initial three doses of infliximab at weeks 0, 2, and 6 were randomized to receive infliximab or placebo every 8 weeks. After 54 weeks, 36% of patients in the infliximab group maintained complete fistula closure compared with 19% in the placebo arm ($P = .009$).

Fistula healing was studied as a secondary endpoint in the adalimumab maintenance trial, CHARM (Crohn trial of the fully Human antibody Adalimumab for Remission Maintenance).[9] The CHARM trial assessed the efficacy of adalimumab in maintaining response and remission in patients with luminal Crohn disease. Complete fistula closure at 56 weeks was seen in 33% of the treated group (ie, total randomized population on therapy who had fistulas at baseline, combined 40 mg weekly and every other week adalimumab dosing arms) compared with 13% in the placebo arm ($P = .016$). The response was very durable. In patients who demonstrated fistula closure at week 26, all maintained fistula closure at week 56. Recently, the results of an open-label extension study continued from the end (week 56) of the CHARM trial were presented.[10] The study population was comprised of patients with fistulas at baseline of CHARM; data from the two adalimumab doses were pooled. In this follow-up study, the 2-year complete fistula response rate was 71%, and the 2-year complete cessation of drainage rate was 60%.

Unlike other monoclonal antibodies, certolizumab pegol does not contain an Fc portion and therefore does not induce in vitro complement activation, antibody-dependent cellular cytotoxicity, or apoptosis. Fistula healing also was examined as a secondary endpoint in one of the certolizumab maintenance trials (PRECISE [Pegylated antibody fragment Evaluation in Crohn disease Safety and Efficacy] 1).[11] In the subset of patients with a baseline C-reactive protein level greater than or equal to 10 mg/L, certolizumab was shown to be equivalent to placebo in healing fistulas after 26 weeks of therapy; 30% of certolizumab-treated patients had fistula closure verssus 31% of placebo patients.

Conversely, the second certolizumab trial, PRECISE 2,[12] which evaluated the efficacy and tolerability of certolizumab in the maintenance of clinical response following successful induction therapy in patients with active Crohn disease, had a small number of patients with draining fistulas at enrollment. Fourteen percent of patients in the intention-to-treat population from this study had draining fistulas at baseline (28 patients in the treatment arm and 30 on placebo).[46] Among these patients, 54% of those treated with certolizumab had fistula closure as compared to 43% of those in the placebo group. At week 26, 67% of patients who received continuous certolizumab were able to maintain complete fistula closure. The study was underpowered to examine the efficacy of certolizumab for fistula closure. Based on the results above, the authors suspect that certolizumab pegol is effective in fistulizing disease; however, given the conflicting results, further studies are needed to look at the efficacy of certolizumab pegol for treating Crohn perianal fistulas.

There are no head-to-head trials comparing the efficacy of these agents in treating Crohn disease or for obtaining fistula closure. Additionally, there are no studies comparing the efficacy of surgical treatment alone with combination surgical intervention plus conventional medical treatment (antibiotics, immunosuppressants). A retrospective study involving 32 patients with perianal fistulizing Crohn disease, however, examined the efficacy of infliximab alone versus infliximab as an adjunct to seton placement.[11] Patients with fistulizing Crohn disease who had EUA with seton placement prior to receiving infliximab had an initial response of 100% versus 82% for patients who only received infliximab (response was defined as complete closure and cessation of drainage from the fistula). Patients who received infliximab after EUA with seton placement also had a lower recurrence rate (44% vs 79%) and longer time to recurrence (13.5 months vs 3.6 months). In another retrospective review, Topstad and colleagues showed that seton placement prior to infliximab resulted in complete response in 67% of patients.[47]

Natalizumab, a recombinant, humanized monoclonal antibody to alpha-4 integrin, which inhibits leukocyte adhesion and migration into inflamed tissue, has demonstrated efficacy in reducing the clinical severity of Crohn disease. It does not appear to be useful in fistulizing disease, however. On the basis of the initial double-blind, placebo-controlled trial by Ghosh and colleagues,[48] natalizumab did not appear to be effective in fistulizing Crohn disease. The subsequent evaluation of *natalizumab* as continuous therapy (ENACT)-1, ENACT-2, and efficacy of natalizumab in Crohn disease response and remission trials specifically excluded patients with active fistulas.[49,50] Therefore, this biologic agent cannot be recommended for patients with fistulizing Crohn disease.

Much has been learned about the treatment of fistulizing Crohn disease since the initial infliximab trials nearly a decade ago. Data indicate that most patients with fistulizing disease will need maintenance therapy, as brief exposure to TNF antagonists does stop drainage of fistulas initially, but reoccurrence is common after cessation of therapy. Indeed, after 1 year of maintenance therapy with infliximab, complete closure of fistula tracks is rare, as evidenced by evidence on MRI or EUS examination of persistent fistula activity even when the fistula drainage stops.[31]

MISCELLANEOUS NONSURGICAL THERAPIES

Additional therapies including hyperbaric oxygen, elemental diets, total parenteral nutrition, mycophenolate mofetil, thalidomide, and granulocyte colony-stimulating factor have been reported in uncontrolled case series and case reports as being effective for treating perianal Crohn disease. No controlled trials, however, exist.[51,52]

One of the newer medical therapies utilizes oral spherical adsorptive carbon (AST-120). A prospective trial from Japan looked at AST-120 versus placebo for treating perianal fistulas in Crohn disease.[53] Patients were randomized and received AST-120 (N = 27) or placebo (N = 30). This study showed improvement in fistulas 37% versus 10% in placebo arm (P = .03), and remission rates were 29.6% and 6.7%, respectively (P = .035). Further studies, however, are needed to verify its efficacy.

THE USE OF IMAGING TO MONITOR FISTULA HEALING

Retrospective and small prospective trials have shown outcomes can be optimized by using imaging (EUS/MRI) to guide combination medical and surgical therapy in these patients.[54,55] Schwartz and colleagues looked at using EUS to assess and guide therapy for fistulas. Twenty one patients with Crohn perianal fistula underwent serial EUS exams. The findings were used to guide therapy (ie, the presence of fistula healing on EUS was used to decide the appropriate time for seton removal). In this study, no abscess developed during treatment in any patient. EUS evidence of persistent fistula activity was seen in 10 patients (48%); this activity would not have been appreciated with physical examination alone. This study showed using EUS to guide therapy for Crohn perianal fistulas resulted in high short- and long-term fistula response rate.[55]

Spradlin and colleagues prospectively studied EUS related to outcomes for patients with perianal fistulizing Crohn disease. In this study, 10 patients with perianal Crohn disease were prospectively enrolled in a randomized study. All patients underwent a rectal EUS to delineate fistula anatomy followed by an EUA by a colorectal surgeon with seton placement or incision and drainage, as indicated. The surgeon was blinded to the initial EUS results of patients in the control group. Patients in the EUS group underwent scheduled EUS and surgical interventions based on the findings. Those in the control group underwent additional interventions at the discretion of the surgeon (without EUS guidance). After 54 weeks, all patients had a repeat EUS performed to determine the fistula status. One of five (20%) in the control group and four of five (80%) in the EUS group had complete cessation of drainage.[56]

In a study by Tougeron and colleagues, MRI was used to assess and follow patients with fistulas. Patients with perianal fistulizing Crohn disease had baseline clinical and MRI characteristics recorded and were treated with infliximab. They did not find a MRI characteristic that was predictive of therapy response. The study did find that the presence of proctitis was associated with a lack of response to treatment.[57]

SURGICAL THERAPY

Surgical treatment is an integral part of treating fistulizing Crohn disease. The reported incidence of perianal fistulas that require surgery in patients with Crohn disease varies from 25% to 30%.[58,59] It has been shown that the combination of medical and surgical therapy results in the best outcome for these patients.[9,11,47,60] Surgical evaluation with EUA and seton placement allows for control of fistula healing during medical treatment. It is thought that the rapid closure of the cutaneous openings of the fistula tracks, which may be seen with anti-TNF drugs, can lead to abscess formation in the middle of the fistula track. In the two infliximab fistula trials, abscess formation during treatment was 11% to 15%.[61,62]

The most common surgical treatment options include EUA, which involves probing of the fistula tract, seton placement, incision, and drainage, or fistulotomy, in which the fistula tract is incised open. The placement of a draining seton maintains fistula drainage until the tract becomes inactive on medical treatment. A noncutting seton or draining seton is threaded through the fistula tract and is tied outside the anal canal. The seton can be removed when the fistula track has healed, or it can remain in situ for an extended period if healing has not occurred.[63]

Patients with superficial or low perianal fistulas who do not have active inflammation in their rectum (ie, simple fistulas) can be treated safely by fistulotomy alone with resolution of fistula symptoms in up to 85% patients.[64] Advancement flap procedures have been attempted as treatment for perianal fistulas with good initial healing rates of up to 89%, but recurrence was found in 34% of these patients during follow up.[65] In a similar study, an initial healing rate of 71% was seen after advancement flap procedure, but recurrence was 50% within 5 years.[66]

Fibrin glue also has been attempted to control fistulas in Crohn disease, and results have been varied; success rates vary from 0% to 80%.[67–70] This variability can be attributed, among other things, to the different types of fistulas treated (simple or complex; cryptoglandular, Crohn, or traumatic etiology) and the adjuvant therapies used with the glue. More studies are needed prior to recommending this as a therapeutic option.

Fistula plugs, bioprosthetic plugs made from porcine intestinal submucosa, also have been used in several studies, with mixed results.[67,71,72]

Abscesses associated with fistula must be drained in order to achieve healing. The surgical approach can include local incision and drainage, catheter drainage, or seton placement. According to the recommendations of the American Society of Colon and

Rectal Surgeons, anal abscesses should be drained in a timely manner. Lack of fluctuance should not be a reason to delay treatment. Perianal abscesses often can develop into a chronic fistula.[73]

In a 20-year review of patients with perianal Crohn disease performed prior to the introduction of anti-TNF antibodies, the rate of protectomy was 14%.[10] Even this drastic operation leaves 23% of patients with persistent perineal sinuses or unhealed perineal wounds.[74] Fecal diversion or proctocolectomy is reserved for patients with the most severe rectal disease that is refractory to other more conservative approaches. Diverting ostomy has been used to control fistulas in patients with severe disease. Ileostomy, however, has not been shown to change the natural progression of the disease and does not reduce the risk of fistula recurrence.[75] Additionally, the fistulas may become active again when the fecal stream is restored.

RECTOVAGINAL FISTULAS

Rectovaginal fistulas occur in 5% to 10% of female patients with Crohn disease.[76] These types of fistulas typically have to be repaired surgically, as medical management alone is not often successful. The surgical repair options include anocutaneous flap, vaginal flap or Martius graft.[77,78] Infliximab has been used as treatment for rectovaginal fistulas; of the 282 patients in the ACCENT II study, 25 of 138 (18.1%) women had a total of 27 draining rectovaginal fistulas at baseline. Of those who received infliximab, only 44.8% (13 of 29) had closure of rectovaginal fistulas at week 14.[79]

In the study by Topstad and colleagues, which primarily looked at the efficacy of infliximab combined with selective seton drainage in the healing of fistulizing anorectal Crohn disease, there were eight patients with rectovaginal fistulas. Of these women, complete response occurred in one, partial response in five, and no response in two. No patient with a combined rectovaginal/perianal fistula had a complete response.[47]

TREATMENT ALGORITHM

In counseling patients about the treatment of fistulizing Crohn disease, the most important decision is when to start biologic therapies. The top-down approach to starting anti-TNF therapy advocates the use of biologic therapy earlier in the disease course in order to prevent the complications associated with the disease.[23] In this paradigm, rather than ramping up therapy in the traditional step-up or sequential approach, proceeding from the weakest (ie, lowest efficacy [eg, 5-aminosalicylic acid or 5-ASA]) to the "strongest" (anti-TNF-alpha agents) therapeutic interventions, with each subsequent therapy being added due to lack of response or toxicity, one would reverse the treatment pyramid and start with the most effective therapy at the beginning (early in the disease course) in order to change the natural history of the disease and prevent complications. This type of treatment schema can be applied to fistulizing Crohn disease also. Indeed, the presence of fistulizing disease is one of the factors predictive of severe disabling Crohn disease.[24]

Because fistulizing disease is one of the predictive markers of severe disease, initiating therapy with anti-TNF agents early on in these patients is preferential for several reasons. Studies have shown that once a fistula becomes complex, the chance for complete closure of that fistula drops dramatically.[55] Therefore, by employing the most efficacious treatment available, one hopes to prevent this transformation. In addition, subanalysis of the certolizumab and adalimumab maintenance trials demonstrates significantly increased response rates to these agents in patients treated earlier in their disease course.[80,81] For instance, in the CHARM trial, patients who

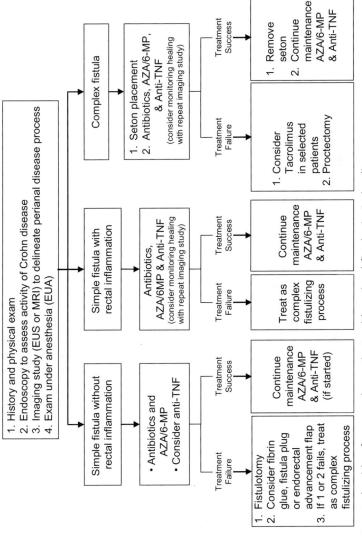

Fig. 3. Current treatment algorithm for managing patients with perianal fistulas in Crohn disease.

had Crohn disease less than 2 years had remission rates with maintenance adalimumab at week 56 of 51%, compared with remission rates of only 35% in patients who had Crohn disease longer than 5 years (P<.001).[81]

Treatment must be individualized for each patient on the basis of the type of fistula present (**Fig. 3**). Thus, the approach to treating patients with fistulas begins by first stratifying the perianal disease into one of three fistula types: simple fistulas without proctitis, simple fistulas with proctitis, or complex fistulas. This stratification generally is done by imaging the perianal disease with either MRI or EUS examination and endoscopy.

In patients with simple fistulas without proctitis, treatment consists of medical therapy and involves a trial of antibiotics and immunosuppressants, with or without anti-TNF-alpha agents. The use of surgical treatment in this subset of patients is not mandatory, as healing rates with isolated medical therapy are generally good. If no response is observed, then a combined surgical and medical approach with an anti-TNF-alpha agent is recommended.[82] Patients with simple fistulas and concomitant proctitis should be treated with a combined surgical and medical approach using anti-TNF-alpha agents as first-line therapy to decrease inflammation and allow fistula closure. A short trial of rectal 5-ASA or rectal steroids to reduce inflammation may represent a reasonable alternative. Clinicians typically begin with a top down approach, using an anti-TNF-alpha agent early to prevent the fistulizing process from becoming complex.

Complex fistulas absolutely require surgical intervention with the placement of draining setons, followed by treatment with a combination of antibiotics, immunosuppresents, and anti-TNF-alpha therapy, as the goal of therapy in this setting changes from complete fibrosis of the tract to control of fistula drainage and prevention of abscess formation.[55]

SUMMARY

Fistulas are a frequent manifestation of Crohn disease and can result in significant morbidity and often lead to the need for surgical intervention. Historically, it has been more difficult to obtain complete fistula closure in patients with perianal Crohn disease. The advent of anti-TNF-alpha agents and the use of more accurate imaging modalities such as MRI and rectal EUS have greatly enhanced the ability to manage fistulizing Crohn disease. A combined medical and surgical approach is usually the best option for most patients.

REFERENCES

1. Schwartz DA, Loftus EV Jr, Tremaine WJ, et al. The natural history of fistulizing Crohn's disease in Olmsted County, Minnesota. Gastroenterology 2002;122: 875–80.
2. Hellers G, Bergstrand O, Ewerth S, et al. Occurrence and outcome after primary treatment of anal fistulae in Crohn's disease. Gut 1980;21:525–7.
3. Tang LY, Rawsthorne P, Bernstein CN. Are perineal and luminal fistulas associated in Crohn's disease? A population-based study. Clin Gastroenterol Hepatol 2006;4:1130–4.
4. Michelassi F, Stella M, Balestracci T, et al. Incidence, diagnosis, and treatment of enteric and colorectal fistulae in patients with Crohn's disease. Ann Surg 1993; 218:660–6.
5. Hughes LE. Clinical classification of perianal Crohn's disease. Dis Colon Rectum 1992;35:928–32.

6. Hughes LE. Surgical pathology and management of anorectal Crohn's disease. J R Soc Med 1978;71:644–51.
7. Parks AG, Gordon PH, Hardcastle JD. A classification of fistula in ano. Br J Surg 1976;63:1–12.
8. American Gastroenterological Association medical position statement: perianal Crohn's disease. Gastroenterology 2003;125:1503–7.
9. Makowiec F, Jehle EC, Becker HD, et al. Perianal abscess in Crohn's disease. Dis Colon Rectum 1997;40:443–50.
10. Williamson PR, Hellinger MD, Larach SW, et al. Twenty-year review of the surgical management of perianal Crohn's disease. Dis Colon Rectum 1995;38:389–92.
11. Regueiro M, Mardini H. Treatment of perianal fistulizing Crohn's disease with infliximab alone or as an adjunct to exam under anesthesia with seton placement. Inflamm Bowel Dis 2003;9:98–103.
12. Bayer I, Gordon PH. Selected operative management of fistula in ano in Crohn's disease. Dis Colon Rectum 1994;37:760–5.
13. Van Beers B, Grandin C, Kartheuser A, et al. MRI of complicated anal fistulae: comparison with digital examination. J Comput Assist Tomogr 1994;18:87–90.
14. Glass RE, Ritchie JK, Lennard-Jones JE, et al. Internal fistulas in Crohn's disease. Dis Colon Rectum 1985;28:557–61.
15. Fazio VW, Wilk P, Turnbull RB Jr, et al. The dilemma of Crohn's disease: ileo-sigmoidal fistula complicating Crohn's disease. Dis Colon Rectum 1977;20:381–6.
16. Kuijpers HC, Schulpen T. Fistulography for fistulain ano. Is it useful? Dis Colon Rectum 1985;28:103–4.
17. Weisman RI, Orsay CP, Pearl RK, et al. The role of fistulography in fistula in ano. Report of five cases. Dis Colon Rectum 1991;34:181–4.
18. Schratter-Sehn AU, Lochs H, Vogelsang H, et al. Endoscopic ultrasonography versus computed tomography in the differential diagnosis of perianorectal complications in Crohn's disease. Endoscopy 1993;25:582–6.
19. Van Outryve MJ, Pelckmans PA, Michielsen PP, et al. Value of transrectal ultraso-nography in Crohn's disease. Gastroenterology 1991;101:1171–7.
20. Fishman EK, Wolf EJ, Jones B, et al. CT evaluation of Crohn's disease: effect on patient management. AJR Am J Roentgenol 1987;148:537–40.
21. Berliner L, Redmond P, Purow E, et al. Computed tomography in Crohn's disease. Am J Gastroenterol 1982;77:548–53.
22. Goldberg HI, Gore RM, Margulis AR, et al. Computed tomography in the evalu-ation of Crohn disease. AJR Am J Roentgenol 1983;140:277–82.
23. Lunniss PJ, Barker PG, Sultan AH, et al. Magnetic resonance imaging of fistula in ano. Dis Colon Rectum 1994;37:708–18.
24. Lunniss PJ, Armstrong P, Barker PG, et al. Magnetic resonance imaging of anal fistulae. Lancet 1992;340:394–6.
25. Barker PG, Lunniss PJ, Armstrong P, et al. Magnetic resonance imaging of fistula in ano: technique, interpretation, and accuracy. Clin Radiol 1994;49:7–13.
26. Haggett PJ, Moore NR, Shearman JD, et al. Pelvic and perineal complications of Crohn's disease: assessment using magnetic resonance imaging. Gut 1995;36:407–10.
27. Rasul I, Wilson SR, MacRae H, et al. Clinical and radiological responses after infliximab treatment for perianal fistulizing Crohn's disease. Am J Gastroenterol 2004;99:82–8.

28. Schwartz DA, Wiersema MJ, Dudiak KM, et al. A comparison of endoscopic ultra-sound, magnetic resonance imaging, and exam under anesthesia for evaluation of Crohn's perianal fistulas. Gastroenterology 2001;121:1064–72.

29. Orsoni P, Barthet M, Portier F, et al. Prospective comparison of endosonography, magnetic resonance imaging, and surgical findings in anorectal fistula and abscess complicating Crohn's disease. Br J Surg 1999;86:360–4.

30. Tio TL, Mulder CJ, Wijers OB, et al. Endosonography of perianal and pericolorec-tal fistula and/or abscess in Crohn's disease. Gastrointest Endosc 1990;36:331–6.

31. Van Assche G, Vanbeckevoort D, Bielen D, et al. Magnetic resonance imaging of the effects of infliximab on perianal fistulizing Crohn's disease. Am J Gastro-enterol 2003;98:332–9.

32. van Bodegraven AA, Sloots CE, Felt-Bersma RJ, et al. Endosonographic evidence of persistence of Crohn's disease-associated fistulas after infliximab treatment, irrespective of clinical response. Dis Colon Rectum 2002;45:39–45 [discussion: 45–6].

33. Bell SJ, Halligan S, Windsor AC, et al. Response of fistulating Crohn's disease to infliximab treatment assessed by magnetic resonance imaging. Aliment Pharma-col Ther 2003;17:387–93.

34. Brandt LJ, Bernstein LH, Boley SJ, et al. Metronidazole therapy for perineal Crohn's disease: a follow-up study. Gastroenterology 1982;83:383–7.

35. Present DH, Korelitz BI, Wisch N, et al. Treatment of Crohn's disease with 6-mercaptopurine. A long-term, randomized, double-blind study. N Engl J Med 1980;302:981–7.

36. Bernstein LH, Frank MS, Brandt LJ, et al. Healing of perineal Crohn's disease with metronidazole. Gastroenterology 1980;79:599.

37. Thia KT, Mahadevan U, Feagan BG, et al. Ciprofloxacin or metronidazole for the treatment of perianal fistulas in patients with Crohn's disease: a randomized, double-blind, placebo-controlled pilot study. Inflamm Bowel Dis 2009;15:17–24.

38. Pearson DC, May GR, Fick GH, et al. Azathioprine and 6-mercaptopurine in Crohn disease. A meta-analysis. Ann Intern Med 1995;123:132–42.

39. Dejaco C, Harrer M, Waldhoer T, et al. Antibiotics and azathioprine for the treat-ment of perianal fistulas in Crohn's disease. Aliment Pharmacol Ther 2003;18:1113–20.

40. Gonzalez-Lama Y, Abreu L, Vera MI, et al. Long-term oral tacrolimus therapy in refractory to infliximab fistulizing Crohn's disease: a pilot study. Inflamm Bowel Dis 2005;11:8–15.

41. Fukushima T, Sugita A, Masuzawa S, et al. Effects of cyclosporin A on active Crohn's disease. Gastroenterol Jpn 1989;24:12–5.

42. Lichtiger S. Cyclosporine therapy in inflammatory bowel disease: open-label experience. Mt Sinai J Med 1990;57:315–9.

43. Hanauer SB, Smith MB. Rapid closure of Crohn's disease fistulas with continuous intravenous cyclosporin A. Am J Gastroenterol 1993;88:646–9.

44. Mahadevan U, Sandborn WJ. Diagnosis and management of pouchitis. Gastro-enterology 2003;124:1636–50.

45. Schroder O, Blumenstein I, Schulte-Bockholt A, et al. Combining infliximab and methotrexate in fistulizing Crohn's disease resistant or intolerant to azathioprine. Aliment Pharmacol Ther 2004;19:295–301.

46. Schreiber S, Thomsen OO, Hanauer S, et al. Cimzia is effective in the treatment of Crohn's disease patients with open fistulas. Inflamm Bowel Dis 2008;14:S1.

47. Topstad DR, Panaccione R, Heine JA, et al. Combined seton placement, infliximab infusion, and maintenance immunosuppressives improve healing rate in fistulizing anorectal Crohn's disease: a single center experience. Dis Colon Rectum 2003;46:577–83.
48. Ghosh S, Goldin E, Gordon FH, et al. Natalizumab for active Crohn's disease. N Engl J Med 2003;348:24–32.
49. Sandborn WJ, Colombel JF, Enns R, et al. Natalizumab induction and maintenance therapy for Crohn's disease. N Engl J Med 2005;353:1912–25.
50. Targan SR, Feagan BG, Fedorak RN, et al. Natalizumab for the treatment of active Crohn's disease: results of the ENCORE Trial. Gastroenterology 2007;132: 1672–83.
51. Lavy A, Weisz G, Adir Y, et al. Hyperbaric oxygen for perianal Crohn's disease. J Clin Gastroenterol 1994;19:202–5.
52. Sandborn WJ, Fazio VW, Feagan BG, et al. AGA technical review on perianal Crohn's disease. Gastroenterology 2003;125:1508–30.
53. Fukuda Y, Takazoe M, Sugita A, et al. Oral spherical adsorptive carbon for the treatment of intractable anal fistulas in Crohn's disease: a multicenter, randomized, double-blind, placebo-controlled trial. Am J Gastroenterol 2008;103: 1721–9.
54. Spradlin N, Wise P, Herline A, et al. A randomized prospective trial of endoscopic ulrasound (EUS) to guide combination medical and surgical treatment for Crohn's perianal fistulas. Am J Gastroenterol 2008;103:2527–35.
55. Schwartz DA, White CM, Wise PE, et al. Use of endoscopic ultrasound to guide combination medical and surgical therapy for patients with Crohn's perianal fistulas. Inflamm Bowel Dis 2005;11:727–32.
56. Spradlin NM, Wise PE, Herline AJ, et al. A randomized prospective trial of endoscopic ultrasound to guide combination medical and surgical treatment for Crohn's perianal fistulas. Am J Gastroenterol 2008;103:2527–35.
57. Tougeron D, Savoye G, Savoye-Collet C, et al. Predicting factors of fistula healing and clinical remission after infliximab-based combined therapy for perianal fistulizing Crohn's disease. Dig Dis Sci 2009;54:1746–52.
58. Fichera A, Michelassi F. Surgical treatment of Crohn's disease. J Gastrointest Surg 2007;11:791–803.
59. Williams JG, Farrands PA, Williams AB, et al. The treatment of anal fistula: ACPGBI position statement. Colorectal Dis 2007;9(Suppl 4):18–50.
60. Fuhrman GM, Larach SW. Experience with perirectal fistulas in patients with Crohn's disease. Dis Colon Rectum 1989;32:847–8.
61. Present DH, Rutgeerts P, Targan S, et al. Infliximab for the treatment of fistulas in patients with Crohn's disease. N Engl J Med 1999;340:1398–405.
62. Sands BE, Anderson FH, Bernstein CN, et al. Infliximab maintenance therapy for fistulizing Crohn's disease. N Engl J Med 2004;350:876–85.
63. van der Hagen SJ, Baeten CG, Soeters PB, et al. Staged mucosal advancement flap for the treatment of complex anal fistulas: pretreatment with noncutting setons and in case of recurrent multiple abscesses a diverting stoma. Colorectal Dis 2005;7:513–8.
64. Levien DH, Surrell J, Mazier WP. Surgical treatment of anorectal fistula in patients with Crohn's disease. Surg Gynecol Obstet 1989;169:133–6.
65. Makowiec F, Jehle EC, Starlinger M. Clinical course of perianal fistulas in Crohn's disease. Gut 1995;37:696–701.
66. Hyman N. Endoanal advancement flap repair for complex anorectal fistulas. Am J Surg 1999;178:337–40.

67. Abel ME, Chiu YS, Russell TR, et al. Autologous fibrin glue in the treatment of rectovaginal and complex fistulas. Dis Colon Rectum 1993;36:447–9.

68. Cintron JR, Park JJ, Orsay CP, et al. Repair of fistulas in ano using fibrin adhesive: long-term follow-up. Dis Colon Rectum 2000;43:944–9 [discussion: 949–50].

69. Lindsey I, Smilgin-Humphreys MM, Cunningham C, et al. A randomized, controlled trial of fibrin glue vs. conventional treatment for anal fistula. Dis Colon Rectum 2002;45:1608–15.

70. Singer M, Cintron J, Nelson R, et al. Treatment of fistulas in ano with fibrin sealant in combination with intra-adhesive antibiotics and/or surgical closure of the internal fistula opening. Dis Colon Rectum 2005;48:799–808.

71. Schwandner O, Stadler F, Dietl O, et al. Initial experience on efficacy in closure of cryptoglandular and Crohn's transsphincteric fistulas by the use of the anal fistula plug. Int J Colorectal Dis 2008;23:319–24.

72. Ky AJ, Sylla P, Steinhagen R, et al. Collagen fistula plug for the treatment of anal fistulas. Dis Colon Rectum 2008;51:838–43.

73. Practice parameters for treatment of fistula in ano—supporting documentation. The Standards Practice Task Force. The American Society of Colon and Rectal Surgeons. Dis Colon Rectum 1996;39:1363–72.

74. Yamamoto T, Bain IM, Allan RN, et al. Persistent perineal sinus after proctocolectomy for Crohn's disease. Dis Colon Rectum 1999;42:96–101.

75. Galandiuk S, Kimberling J, Al-Mishlab TG, et al. Perianal Crohn disease: predictors of need for permanent diversion. Ann Surg 2005;241:796–801 [discussion: 801–2].

76. Singh B, Mc CMNJ, Jewell DP, et al. Perianal Crohn's disease. Br J Surg 2004;91:801–14.

77. Bauer JJ, Sher ME, Jaffin H, et al. Transvaginal approach for repair of rectovaginal fistulae complicating Crohn's disease. Ann Surg 1991;213:151–8.

78. Songne K, Scotte M, Lubrano J, et al. Treatment of anovaginal or rectovaginal fistulas with modified Martius graft. Colorectal Dis 2007;9:653–6.

79. Sands BE, Blank MA, Patel K, et al. Long-term treatment of rectovaginal fistulas in Crohn's disease: response to infliximab in the ACCENT II Study. Clin Gastroenterol Hepatol 2004;2:912–20.

80. Schreiber S, Colombel JF, Panes J, et al. Recent-onset Crohn's disease shows higher remission rates and durability of response to treatment with subcutaneous monthly certolizumab pegol: results from the analysis of the PRECISE 2 phase III study [abstract]. Gut 2006;55:A131.

81. Schreiber S, Colombel JF. Early Crohn's disease shows high levels of remission to therapy with adalimumab: sub-analysis of CHARM [abstract]. Gastroenterology 2007;132(Suppl 2):A985.

82. Sandborn WJ, Present DH, Isaacs KL, et al. Tacrolimus for the treatment of fistulas in patients with Crohn's disease: a randomized, placebo-controlled trial. Gastroenterology 2003;125:380–8.

Pediatric Inflammatory Bowel Disease: Highlighting Pediatric Differences in IBD

Cary G. Sauer, MD, MSc[a], Subra Kugathasan, MD[b],*

KEYWORDS

- Crohn disease • Ulcerative colitis
- Inflammatory bowel disease • Pediatric
- Evidence-based treatment algorithms

Inflammatory bowel disease (IBD) includes Crohn disease (CD) and ulcerative colitis (UC), and is often diagnosed in late childhood and early adulthood. IBD is thought to develop as a result of dysregulation of the immune response to normal gut flora in a genetically susceptible host. Approximately 25% of incident cases of IBD occur during childhood and the rest occur throughout adulthood, peaking in the second and third decades of life. What determines the age of onset remains unexplained. Studying early-onset presentation and epidemiology of complex predominately adult diseases such as IBD is particularly necessary, as the early onset may represent the "pure" form of the disease process and hence may hold secrets of the initiating events of IBD pathogenesis. Basic, translational, and clinical scientists continue to focus on pediatric IBD, because it may shed light not only on the cause but also the prevention of this lifelong disease. Over the last decade, data from pediatric IBD studies have demonstrated many similarities and differences between pediatric and adult onset, which continue to add pieces to an increasingly complex IBD puzzle. The mechanism responsible for these similarities and differences remains unanswered.

The purpose of this article is to discuss clinically relevant epidemiology and treatment aspects of pediatric IBD, with a special focus on similarities and differences in pediatric and adult IBD. Epidemiologic similarities and differences may ultimately provide the link to a better understanding of the pathogenesis of IBD. This article

This article originally appeared in *Gastroenterology Clinics of North America,* Volume 38, Issue 4.
[a] Department of Pediatrics, Emory University School of Medicine, Emory Children's Center, 2015 Uppergate Drive, Atlanta, GA 30322, USA
[b] Division of Pediatric Gastroenterology, Emory University School of Medicine, Emory Children's Center, 2015 Uppergate Drive, Suite 248, Atlanta, GA 30322, USA
* Corresponding author.
E-mail address: subra.kugathasan@emory.edu (S. Kugathasan).

Med Clin N Am 94 (2010) 35–52
doi:10.1016/j.mcna.2009.10.002
0025-7125/09/$ – see front matter © 2010 Elsevier Inc. All rights reserved.

also highlights evidence-based treatment algorithms, with special focus on pediatric studies and care for children.

EPIDEMIOLOGY
Gender Differences

The male to female ratio of IBD differs in multiple studies when comparing pediatric IBD to adult IBD. Whereas in adult IBD there is an equal ratio of male to female disease or perhaps more women with disease, prepubertal males seem to be more affected by pediatric CD. Van Limbergen and colleagues[1] demonstrated that in pediatric CD there is a strong trend toward males, with a male to female ratio of 1.5:1. Vernier-Massouille and colleagues[2] also confirmed a male predilection, with a similar ratio of 1.4:1 in children younger than 15 years. This figure directly compares with a ratio nearing 1:1 in patients older than 15 years in the same population. Other adult epidemiologic studies similarly have shown a gender ratio of approximately 1:1. A summary of recent epidemiologic studies demonstrating a male preponderance in pediatric CD is provided in **Table 1**.

Pediatric UC does not demonstrate the male predominance seen in pediatric CD. In fact, similar to adult UC, males and females are equally affected in pediatric UC in multiple studies. **Table 2** demonstrates the equal distribution of males and females in pediatric UC.

Very early onset IBD (age <5–8 years) has been recently suggested as perhaps a different spectrum of IBD. Multiple epidemiologic studies have demonstrated a male preponderance of very early onset IBD. It is unclear whether this male preponderance is only seen in CD or in both CD and UC, as many of the studies do not provide specific gender information based on specific diagnosis.[3]

Together, these gender differences generate more questions than they answer. The effect of puberty and sex hormones on disease pathogenesis continues to be unanswered. Further study will continue to explore these interesting epidemiologic findings and may ultimately provide important information as to the cause of pediatric IBD.

Table 1
Male preponderance in pediatric CD compared to adult CD

| | CD | | | |
	Male	Female	Male:Female Ratio	
Van Limbergen et al[1]	164	112	1.464285714	Childhood
	216	380	0.568421053	Adult
Kugathasan et al[50]	80	49	1.632653061	Childhood
Vernier-Massouille et al[2]	256	216	1.185185185	Childhood
Kappelman et al[51]	47	38	1.236842105	Childhood
(per 100,000)	183	216	0.847222222	Adult
Herrinton et al[52]	40	27	1.481481481	Childhood
(per 100,000)	184	188	0.978723404	Adult
Sawczenko et al[53]	62	38	1.631578947	Childhood
(per 100 diagnoses)				
Newby et al[54]	83	33	2.515151515	Childhood

Table 2
Equal distribution of males and females in pediatric and adult UC

	UC			
	Male	Female	Male:Female Ratio	
Van Limbergen et al[1]	48	51	0.941176471	Childhood
	342	359	0.95264624	Adult
Kugathasan et al[50]	33	27	1.222222222	Childhood
Kappelman et al[51]	29	26	1.115384615	Childhood
(per 100,000)	238	237	1.004219409	Adult
Herrinton et al[52]	28	29	0.965517241	Childhood
(per 100,000)	312	283	1.102473498	Adult
Sawczenko et al[53]	51	49	1.040816327	Childhood
(per 100 diagnoses)	—	—	—	—
Newby et al[54]	45	29	1.551724138	Childhood

Crohn Disease:Ulcerative Colitis Ratio

The ratio of CD:UC significantly differs in children and adults. Van Limbergen and colleagues[1] demonstrated a significant predilection for CD in children, with a ratio of 2.8:1. Adult IBD demonstrated a ratio of 0.85:1. Other epidemiologic studies that have been performed using various methods (ie, population based, insurance claims, and so forth) have suggested a similar higher ratio of CD than UC in children. This directly differs from adult studies that have demonstrated more UC than CD diagnoses. **Table 3** illustrates recent studies that reveal this significant difference in CD:UC ratios in children and adults.

There is clearly a significantly higher CD:UC ratio in children than in adults. Similar to gender differences, this observation clearly requires further investigation, with few data available to suggest a mechanism for this significant difference between pediatric and adult IBD.

Table 3
CD preponderance in pediatric IBD and UC preponderance in adult IBD

	CD	UC	CD:UC Ratio	
Van Limbergen et al[1]	276	99	2.79	Childhood
	596	701	0.85	Adult
Kugathasan et al[50]	129	60	2.15	Childhood
Vernier-Massouille et al[2]	472	151	3.13	Childhood
Kappelman et al[51]	1118	722	1.55	Childhood
(per 100,000 prevalence)	12800	15151	0.84	Adult
Herrinton et al[52]	67	57	1.18	Childhood
(per 100,000 period prevalence)	186	299	0.62	Adult
Sawczenko et al[55]	431	211	2.04	Childhood
Auvin et al[56]	367	122	3.01	Childhood
Newby et al[54]	116	74	1.57	Childhood
Heyman et al[57]	798	393	2.03	Childhood

Disease Location

Disease location at presentation differs in pediatric IBD compared with adult IBD. In pediatric CD a majority of patients have ileocolonic disease or colonic disease, whereas adults more often present with terminal ileal disease without colonic involvement. During follow-up of pediatric CD, Vernier-Massouille and colleagues[2] and Van Limbergen and colleagues[1] both demonstrated a progression of disease location with increasing ileocolonic disease at follow-up. Meanwhile, Van Limbergen and colleagues showed that more than one-third of adults had terminal ileal disease only. In multiple pediatric studies, up to 80% to 90% of children experience colonic disease (colon only or ileocolonic) whereas only approximately 50% of adults experience colonic CD. It is unclear why there is an increased ileocolonic/colonic disease in children and no accepted theory has been offered as to this observation. No treatment studies have suggested that children with ileocolonic disease require different treatment from terminal ileal disease alone. **Table 4** demonstrates the high rate of ileocolonic disease in children at both diagnosis and follow-up in 2 studies.

Pediatric UC location also differs from that of adult disease. Pediatric UC presents more often with pancolitis versus left-sided colitis/proctitis. In fact, most pediatric UC studies demonstrate up to 80% to 90% of children present with pancolitis, and a recent study by Van Limbergen and colleagues[1] suggested that pediatric UC progresses with increasing percentage of pancolitis at follow-up. The significance of the high percentage of pancolitis at presentation is unknown. **Table 5** demonstrates an increased pancolitis presentation in pediatric UC.

In summary, pediatric CD more often involves the ileocolonic/colonic regions whereas adult CD does not demonstrate a high proportion of colonic disease. Meanwhile, pediatric UC more often presents with pancolitis whereas adult UC more often presents with left-sided colitis. The mechanism behind these observations is not well understood and no data are available to support any concrete hypotheses.

Table 4
Higher ileocolonic disease prevalence in pediatric CD compared to adult CD

	CD Location				
	Terminal Ileum (L1)	Colon Only (L2)	Ileocolonic (L3)	Upper Gastrointestinal Disease (L4)	
Vernier-Massouille et al[2]	14%	17%	69%	34%	Childhood diagnosis
	9%	9%	82%	48%	Childhood follow-up (10 y)
Van Limbergen et al[1]	6%	36%	51%	51%	Childhood diagnosis
	5%	36%	54%	61%	Childhood follow-up (4 y)
	36%	38%	23%	12%	Adult
Kugathasan et al[50]	25%	32%	29%	14%	Childhood diagnosis
Sawczenko et al[58]	9%	7%	84%	50%	Childhood diagnosis
Auvin et al[56]	19%	10%	71%	—	Childhood diagnosis

Table 5
Pancolitis predominance in pediatric UC

	UC Location			
	Proctitis (E1)	Distal Disease (Left-sided) (E2)	Pancolitis (E3)	
Van Limbergen et al[1]	4%	21%	75%	Childhood diagnosis
	1%	16%	82%	Childhood follow-up
	17%	35%	48%	Adult follow-up
Hyams et al[59]	22%	39%	43%	Childhood diagnosis
Kugathasan et al[50]	—	10%	90%	Childhood diagnosis
Hyams et al[60]	—	—	80%	—
Sawczenko et al[58]	4%	—	81%	Childhood diagnosis
Auvin et al[56]	11%	57%	32%	Childhood diagnosis

Disease Phenotype

Disease phenotype in both CD and UC differs when comparing children with adults. Pediatric CD presents predominantly with inflammatory or nonstricturing, nonpenetrating disease. Stricturing and penetrating disease is relatively uncommon at presentation in pediatric CD. However, even with treatment, multiple studies have shown that CD progresses to stricturing and penetrating disease in many children. Adult disease presents more often with stricturing and penetrating disease. Two recent natural history articles reveal a significant progression of pediatric CD from inflammatory disease to sticturing disease, as illustrated in **Table 6**.

Pediatric UC more often presents with pancolitis, and has been suggested to be a more severe phenotype in children than in adults. Recent epidemiologic data demonstrate that indeed, time from diagnosis to first surgery in UC is significantly shorter in children than in adults. By 10 years after diagnosis more than 40% of children had undergone colectomy, whereas only 20% of adult-onset UC patients had undergone colectomy.[1]

In summary, pediatric CD frequently displays an inflammatory phenotype at diagnosis that progresses to fistulizing/stricturing disease in some patients, whereas adult CD more often presents with fistulizing/stricturing disease. Although some investigators have suggested disease duration and a delay in diagnosis may be the reason for this difference in CD, no data have been published to support this hypothesis.

Table 6
CD phenotype demonstrates progression of disease from inflammatory to structuring and penetrating disease

	CD Phenotype			
	B1: Inflammatory (NS, NP)	B2: Stricturing	B3: Penetrating	
Van Limbergen et al[1]	91%	4%	5%	Childhood diagnosis
	76%	13%	11%	Childhood 4 y follow-up
	66%	14%	20%	Adult follow-up
Vernier-Massouille et al[2]	71%	25%	4%	Childhood diagnosis
	41%	44%	15%	Childhood 10 y follow-up

Pediatric UC frequently displays an aggressive phenotype, with pancolitis and early time to first surgery compared with adult UC, which is more often limited to the left colon.

Genetics

When studying early-onset presentations of disease, there is an assumption that these represent a more severe, more genetically influenced group of patients. It is appealing to geneticists to study these patients because of the increased chance of finding novel risk variants. One of the most compelling hypotheses is that pediatric-onset IBD is more likely to be influenced by genetics compared with late- or adult-onset IBD, as there is less time for environmental modifiers to have influenced the disease.

IBD is highly heritable. This concept is strongly supported by family, twin, and phenotype concordance studies, and now is confirmed by the discoveries of many susceptibility genes.[4] Initial family-based linkage studies of IBD implicated the NOD2 gene in CD and the MHC region on chromosome 6p in UC for increased susceptibility.[5] Genome-wide association scanning (GWAS), which employs high-density single nucleotide polymorphism (SNP) array technology, has recently increased the possible genetic factors linked to IBD pathogenesis. This method of broad, unbiased screening for the contribution of common genetic variation for disease susceptibility has provided strong evidence for many CD and UC suscepti-bility loci.[6] GWAS has identified loci in both UC and CD that are already known to be involved in adaptive immunity genes such as IL23R, IL12B, STAT3, loci on 3p21 (MST1), and 10q24 (NKX2-3). Variants in innate immunity genes, particularly those mediating autophagy and bacterial sensing (ATG16L1, IRGM, and NOD2) have also been discovered through these methods in CD. To date, the majority of this genetic analysis in IBD has been done in adult cohorts with adult-onset disease as the primary phenotype, therefore even less is known about early-onset variants.

Several CD susceptibility alleles have been confirmed in both pediatric and adult populations. However, most of the genetic variation seen in adults has not been studied in children in a large cohort with adequate power. Two pediatric studies at-tempting to replicate the effect of adult-onset IBD loci in children have been performed recently. These studies have demonstrated that autophagy genes play a role in pedi-atric CD but also that known genetic risk factors found in adults may not distinguish early- and late-onset IBD.[7,8]

The first pediatric GWAS IBD scan was performed recently, revealing 2 risk variants not previously reported in adults, in addition to confirming the most significant adult risk variants. Two novel loci, the TNFRSF6B and PSMG1 genes, were discovered using more than 1000 cases of pediatric IBD.[9] The gene TNFRS6B, which encodes a decoy receptor for the FasL pathway (DCR3), was found to increase the risk for pedi-atric-onset CD and UC. On comparison with adult GWAS scans these same loci were identified, but were below the expected threshold when correcting for multiple tests. However, until a GWAS is performed in an exclusively pediatric-onset IBD cohort, it is very difficult to deny that additional pediatric-onset IBD susceptibility genes do not exist. As such, GWAS studies involving larger pediatric-onset CD cohorts and early-onset UC are presently underway.

Adult and pediatric GWAS studies have yet to discover risk variants that are specific to pediatric or adult IBD. Instead, all risk variants that have been discovered are present in both adult and pediatric scans, although not necessarily in the statistically significant range. This observation, if confirmed in additional larger GWAS studies, may further suggest that pediatric and adult IBD have similar genetics and thus are the same disease with different age of presentation.

More detailed functional exploration of genes associated with susceptibility loci reported in GWAS will be instrumental in shedding light on their role in IBD pathogenesis. Taken together, recent pediatric GWAS results substantially advance the current understanding of pediatric-onset IBD by highlighting key pathogenetic mechanisms, and allowing for the first time a comparison between genetic susceptibility in an exclusively pediatric cohort and the previously described populations with predominantly adult-onset disease.

Clinical Presentation

Clinical presentation is similar in adult and pediatric IBD, and for the most part correlates with disease location. Pediatric CD presents with more ileal and colonic disease than adult CD, and therefore more often presents with hematochezia. Small bowel disease presents with diarrhea regardless of childhood or adult onset. Pediatric and adult IBD share many of the same gastrointestinal symptoms which, as one would expect, are associated more with mucosal disease than with age.

Extraintestinal manifestations similarly are present in both children and adults in similar numbers. Extraintestinal manifestations are present in 6% of children prior to diagnosis in one recent study, and cumulative incidence approaches 25%, similar to adult data.[10]

Growth is the most significant difference in presentation between adult and pediatric IBD. Poor growth prior to diagnosis has been documented in multiple studies examining growth in pediatric IBD.[11–14] Furthermore, puberty has been shown to be delayed[12] and some patients have decreased final adult height.[14,15] In addition, a recent study has demonstrated that despite new treatments, catch-up growth does not occur in patients diagnosed with IBD, although it remains to be seen whether these patients have delayed puberty and ultimately achieve their expected adult height.[16] Persistent poor growth may also be one of the only signs of increased disease activity, thus it is important not only in presentation but also in disease activity during treatment.

TREATMENT

Pediatric IBD treatment employs many of the same treatment paradigms as adult IBD. Most medication clinical trials have largely been performed only on adults, and therefore much of the evidence given here is based on adult data. Only a few well-designed clinical trials have been performed in children, and most of those show similar efficacy to adult trials.

The authors have chosen to separate the Treatment section into Induction and Maintenance of remission. What follows is not meant to be an exhaustive review of current literature; rather a review some of the current data and a report on any additional data specific to children.

Corticosteroids

Crohn disease

Induction of remission Two recent Cochrane review articles examined budesonide and conventional corticosteroids (prednisone) as therapy for the induction of remission in CD. A majority of these were adult studies, although in some studies children older than 16 years were included. The reviews clearly show efficacy for induction of remission with both budesonide and conventional steroids, and show slightly less efficacy of budesonide compared with conventional steroids, at least in severe disease.[17,18]

Maintenance of remission Corticosteroids, including both conventional steroids and budesonide, are not recommended for maintenance of remission. Any benefits in maintenance of remission are offset by treatment-related adverse events and thus these medications should be avoided for maintenance of remission, especially in children in whom corticosteroids can significantly affect growth.[19]

Ulcerative colitis
Induction of remission The use of corticosteroids for induction of remission in UC was first described in 1974,[20] and has been the mainstay for induction of remission in moderate to severe UC. More recently, approximately 84% of adults with UC demonstrated a complete or partial improvement of disease activity with corticosteroids, and approximately 49% had prolonged response at 1 year.[21] Budesonide, which has significant first-pass metabolism, is delivered to the distal ileum and proximal colon and thus likely has little efficacy in UC, although a randomized controlled trial has never been published.

Maintenance of remission As with CD, corticosteroids are not recommended for the maintenance of remission in UC as any benefits are more than offset by side effects, especially in growing children.

Summary
In practice, corticosteroids are often used in induction of remission in CD and UC but are often avoided if possible after induction, due to growth side effects and other morbidity associated with persistent corticosteroid usage. Studies have clearly shown that morbidity in CD is associated with corticosteroid use. Therefore, children with new diagnosis CD and UC are often started on corticosteroids with a taper over 2 months. Corticosteroids are avoided, if possible at all other times other than induction of remission.

Nutritional Therapy

Crohn disease
Induction of remission A recent Cochrane review compared nutritional therapy (liquid formula by mouth or via tube) to corticosteroid therapy for induction of remission. Although sole nutritional therapy has been shown to be effective in induction of remission in CD, it remains inferior to corticosteroids in induction of remission. In addition, the same review concluded that protein composition (ie, elemental or nonelemental protein) has no effect on efficacy of nutritional therapy.[22] The only study that favors enteral nutrition over corticosteroids was a pediatric study.[23]

However, practically speaking, the induction of remission with sole nutritional therapy remains difficult due to adherence in children. Most parents are reluctant to commit total enteral nutrition for their children for 6 to 8 weeks as required. In addition, few children are able to consume adequate formula volume by mouth, and thus would require insertion of nasogastric tubes or possibly a gastrostomy tube.

Maintenance of remission Only 2 randomized studies have been published regarding maintenance of remission in CD with nutrition in adults, and no studies have examined this in children. Takagi and colleagues[24] conducted a randomized controlled trial of 51 adults in remission, assigning one group a half-elemental diet and another group a regular diet with no instructions or limitations, with all patients taking mesalamine. The study demonstrated a significantly lower relapse rate in the half-elemental diet group (34.6% vs 64.0%). A recent Cochrane review suggested that there may be some efficacy in enteral nutrition for maintenance therapy, although larger studies are needed to confirm this possibility.[25]

Ulcerative colitis
No studies have been reported for the induction or maintenance of remission with enteral therapy for UC.

Summary
Although both the European Society for Pediatric Gastroenterology, Hepatology, and Nutrition and the Japanese Society for Pediatric Gastroenterology, Hepatology, and Nutrition recommend nutritional therapy as sole primary therapy for CD, it is often a difficult treatment to initiate in the United States. The most significant deterrent continues to be the resistance by many parents and children to commit to 8 weeks of specialized formula alone (either by mouth or through a feeding tube such as a nasogastric tube) without taking any other food by mouth. Furthermore, it is unclear whether a child can be maintained on nutritional therapy alone and therefore, other maintenance medications need to be initiated. In addition, the short-term side effects with corticosteroid induction are debatably minimal.

5-Aminosalicylate

Crohn disease
Induction of remission No randomized controlled studies have been performed examining the induction of remission by aminosalicylates in pediatric CD. Hanauer and colleagues[26] published a meta-analysis examining aminosalicylates in active CD and showed a modest effect (if any) on improvement of Crohn Disease Activity Index (CDAI).

Although some pediatric gastroenterologists continue to use aminosalicylates for the induction of remission in CD, there are no good data to support the use for induction of remission, although there may be modest beneficial effects.

Maintenance of remission No randomized studies have been published for maintenance of remission in pediatric CD. A recent Cochrane review examined aminosalicylates in the maintenance of remission in CD. The results do not show any benefit of aminosalicylates compared with placebo.[27]

Ulcerative colitis
Induction of remission A recent Cochrane review that includes only adult studies demonstrated a benefit from high-dose aminosalicylates (>3 g) in the induction of remission in UC, although remission rates remain significantly lower than in those using corticosteroids.[28]

Most importantly in pediatric UC, a majority of patients present with moderate to severe disease, as demonstrated by the high percentage of pancolitis. Whereas aminosalicylates can be used for induction of remission, due to severity of disease in pediatric UC they are rarely used as sole induction, but rather in conjunction with corticosteroids for induction of remission.

Maintenance of remission As with many of the medications mentioned here, no randomized trials have been conducted in children examining the use of aminosalicylates in maintenance of remission in children. A Cochrane review has demonstrated efficacy of aminosalicylates in maintaining remission in UC compared with placebo.[29]

Summary

There are no randomized controlled trials for the induction or maintenance of remission of aminosalicylates in pediatric IBD. Aminosalicylates are still often used in pediatric IBD. These agents are well tolerated in children, have few side effects, and thus have continued to be used by pediatric gastroenterologists despite the lack of evidence in CD and efficacy only in mild to moderate UC. Even though aminosalicylates are well tolerated, the most significant "side effect" is decreased quality of life due to the number of pills or capsules ingested each day, which often is considered in treatment of children with IBD.

However, it should be noted that aminosalicylates likely have most efficacy in colonic disease regardless of whether the diagnosis is CD or UC. Given the data demonstrating more colonic disease in children (up to 80%), the use of aminosalicylates in colonic CD may be of some benefit, although there are no data examining this question. Whether aminosalicylates could be used as sole therapy in colonic CD has never been examined.

Based on the current data, the authors cannot support the usage of aminosalicylates in ileal CD, as there seem to be no compelling data to support their use. However, there are data to support the use of high-dose aminosalicylates in the management of UC, and there may be some efficacy in colonic CD, although there are no data for this possibility.

Immunomodulators (6-Mercaptopurine, Azathioprine, Methotrexate)

Crohn disease

Induction of remission Because of its delay in efficacy, 6-mercaptopurine (6-MP) and azathioprine (AZA) are not used for induction of remission; however, they are often used in conjunction with corticosteroids or other therapy used to induce remission with the knowledge that by the time corticosteroids are weaned, 6-MP and AZA will be effective in maintaining remission (**Table 7**).

A Cochrane review concluded efficacy for methotrexate in induction of remission in CD based on one study.[30] Methotrexate has demonstrated efficacy in inducing remission after failure of induction therapy with steroids in one large double-blind, placebo-controlled multicenter study (n = 141) when compared with placebo.[31] Other smaller studies did not show a significant difference. In children, only retrospective studies

Table 7
Immunomodulators in pediatric IBD

			Induction of Remission	Maintenance of Remission
Markowitz et al[35] n = 75	Prospective	Steroids Steroids + 6-MP	89% 89%	53% at 548 d 91% at 548 d
Uhlen et al[32] n = 61	Retrospective	MTX after failed 6-MP/AZA	39% at 3 mo	45% at 12 mo
Weiss et al[36] n = 25	Retrospective	MTX after failed 6-MP/AZA	64%	60% at 12 mo
Turner et al[33] n = 60	Retrospective	MTX after failed 6-MP/AZA	42% at 6 mo	42% at 6 mo

have been conducted. One retrospective, multicenter study (n = 61) demonstrated improvement in disease or complete remission in 80% of children who were not responding to AZA.[32] A second retrospective study (n = 60) demonstrated remission at 6 and 12 months in 42% of children placed on methotrexate after 6-MP/AZA failure.[33]

Maintenance of remission 6-MP and AZA have demonstrated efficacy in maintaining remission in CD in multiple studies, and a recent Cochrane review confirms significant efficacy compared with placebo.[34]

In children, one prospective multicenter, double-blind, placebo-controlled trial demonstrated induction of remission with prednisone and 6-MP, and maintenance of remission with 6-MP. Seventy-five children were randomized to prednisone and 6-MP or prednisone alone, with similar induction of remission rates (89%). At 548 days after remission, 91% of the 6-MP group continued to be in remission whereas only 53% of the steroid only group remained in remission. Initiation of 6-MP at diagnosis also has a significant steroid-sparing effect.[35]

Ulcerative colitis
Induction of remission Similar to CD, due to the slow onset of action of 6-MP and AZA these medications are rarely used as primary therapy for induction. No studies evaluating methotrexate in adults or children are available for the induction of remission. A recent Cochrane review concluded that there are no published reports to demonstrate efficacy of methotrexate in the induction of remission in UC.[37]

Maintenance of remission No large studies have examined the use of 6-MP and AZA for the maintenance of remission in UC. A Cochrane review identified 4 studies that showed efficacy of 6-MP/AZA compared with placebo. Another Cochrane review concluded no efficacy in methotrexate in maintaining remission in UC.[38]

In children, one retrospective study of 20 corticosteroid dependent or refractory patients revealed efficacy, with discontinuation of corticosteroids in 75% and 67% continuing to be steroid free at follow-up.[39]

Summary
6-MP and AZA clearly show efficacy in maintaining remission in pediatric CD in a well-designed pediatric study. In addition, these medications have a significant steroid-sparing affect. Because of these data they are often initiated at diagnosis for the management of moderate to severe CD. 6-MP and AZA also have a role in the maintenance of remission in moderate to severe pediatric UC.

Methotrexate induced and maintained remission in one pediatric trial. Methotrexate is often used due to its quick action, unlike 6-MP and AZA that have slow onset of action. The most significant issue with methotrexate is its bioavailability, as oral medication may not be as efficacious as subcutaneous injections. Despite this, methotrexate is an excellent option when immediate action is necessary and when one wants to avoid biologics.

Biologics

Crohn disease
Induction and maintenance of remission A Cochrane review clearly shows efficacy for the use of infliximab in the induction and maintenance of remission in CD.[40,41] In addition, there are multiple pediatric studies that demonstrate efficacy in induction of remission in children with CD. The first pediatric trial of infliximab in moderate to severe CD demonstrated clinical remission at 30 weeks in 60% of patients, and

prolonged remission in 56% of patients at 54 weeks when continued on an every 8 week course.[42] Although these results are significantly higher than the adult studies, it should be mentioned that 90% of patients in this study were on concomitant immunomodulators. Therefore, the results may be higher than seen in clinical practice. A recent study evaluated maintenance of remission in children receiving infliximab for more than 1 year, and demonstrated withdrawal of corticosteroids and clinically inactive disease in 30% to 40% of children who were maintained on infliximab.[43] A recent French study confirms the necessity of scheduled and not random infliximab doses in children.[44]

Ulcerative colitis

Induction and maintenance of remission As with many of the other therapeutic agents for IBD, there are no randomized controlled trials of biologics in children with IBD. There are several retrospective studies that demonstrate efficacy in inducing and maintaining remission in children with moderate to severe UC. Data are available in adults with moderate to severe UC, demonstrating efficacy of infliximab in inducing remission, promoting mucosal healing, and reducing the need for colectomy.[45]

Summary

Biologics clearly demonstrate efficacy in inducing and maintaining remissions in pediatric IBD. Perhaps the more pressing debate is the proper use of biologics and the results of more long-term follow-up. Although it is clear that some children fail other treatments for IBD and require biologics, it is difficult to recommend biologics as first-line therapy given the paucity of long-term follow-up data. With no current "exit strategy," biologic initiation requires treatment for an indefinite period of time.

Special Considerations in the Treatment of Inflammatory Bowel Disease in Children

Children with IBD require special consideration in their treatment, specifically regarding growth, hepatosplenic T-cell lymphoma, and goals of therapy.

Growth

In children, growth remains one of the most significant outcomes, as poor growth often can be the only "symptom" of disease. As discussed in the Presentation section, growth is poor prior to diagnosis, children with CD have delayed puberty and decreased final adult height, and many do not exhibit catch-up growth after diagnosis. Growth parameters are included in the Pediatric CDAI, as poor growth remains a clinical sign. Close attention to both height velocity and weight are necessary during the treatment of pediatric CD, as this may be the only clinical sign of persistent disease activity.

No specific treatment paradigms have been shown to be superior in improving growth. Biologics and surgical resection have been shown to improve growth; however, these may not be superior to immunomodulators.[46] No other treatments such as growth hormone have shown superiority. Regarding growth, treatment should thus focus on controlling disease activity and providing sufficient calories, which may require supplementation with high-calorie formula.

Hepatosplenic T-cell lymphoma

Although overall increased risk of lymphoma has been reported in patients with IBD who have been exposed to biologic or immunomodulator therapy, a rare fatal form of lymphoma, hepatosplenic T-cell lymphoma (HSTCL), is now linked only in children and young adults with IBD. Cases of HSTCL have been reported with both combination therapy with 6-MP/AZA and monotherapy with 6-MP/AZA, but not with infliximab monotherapy alone. There are now approximately 18 cases of HSTCL with individuals on both 6-MP/AZA and infliximab. These cases reveal preponderance for young male patients, although the mechanism of this observation is unknown. Due to this potential risk of this fatal disease, the treatment of pediatric IBD does not currently include combination therapy with biologics and immunomodulators. However, with recent data from the SONIC trial showing superior efficacy of combination immunomodulator and biologic therapy compared with either therapy alone, there is considerable debate regarding combination therapy, at least in young females.

Goals of therapy

Growth and clinical remission remain the most important goals of therapy. Clinical remission may be best defined by the appropriate activity index. A Pediatric Crohn Disease Activity Index (PCDAI)[47] and a Pediatric Ulcerative Colitis Activity Index (PUCAI)[48] have been developed and validated, and are currently in use both clinically and for research purposes. These indices are similar to adult indices, with some specific differences. In children, the PCDAI includes growth measures in addition to symptoms, physical examination, and laboratory measures. The PUCAI was more recently developed and is completely symptom based, as growth abnormalities are less likely to be observed in pediatric UC. Endoscopic healing remains a debated topic, although repeated endoscopy is not recommended in children.

Treatment Conclusions

Crohn disease

The treatment paradigm for CD remains similar to adult treatment of IBD. Prednisone remains the most effective medication for induction of remission and is often used as a short course for induction only purposes, then avoided due to growth side effects. Although nutritional therapy has proven to be effective in inducing remission, no well-performed studies have shown efficacy in maintaining remission, and sole nutritional therapy remains an option for induction of remission for those willing to commit to this treatment. Research demonstrates a minimal (if any) benefit for aminosalicylates in the induction of remission in CD, and no benefit in the maintenance of remission. However, more children with CD have colonic disease and therefore aminosalicylates may be of some benefit, given their proven efficacy in UC. Due to the high frequency of moderate to severe CD disease in children, immunomodulators are frequently used at or shortly after diagnosis. Markowitz and colleagues demonstrated a steroid-sparing effect and maintenance of remission in children treated with immunomodulators, and a short course of prednisone at diagnosis. Biologics remain an option although given the high efficacy of immunomodulators, biologics are most often reserved for children who fail immunomodulator therapy. At this time, biologics cannot be recommended as first-line therapy. However, continued research may predict those children with more severe disease, and at that point biologics may be suggested as first-line therapy for those with severe disease.

Ulcerative colitis

Ulcerative colitis treatment continues to be similar for children and adults, although research has demonstrated more pancolitis and shorter time to surgery in pediatric UC, perhaps supporting more aggressive treatment for children with UC. Prednisone remains the most effective induction of remission therapy, but is only recommended at diagnosis with a short course due to growth effects. Aminosalicylates show efficacy in induction and maintenance of remission, but are reserved as sole treatment only in the mildest cases of pediatric UC. Immunomodulators are often necessary in pediatric UC due to its moderate to severe presentation in children, and are effective in maintaining remission. Biologics are effective in inducing and maintaining remission in pediatric UC but are reserved at this time primarily for immunomodulator failures.

The Future of IBD Treatment in Children

Perhaps the most pressing issue in the treatment of IBD in children is the identification of a more severe phenotype that would respond best to biologics at diagnosis and thus prevent the need for surgical therapy. Over the next decade, determining which patients are at most risk for surgery and other complications may reveal a tool to predict disease severity and potentially prove that these individuals fare better with top-down therapy. However, at this time it is difficult to argue the top-down approach, given the unknown effects of biologic therapy used for decades in children diagnosed at an early age.

SUMMARY

While this question about differing age of onset among the chronic complex inflammatory disorders such as IBD encourages debate, a fundamental issue in IBD remains unanswered. Does pediatric IBD represent the same disease process occurring in adults but merely at an earlier age (ie, age of onset is a random event), or does pediatric IBD display different pathogenesis (hence different natural history) but simply with the same clinical presentation as adults? An argument can be made suggesting a different spectrum of the same disease or different pathogenesis that leads to similar disease phenotypes.

Although no hard scientific evidence exists regarding differing etiology, pediatric-onset IBD does "differ" from adult IBD in many aspects.[49] As highlighted in this article, there is growing evidence from clinical observations as well as epidemiologic and natural history studies that pediatric-onset IBD represents a distinct disease with differences in disease type, disease location, disease behavior, gender preponderance, and genetically attributable risk compared with its adult counterpart.[50] These differences need to be further explored, as they may someday hold the key to understanding the pathogenesis of IBD.

More specifically, children are more likely to be diagnosed with CD versus UC, and there is a predilection for males in pediatric CD but not pediatric UC. In addition, pediatric CD more often presents with ileocolonic disease and inflammatory phenotype, which progresses in some to structuring and fistulizing phenotype, although predicting this progression is difficult. Pediatric UC presents with more pancolitis and may be more severe, as suggested by an earlier time to first surgery.

Very early onset IBD (age <5–8 years) also exhibits a male preponderance and presents with colonic disease more often than when diagnosed in later childhood or adulthood. It remains unclear whether very early onset IBD has different genetic variations or other differences in pathogenesis.

Treatment paradigms are similar in adult and pediatric IBD, with only a few prospective trials available in pediatrics, but all with similar results to adult trials. Outcome remains the most significant driver of treatment options, and in children disease activity, and specifically growth, are important outcome measures. There are some important risks that seem to affect children more than adults including HSTCL, which has a predilection for younger males. These factors affect treatment paradigms, and further study is necessary to determine the precise risk (if any) for and to better understand the pathology of this serious lymphoma.

Overall, pediatric IBD may hold the key to understanding the pathogenesis of IBD, with the hopes of leading to prevention. As expected, highlighting the differences and similarities between pediatric and adult IBD has generated more questions than answers. It is important that these specific differences are further explored through high-quality research in the search for the cause and cure of IBD.

REFERENCES

1. Van Limbergen J, Russell RK, Drummond HE, et al. Definition of phenotypic characteristics of childhood-onset inflammatory bowel disease. Gastroenterology 2008;135:1114–22.
2. Vernier-Massouille G, Balde M, Salleron J, et al. Natural history of pediatric Crohn's disease: a population-based cohort study. Gastroenterology 2008;135:1106–13.
3. Mamula P, Telega GW, Markowitz JE, et al. Inflammatory bowel disease in children 5 years of age and younger. Am J Gastroenterol 2002;97:2005–10.
4. Biank V, Broeckel U, Kugathasan S. Pediatric inflammatory bowel disease: clinical and molecular genetics. Inflamm Bowel Dis 2007;13:1430–8.
5. Satsangi J. Gene discovery in IBD: a decade of progress. J Pediatr Gastroenterol Nutr 2008;46(suppl 1):E1–2.
6. Barrett JC, Hansoul S, Nicolae DL, et al. Genome-wide association defines more than 30 distinct susceptibility loci for Crohn's disease. Nat Genet 2008;40:955–62.
7. Peterson N, Guthery S, Denson L, et al. Genetic variants in the autophagy pathway contribute to paediatric Crohn's disease. Gut 2008;57:1336–7 [author reply 1337].
8. Essers JB, Lee JJ, Kugathasan S, et al. Established genetic risk factors do not distinguish early and later onset Crohn's disease. Inflamm Bowel Dis 2009;15(10):1508–14.
9. Kugathasan S, Baldassano RN, Bradfield JP, et al. Loci on 20q13 and 21q22 are associated with pediatric-onset inflammatory bowel disease. Nat Genet 2008;40:1211–5.
10. Jose FA, Garnett EA, Vittinghoff E, et al. Development of extraintestinal manifestations in pediatric patients with inflammatory bowel disease. Inflamm Bowel Dis 2009;15:63–8.
11. Griffiths AM, Nguyen P, Smith C, et al. Growth and clinical course of children with Crohn's disease. Gut 1993;34:939–43.
12. Hildebrand H, Karlberg J, Kristiansson B. Longitudinal growth in children and adolescents with inflammatory bowel disease. J Pediatr Gastroenterol Nutr 1994;18:165–73.
13. Kanof ME, Lake AM, Bayless TM. Decreased height velocity in children and adolescents before the diagnosis of Crohn's disease. Gastroenterology 1988;96:1523–7.
14. Markowitz J, Grancher K, Rosa J, et al. Growth failure in pediatric inflammatory bowel disease. J Pediatr Gastroenterol Nutr 1993;16:368–9.
15. Kirschner BS. Growth and development in chronic inflammatory bowel disease. Acta Paediatr Scand Suppl 1990;366:98–104.
16. Pfefferkorn M, Burke G, Griffiths A, et al. Growth abnormalities persist in newly diagnosed children with Crohn disease despite current treatment paradigms. J Pediatr Gastroenterol Nutr 2009;48:168–74.
17. Benchimol EI, Seow CH, Steinhart AH, et al. Traditional corticosteroids for induction of remission in Crohn's disease. Cochrane Database Syst Rev 2008;(2):CD006792. DOI: 10.1002/14651858.
18. Seow CH, Benchimol EI, Griffiths AM, et al. Budesonide for induction of remission in Crohn's disease. Cochrane Database Syst Rev 2008;(3):CD000296. DOI: 10.1002/14651858.

19. Benchimol EI, Seow CH, Otley AR, et al. Budesonide for maintenance of remission in Crohn's disease. Cochrane Database Syst Rev 2009;(1):CD002913. DOI: 10.1002/14651858.

20. Truelove SC, Jewell DP. Intensive intravenous regimen for severe attacks of ulcerative colitis. Lancet 1974;1:1067–70.

21. Faubion WA Jr, Loftus EV Jr, Harmsen WS, et al. The natural history of corticosteroid therapy for inflammatory bowel disease: a population-based study. Gastroenterology 2001;121:255–60.

22. Zachos M, Tondeur M, Griffiths AM. Enteral nutritional therapy for induction of remission in Crohn's disease. Cochrane Database Syst Rev 2007;(1):CD000542. DOI: 10.1002/14651858.

23. Borrelli O, Cordischi L, Cirulli M, et al. Polymeric diet alone versus corticosteroids in the treatment of active pediatric Crohn's disease: a randomized controlled open-label trial. Clin Gastroenterol Hepatol 2006;4:744–53.

24. Takagi S, Utsunomiya K, Kuriyama S, et al. Effectiveness of an 'half elemental diet' as maintenance therapy for Crohn's disease: a randomized-controlled trial. Aliment Pharmacol Ther 2006;24:1333–40.

25. Akobeng AK, Thomas AG. Enteral nutrition for maintenance of remission in Crohn's disease. Cochrane Database Syst Rev 2007;(3):CD005984. DOI: 10.1002/14651858.

26. Hanauer SB, Stromberg U. Oral Pentasa in the treatment of active Crohn's disease: a meta-analysis of double-blind, placebo-controlled trials. Clin Gastroenterol Hepatol 2004;2:379–88.

27. Akobeng AK, Gardener E. Oral 5-aminosalicylic acid for maintenance of medically-induced remission in Crohn's Disease. Cochrane Database Syst Rev 2005;(1):CD003715. DOI: 10.1002/14651858.

28. Sutherland L, MacDonald JK. Oral 5-aminosalicylic acid for induction of remission in ulcerative colitis. Cochrane Database Syst Rev 2003;(2):CD000543. DOI: 10.1002/14651858.

29. Sutherland L, Macdonald JK. Oral 5-aminosalicylic acid for maintenance of remission in ulcerative colitis. Cochrane Database Syst Rev 2006;(2):CD000544. DOI: 10.1002/14651858.

30. Alfadhli AA, McDonald JW, Feagan BG. Methotrexate for induction of remission in refractory Crohn's disease. Cochrane Database Syst Rev 2005;(4):CD003459. DOI: 10.1002/14651858.

31. Feagan BG, Rochon J, Fedorak RN, et al. Methotrexate for the treatment of Crohn's disease. The North American Crohn's Study Group Investigators. N Engl J Med 1995;332:292–7.

32. Uhlen S, Belbouab R, Narebski K, et al. Efficacy of methotrexate in pediatric Crohn's disease: a French multicenter study. Inflamm Bowel Dis 2006;12:1053–7.

33. Turner D, Grossman AB, Rosh J, et al. Methotrexate following unsuccessful thiopurine therapy in pediatric Crohn's disease. Am J Gastroenterol 2007;102: 2804–12 [quiz 2803, 2813].

34. Prefontaine E, Sutherland LR, Macdonald JK, et al. Azathioprine or 6-mercaptopurine for maintenance of remission in Crohn's disease. Cochrane Database Syst Rev 2009;(1):CD000067. DOI: 10.1002/14651858.

35. Markowitz J, Grancher K, Kohn N, et al. A multicenter trial of 6-mercaptopurine and prednisone in children with newly diagnosed Crohn's disease. Gastroenterology 2000;119:895–902.

36. Weiss B, Lerner A, Shapiro R, et al. Methotrexate treatment in pediatric Crohn disease patients intolerant or resistant to purine analogues. J Pediatr Gastroenterol Nutr 2009;48:526–30.

37. Chande N, MacDonald JK, McDonald JW. Methotrexate for induction of remission in ulcerative colitis. Cochrane Database Syst Rev 2007;(4):CD006618. DOI: 10.1002/14651858.

38. Ei-Matary W, Vandermeer B, Griffiths AM. Methotrexate for maintenance of remission in ulcerative colitis. Cochrane Database Syst Rev 2009;(3):CD007560. DOI: 10.1002/14651858.

39. Kader HA, Mascarenhas MR, Piccoli DA, et al. Experiences with 6-mercaptopurine and azathioprine therapy in pediatric patients with severe ulcerative colitis. J Pediatr Gastroenterol Nutr 1999;28:54–8.

40. Behm BW, Bickston SJ. Tumor necrosis factor-alpha antibody for maintenance of remission in Crohn's disease. Cochrane Database Syst Rev 2008;(1):CD006893. DOI: 10.1002/14651858.

41. Akobeng AK, Zachos M. Tumor necrosis factor-alpha antibody for induction of remission in Crohn's disease. Cochrane Database Syst Rev 2004;(4):CD003574. DOI: 10.1002/14651858.

42. Hyams J, Crandall W, Kugathasan S, et al. Induction and maintenance infliximab therapy for the treatment of moderate-to-severe Crohn's disease in children. Gastroenterology 2007;132:863–73 [quiz 1165–6].

43. Hyams JS, Lerer T, Griffiths A. Long-term outcome of maintenance infliximab therapy in children with Crohn's disease. Inflammatory Bowel Dis 2009;15:816–22.

44. Ruemmele FM, Lachaux A, Cezard JP, et al. Efficacy of infliximab in pediatric Crohn's disease: a randomized multicenter open-label trial comparing scheduled to on demand maintenance therapy. Inflamm Bowel Dis 2009;15:388–94.

45. Lawson MM, Thomas AG, Akobeng AK. Tumour necrosis factor alpha blocking agents for induction of remission in ulcerative colitis. Cochrane Database Syst Rev 2006;(3):CD005112.

46. Heuschkel R, Salvestrini C, Beattie RM, et al. Guidelines for the management of growth failure in childhood inflammatory bowel disease. Inflamm Bowel Dis 2008; 14:839–49.

47. Hyams JS, Ferry GD, Mandel FS, et al. Development and validation of a pediatric Crohn's disease activity index. J Pediatr Gastroenterol Nutr 1991;12:439–47.

48. Turner D, Otley AR, Mack D, et al. Development, validation, and evaluation of a pediatric ulcerative colitis activity index: a prospective multicenter study. Gastroenterology 2007;133:423–32.

49. Kugathasan S, Cohen S. Searching for new clues in inflammatory bowel disease: tell tales from pediatric IBD natural history studies. Gastroenterology 2008;135: 1038–41.

50. Kugathasan S, Judd RH, Hoffmann RG, et al. Epidemiologic and clinical characteristics of children with newly diagnosed inflammatory bowel disease in Wisconsin: a statewide population-based study. J Pediatr 2003;143:525–31.

51. Kappelman MD, Rifas-Shiman SL, Kleinman K, et al. The prevalence and geographic distribution of Crohn's Disease and ulcerative colitis in the United States. Clin Gastroenterol Hepatol 2007;5:1424–9.

52. Herrinton LJ, Liu L, Lafata JE, et al. Estimation of the period prevalence of inflammatory bowel disease among nine health plans using computerized diagnoses and outpatient pharmacy dispensings. Inflamm Bowel Dis 2007;13:451–61.

53. Sawczenko A, Sandhu BK, Logan RFA, et al. Prospective survey of childhood inflammatory bowel disease in the British Isles. Lancet 2001;357:1093–4.

54. Newby EA, Croft NM, Green M, et al. Natural history of paediatric inflammatory bowel diseases over a 5-year follow-up: a retrospective review of data from the register of paediatric inflammatory bowel diseases. J Pediatr Gastroenterol Nutr 2008;46:539–45.

55. Sawczenko A, Lynn R, Sandhu BK. Variations in initial assessment and management of inflammatory bowel disease across Great Britain and Ireland. Arch Dis Child 2003;88:990–4.

56. Auvin S, Molinie F, Gower-Rousseau C, et al. Incidence, clinical presentation and location at diagnosis of pediatric inflammatory bowel disease: a prospective population-based study in northern France (1988–1999). J Pediatr Gastroenterol Nutr 2005;41:49–55.

57. Heyman MB, Kirschner BS, Gold BD, et al. Children with early-onset inflammatory bowel disease (IBD): analysis of a pediatric IBD consortium registry. J Pediatr 2005;146:35–40.

58. Sawczenko A, Sandhu BK. Presenting features of inflammatory bowel disease in Great Britain and Ireland. Arch Dis Child 2003;88:995–1000.

59. Hyams JS, Davis P, Grancher K, et al. Clinical outcome of ulcerative colitis in children. J Pediatr 1996;129:81–8.

60. Hyams J, Markowitz J, Lerer T, et al. The natural history of corticosteroid therapy for ulcerative colitis in children. Clin Gastroenterol Hepatol 2006;4:1118–23.

Pregnancy and Inflammatory Bowel Disease

Uma Mahadevan, MD

KEYWORDS

- Crohn disease • Ulcerative colitis
- Inflammatory bowel disease • Pregnancy • Infliximab

Inflammatory bowel disease (IBD) often affects women during their peak reproductive years.[1] As medical therapy for IBD advances, more patients are in a position to consider pregnancy; however, striking the balance between optimal medical therapy and fetal health has become increasingly complex. The ability to conceive and carry a healthy child to term, medications compatible with use during conception, pregnancy and lactation, and appropriate management of an IBD flare during pregnancy are questions for which highly charged decisions must be made with limited data. **Box 1** summarizes key questions and answers discussed in this article on the management of ulcerative colitis (UC) and Crohn disease (CD) during pregnancy.

INHERITANCE

Patients are often concerned about passing their disease on to their offspring, as family history is the strongest predictor for developing IBD. If one parent is affected, the risks of the offspring developing IBD are 2 to 13 times higher than in the general population.[2,3] One study estimated that the risk of IBD in first-degree relatives of probands with UC and CD were 1.6% and 5.2% respectively.[4] If both parents have IBD, the risk of their offspring developing IBD over their lifetime was estimated to be as high as 36%.[5,6]

FERTILITY AND SEXUAL FUNCTION

Infertility is defined as the diminished ability or inability to conceive and have offspring. It is also defined in specific terms as the failure to conceive after a year of regular intercourse without contraception. In general, women with CD appear to have similar fertility rates to the general population. Older, referral center studies estimated infertility rates between 32% and 42% in women with CD[7,8]; however, community-based and population-based studies suggest infertility rates (5%–14%) similar to the general

This article originally appeared in *Gastroenterology Clinics of North America*, Volume 38, Issue 4.
Center for Colitis and Crohn's Disease, University of California, San Francisco, 2330 Post Street 610, San Francisco, CA 94115, USA
E-mail address: uma.mahadevan@ucsf.edu

Box 1
Common patient questions and answers

1. Will my child get IBD?

   a. 1.6% if mother has UC

   b. 5.2% if mother has CD

   c. 36.0% if both spouses are affected

2. What are my chances of getting pregnant?

   a. Fertility is similar to the general population for presurgical UC and CD

   b. Ileal pouch anal anastomosis reduces fertility by 50% to 80%

   c. Surgery for Crohn may also slightly reduce fertility

3. Do women with IBD have higher rates of sexual dysfunction?

   a. Yes. Depression and surgery are predictors

4. What are my expected pregnancy outcomes?

   a. Increased spontaneous abortion and stillbirth

   b. Increased preterm birth, low birth weight, small for gestational age infants

   c. Increased complications of labor and delivery

   d. Congenital anomalies—data mixed, but no clear increased risk

   e. Even if disease is under good control, increased risk of adverse outcomes compared with the general population

5. What will pregnancy do to my IBD?

   a. The risk of flaring during pregnancy is the same as if not pregnant—34% at 1 year

6. What medications can I use? (Food and Drug Administration Category)

   a. Mesalamine (B): conception, pregnancy, lactation

      i. Sulfasalazine—increase folic acid to 2 mg daily

   b. Corticosteroids (C) and budesonide (C):

      i. Use if needed, but avoid use in first trimester

         1. increased risk of cleft palate

      ii. Increased risk of gestational diabetes

   c. Azathioprine/6Mercaptopurine (D)

      i. Low risk. Benefits of maintaining remission outweigh risk

      ii. Compatible with use in conception, pregnancy and lactation

      iii. Wait 4 hours after taking dose to breastfeed

   d. Infliximab and Adalimumab (B)

      i. Low risk. Compatible with use in conception, pregnancy, lactation

      ii. Transfers across placenta. Avoid use in late third trimester

      iii. Consider holding rotavirus vaccination in infant (live virus)

---

e. Certolizumab (B)

    i. Low risk. Compatible with use in conception, pregnancy, lactation

    ii. Limited transfer across placenta in third trimester so dose on schedule

f. Natalizumab (C)

    i. Limited data. No reports of congenital anomalies

g. Methotrexate (X)

    i. Contraindicated. Discontinue 6 months before attempting conception

---

population.[1,9] Surgery for CD may decrease fertility compared with medical therapy alone.[10]

Women with UC have fertility rates similar to the general population before surgery.[10–12] A study by Ording Olsen and colleagues[13] of 290 women with UC versus 661 non-IBD controls found that women with UC had fecundability ratios (FR) (the ability to conceive per menstrual cycle with unprotected intercourse) equal to the general population (FR = 1.01). However, after surgery for an ileal pouch anal anastomosis (IPAA), the FR dropped to 0.20 ($P<.001$). The reduction in fertility may be attributable to surgery in the pelvis and the consequent adhesions and damage to the reproductive organs. Patients who undergo a proctocolectomy with ileostomy also experience a reduction in fertility,[14] as do patients with familial adenomatous polyposis who undergo IPAA.[15]

This finding has been confirmed by a meta-analysis as well as a systemic review. In a meta-analysis[16] of 7 studies, IPAA increased the risk of infertility in women with UC by approximately threefold. Infertility, defined as failure to achieve pregnancy in 12 months of attempting conception, increased from 15% to 48% in women post-IPAA. The relative risk of infertility after IPAA was 3.17 (2.41–4.18), with nonsignificant heterogeneity. The weighted average infertility rate in medically treated UC was 15% for all seven studies, and the weighted average infertility rate was 48% after IPAA. In the systematic review,[17] a total of 22 studies, with 1852 females, were included. The infertility rate was 12% before restorative proctocolectomy and 26% after IPAA, among 945 patients in seven studies.

With respect to sexual dysfunction, a German survey of 1000 patients[18] found that women with IBD showed impaired function irrespective of disease activity as compared with healthy controls. High socioeconomic status was a protective factor for several subscores in women; depression was the most important predictor of dysfunction.[18] In the systematic review stated in the preceding paragraph, an incidence of sexual dysfunction of 8% preoperatively and 25 % postoperatively (7 studies, n = 419) was reported in women undergoing IPAA.

The risk of infertility and sexual dysfunction should be discussed with the patient before surgery as part of the potential risks of the operation. It is unclear if techniques such as laparoscopic IPAA or a subtotal colectomy with rectal stump and ileostomy during the childbearing years are helpful in reducing infertility and sexual dysfunction rates. The drawbacks of the latter procedure include rare ileostomy complications during pregnancy such as obstruction and stoma-related problems,[19] technical difficulties in creating a functioning pouch several years after the initial surgery, and the patient's reluctance to have a long-term stoma.

Cervical dysplasia, another factor for reduced fertility, has been reported to be increased among women with IBD, particularly if they use immunosuppressants[20] or infliximab.[21] Although larger population-based studies[22] and referral center studies[23] have not confirmed these findings, it is recommended that women with

IBD, regardless of medication status, have annual papanicolau smears and young women should receive the human papilloma virus vaccine.

PREGNANCY OUTCOMES

Population-based studies have clearly shown an increased risk of preterm birth, low birth weight (LBW), and small for gestational age infants among the offspring of women with IBD.[24–26] Cesarean sections are also more common.[25] Whether there is an increase in congenital anomalies is unclear and may be related to medication use (see section on medication below).

A population-based cohort study by Dominitz and colleagues[27] used the computerized birth records of Washington State to compare pregnancy outcomes in 107 UC and 155 CD patients with 1308 controls. Women with CD had significantly higher rates of preterm delivery, low birth weight, and small for gestational age infants compared with controls. Women with UC, on the other hand, had similar rates to controls, but a significantly higher rate of congenital malformations (7.9% vs 1.7%). The study did not account for medication use and the results have not been replicated in other studies. The Hungarian Case Control Surveillance of congenital anomalies was queried from 1980 to 1996.[28] The odds ratio (OR) of congenital anomalies in UC patients versus controls was 1.3 (95% CI = 0.9,1.8), adjusted for parity, age, and medication use. However, the risk of limb deficiencies, obstructive urinary congenital abnormalities, and multiple congenital abnormalities were increased with OR = 6.2 (95% confidence interval [CI] = 2.9–13.1), OR = 3.3 (95% CI = 1.1–9.5), and OR = 2.6 (95% CI = 1.3–5.4), respectively.

A population representative cohort study of women with IBD in the Northern California Kaiser population[29] compared women with IBD (n = 461) matched to controls (n = 495) by age and hospital of delivery. Women with IBD were more likely to have a spontaneous abortion, OR = 1.65 (95% CI = 1.09, 2.48); an adverse pregnancy outcome (stillbirth, preterm birth, or small for gestational age (SGA) infant), OR = 1.54 (95% CI = 1.00, 2.38); or a complication of labor, OR = 1.78 (95% CI = 1.13, 2.81). However, there was no difference in the rate of congenital malformations in IBD patients versus controls or individually among CD and UC patients. Independent predictors of an adverse outcome included a diagnosis of IBD, a history of surgery for IBD, and non-White ethnicity. Severity of disease and medical treatments were not associated with an adverse outcome suggesting that even women in remission with IBD were more likely to have complications of pregnancy than their general population counterparts.

A meta-analysis by Cornish and colleagues[30] combined 12 studies totaling 3907 patients with IBD. A clear increase in preterm birth, OR =1.87 (95% CI = 1.52, 2.31); low birth weight, OR = 2.1 (95% CI = 1.38, 3.19); and cesarean section, OR = 1.5 (95% CI = 1.26, 1.79) was seen. The risk of congenital anomalies was increased as well with an OR of 2.37 (95% CI = 1.47, 3.82). The difference was seen in patients with UC, not CD, and was primarily based on the Dominitz and colleagues[27] study reported earlier and an older study by Larzilliere and Beau.[31] Overall, the studies regarding the risk of congenital anomalies among the progeny of women with UC are mixed, with some suggesting an increased risk overall[27,31] or for particular anomalies,[28] whereas other studies do not suggest an increased risk at all.[29] If there is a risk, the role of medications, disease activity, and other possible contributing factors needs to be more clearly defined.

DISEASE ACTIVITY
Effect of Pregnancy on IBD

In general, women with IBD are as likely to flare during pregnancy, as they are to flare when not pregnant. Nielsen and colleagues[32] reported an exacerbation rate of 34%

per year during pregnancy and 32% per year when not pregnant in women with UC. Pregnant women with CD also had similar rates of disease exacerbation.[33] In the Kaiser population,[29] most patients had inactive disease throughout their pregnancy with no sudden increase in the postpartum. This is consistent with other published studies that found the rate of disease flare during pregnancy (26%–34%) to be similar to the rate of flare in the nonpregnant IBD population.[32,34,35] Although breastfeeding has anecdotally been associated with an increase in disease activity in the post-partum, this has not been shown to be a contributing factor independent of medication cessation to facilitate breastfeeding.[36]

Disease activity may even be slightly lower during pregnancy.[37] One study found that the rate of relapse may decrease in the 3 years following pregnancy.[38] This was further supported by a study from a 10-year follow up of a European cohort of patients with 580 pregnancies.[39] Patients with CD who were pregnant during the course of their disease had lower rates of stenosis (37% vs 52%, $P = .13$) or resection (0.52 vs 0.66, $P = .37$). The rates of relapse decreased in the years following preg-nancy in both UC (0.34 vs 0.18 flares/year, $P = .008$) and CD patients (0.76 vs 0.12 flares/year, $P = .004$). Although the etiology for this is not understood, a possible factor inducing quiescent disease may be disparity in HLA class II antigens between mother and fetus, suggesting that the maternal immune response to paternal HLA antigens may result in immunosuppression that affects maternal immune-mediated disease. This has been demonstrated in rheumatoid arthritis[40] as well as in IBD.[41]

Effect of Disease Activity on Pregnancy

Earlier studies suggested that disease activity was a predictor of adverse outcome in pregnancy. Disease activity at conception has been associated with a higher rate of fetal loss[35] and preterm birth[32]; disease activity during pregnancy was associated with low birth weight and preterm birth.[42,43] Other potential predictors of an adverse outcome include ileal CD[44] and prior bowel resection.[29,44]

However, in the Kaiser population,[29] disease activity was not predictive of an adverse outcome in any category. Even when limited to the presence of moderate to severe disease activity, there was still no association with an adverse outcome. Most patients with both UC and CD, however, did have inactive or mild disease throughout pregnancy. Similarly, a population-based study from Denmark[45] reported that women with active disease had adjusted risks of LBW, LBW at term, preterm birth, and congenital anomalies of 0.2 (0.0–2.6), 0.4 (0.0–3.7), 2.4 (0.6–9.5), and 0.8 (0.2–3.8), respectively. However, the crude risk of preterm birth was 3.4 (1.1–10.6) in those with moderate-high disease activity. Overall, these two population-based studies suggest that IBD patients have higher rates of adverse pregnancy outcomes regardless of disease activity.

LABOR AND DELIVERY

There is an increased rate of cesarean sections in women with IBD.[25] In general, the decision to have a cesarean section should be made on purely obstetric grounds. The two exceptions are active perianal disease and the presence of an ileoanal pouch. If a patient has inactive perianal disease or no history of perianal disease, she is not at increased risk for perianal disease after a vaginal delivery.[46] However, if the patient has active perianal disease, she can risk aggravating the injury with a vaginal delivery. One report noted an increased incidence of perianal disease following episiotomy,[47] but this has not been replicated in other studies.

Patients who have an IPAA can have a normal vaginal delivery without fears of damaging the pouch.[48] However, the concern with vaginal delivery is for damage to the anal sphincter. Although pouch function may deteriorate during pregnancy, after pregnancy it reverts to the prepregnancy state.[48] However, over time damage to the anal sphincter may be compounded by aging and the effects on the pouch will not be seen for several years when incontinence and number of bowel movements may increase significantly. The patient, her obstetrician, and her surgeon should discuss the theoretical risk to long-term pouch function before making a decision on mode of delivery.

MEDICATIONS

The use of medications during the conception period and pregnancy is a cause of great concern for patients and the physicians caring for them. Overall, most medications used for the treatment of IBD are not associated with significant adverse effects and maintaining the health of the mother remains a priority in the management of these patients. The US Food and Drug Administration (FDA) classification of drugs offers a guide to the use of medications during pregnancy. The FDA categories are listed in **Table 1** and are noted for each drug discussed. **Table 2** summarizes the safety of IBD medications for pregnancy and breastfeeding.

Women

Aminosalicylates
All aminosalicylates (sulfasalazine, mesalamine, balsalazide) are pregnancy category B except olsalazine, which is pregnancy category C. Sulfasalazine is composed of 5-aminosalicylic acid azo-bonded to sulfapyridine. Initial case reports suggested sulfasalazine teratogenicity with evidence of cardiovascular, genitourinary, and neurologic defects.[49–51] However, a larger series of 181 pregnant women did not note an increase in congenital anomalies.[52] A population-based study using the Hungarian Case Control Surveillance of Congenital Abnormalities database[53] also did not find a significant increase in the prevalence of congenital abnormalities in the children of women treated with sulfasalazine. Given the concern over potential antifolate effects of the drug, it is recommended that women take folic acid 2 mg daily in the prenatal

Table 1	
Food and drug administration categories for the use of medications in pregnancy	
FDA Category	**Definition**
A	Controlled studies in animals and women have shown no risk in the first trimester, and possible fetal harm is remote.
B	Either animal studies have not demonstrated a fetal risk but there are no controlled studies in pregnant women, or animal studies have shown an adverse effect that was not confirmed in controlled studies in women in the first trimester.
C	No controlled studies in humans have been performed, and animal studies have shown adverse events, or studies in humans and animals not available; give if potential benefit outweighs the risk.
D	Positive evidence of fetal risk is available, but the benefits may outweigh the risk if life-threatening or serious disease.
X	Studies in animals or humans show fetal abnormalities; drug contraindicated

Data from Food and Drug Administration. Regulations 1980;44:37, 434–7, 467.

Table 2
Medications used in the treatment of inflammatory bowel disease

Drug	FDA Category	Recommendations for Pregnancy	Breastfeeding[71]
Adalimumab	B	Limited human data: low risk[a] Likely cross placenta	No human data: probably compatible
Alendronate	C	Limited human data; long half life: Animal data suggest risk.	No human data: probably compatible
Azathioprine/ 6-mercaptopurine	D	Data in IBD, transplant literature suggest some risk, but low	Limited transfer. Likely compatible
Balsalazide	B	Low risk	No human data: potential diarrhea
Budesonide	C	Data with inhaled drug low risk. Limited human data for oral drug	No human data
Certolizumab	B	Limited human data: low risk Limited transfer across placenta	No evidence of transfer. Likely compatible
Ciprofloxacin	C	Avoid: Potential toxicity to cartilage	Limited human data: probably compatible
Corticosteroids	C	Low risk: possible small risk of cleft palate, adrenal insufficiency, premature rupture of membranes	Compatible
Cyclosporine	C	Low risk	Limited human data: potential toxicity
Fish oil supplements	—	Low risk. Possibly beneficial	No human data
Infliximab	B	Low risk: limited human data: crosses placenta and detectable in infant after birth	No evidence of transfer. Likely compatible
Mesalamine	B	Low risk	Limited human data: potential diarrhea
Methotrexate	X	Contraindicated: teratogenic	Contraindicated
Metronidazole	B	Given limited efficacy in IBD, would avoid in first trimester	Limited human data: potential toxicity
Olsalazine	C	Low risk	Limited human data: potential diarrhea
Risedronate	C	Limited human data. Long half life	Safety unknown
Rifaximin	C	No human data. Animal data report some risk	Safety unknown
Sulfasalazine	B	Low risk. Give folate 2 mg daily	Limited human data: potential diarrhea
Tacrolimus	C	Low risk	Limited human data: potential toxicity
Thalidomide	X	Contraindicated: teratogenic	No human data: potential toxicity

Abbreviations: FDA, Food and Drug Administration; IBD, inflammatory bowel disease.[71]

[a] Low risk is defined as "the human pregnancy data do not suggest a significant risk of embryo or fetal harm."

Data from Mahadevan U, Kane S. American gastroenterological association institute medical position statement on the use of gastrointestinal medications in pregnancy. Gastroenterology 2006;131(1):278–82.

period and throughout pregnancy. Breast-feeding is also considered low risk with sulfasalazine. Unlike other sulfonamides, bilirubin displacement, and therefore kernicterus, does not occur in the infant.[54] This may be due to negligible transfer via breast milk.

Case series of mesalamine use in pregnancy do not suggest an increased risk to the fetus.[55–57] This has been supported by a prospective controlled trial of 165 women exposed to mesalamine compared with matched controls with no exposure[58] and a population-based cohort study from Denmark.[59] Breastfeeding while on aminosalicylates has been rarely associated with diarrhea in the infant.[60] Women can breastfeed while being treated with 5-aminosalicylates, but infants should be observed for a persistent change in stool frequency.

Antibiotics

Metronidazole is a pregnancy category B drug. Multiple studies have suggested that prenatal use of metronidazole is not associated with birth defects. These studies include two meta-analyses,[61,62] two retrospective cohort studies,[63,64] and a prospective controlled study of 228 women exposed to metronidazole during pregnancy.[65] A population-based case-control study found that overall teratogenic risk was low, but infants of women exposed to metronidazole in the second to third months of pregnancy had higher rates of cleft lip with or without cleft palate.[66] This increase was slight and not believed to be clinically significant.

Metronidazole is excreted in breast milk. If a single dose of metronidazole is given, the American Academy of Pediatrics recommends that breastfeeding should be suspended for 12 to 24 hours.[67] Potential toxicity exists for longer-term use of metronidazole, and it is not compatible with breastfeeding.

Quinolones (eg, ciprofloxacin, levofloxacin, norfloxacin) are pregnancy category C drugs. Quinolones have a high affinity for bone tissue and cartilage and may cause arthropathies in children.[68] The manufacturer reports damage to cartilage in weight-bearing joints after quinolone exposure in immature rats and dogs. However, a prospective controlled study of 200 women exposed to quinolones[69] and a population-based cohort study of 57 women exposed to quinolones[70] did not find an increased risk of congenital malformations. Overall, the risk is believed to be minimal, but given safer alternatives, the drug should be avoided in pregnancy. The data in breastfeeding are limited, but quinolones are probably compatible with use.[71,72]

In general, given the limited evidence of benefit of these agents in IBD and the extended duration of use in the treatment of CD and UC, they should be avoided during pregnancy. Short courses for the treatment of pouchitis can be considered based on the safety data presented previously. An alternative antibiotic for pouchitis is amoxicillin/clavulanic acid, a pregnancy category B drug. A population-based case-control study[73] and a prospective controlled study[74] did not show evidence of increased teratogenic risk, and it is compatible with breastfeeding.

Corticosteroids

Corticosteroids are pregnancy category C drugs. A case-control study of corticosteroid use during the first trimester of pregnancy noted an increased risk of oral clefts in the newborn.[75] This was confirmed by a large case-control study[76] and a meta-analysis that reported a summary OR for case-control studies examining the risk of oral clefts (3.35 [95% CI, 1.97–5.69]).[77] However, the overall risk of major malformations was low (1.45 [95% CI, 0.80–2.60]). A prospective controlled study of 311 women who received glucocorticosteroids during the first trimester did not note an increased rate of major anomalies and no cases of oral cleft were noted.[78] The study was powered to find a 2.5-fold increase in the overall rate of major anomalies. An increased risk of premature rupture of membranes and adrenal insufficiency in the newborn has been reported in the transplant setting[79] and gestational diabetes is a concern as well. Overall, the use of corticosteroids poses a small risk to the developing infant but the mother needs to be informed of both the benefits and the risks of therapy. Prednisone and prednisolone are compatible with breastfeeding.

A case series of eight patients with CD treated with budesonide did not find an increased risk of adverse outcomes.[80] Inhaled or intranasal budesonide is not associated with adverse fetal outcomes based on large clinical series.[81–85] Safety in lactation is not known.

Immunomodulators

The immunomodulators are the most controversial agents used in the treatment of the pregnant woman with IBD.

Methotrexate

Methotrexate, a pregnancy category X drug, is clearly teratogenic and should not be used in women considering conception. Methotrexate is a folic acid antagonist, and use during the critical period of organogenesis (6–8 weeks postconception) is associated with multiple congenital anomalies collectively called methotrexate embryopathy or the fetal aminopterin-methotrexate syndrome.[71] The syndrome is characterized by intrauterine growth retardation; decreased ossification of the calvarium; hypoplastic supraorbital ridges; small, low-set ears; micrognathia; limb abnormalities; and sometimes mental retardation.[85] Exposure in the second and third trimesters may be associated with fetal toxicity and mortality.[71] Methotrexate may persist in tissues for long periods, and it is suggested that patients wait at least 6 months from the discontinuation of the drug before attempting conception.

Methotrexate is excreted in breast milk and may accumulate in neonatal tissues. The AAP classifies methotrexate as a cytotoxic drug with the potential to interfere with cellular metabolism.[86] It is contraindicated in breastfeeding.

Azathioprine/6-mercaptopurine

6-mercaptopurine (6-MP) and its prodrug azathioprine (AZA) are pregnancy category D drugs. Animal studies have demonstrated teratogenicity with increased frequencies of cleft palate, open-eye, and skeletal anomalies seen in mice exposed to AZA and cleft palate, skeletal anomalies, and urogenital anomalies seen in rats.[87] Transplacental and transamniotic transmission of AZA and its metabolites from the mother to the fetus can occur.[88] The oral bioavailability of AZA (47%) and 6-MP (16%) is low,[87] and the early fetal liver lacks the enzyme inosinate pyrophosphorylase needed to convert AZA to 6-MP. Both features may protect the fetus from toxic drug exposure during the crucial period of organogenesis.

The largest evidence on safety comes from transplantation studies where rates of anomalies ranged from 0.0% to 11.8% and no evidence of recurrent patterns of congenital anomalies emerged.[87] A population-based cohort study from Denmark compared 11 women exposed to AZA or 6-MP with the general population.[89] The adjusted OR for congenital malformations was 6.7 (95% CI, 1.4–32.4). However, when a single severely ill patient with autoimmune hepatitis and multiple other medications was removed from the cohort, the OR was 3.4 (95% CI, 0.4–27.3).

In IBD, multiple case series have not noted an increase in congenital anomalies,[9,90–92] although one study did report a higher incidence of fetal loss in women with IBD with *prior* treatment on 6-MP compared with those who never had 6-MP exposure.[93] However, a Danish nationwide cohort study[94] found that women with CD exposed to corticosteroids and AZA/6-MP were more likely to have preterm birth (12.3% and 25.0% respectively) compared with non-IBD controls (6.5%). Congenital anomalies were also more prevalent among AZA/6-MP exposed cases compared with the reference group (15.4% vs 5.7%) with an odds ratio of 2.9 (95% CI 0.9–8.9). However, only 26 women were exposed to AZA/6-MP during conception versus 628 patients in the reference group, and the authors controlled for "disease activity," which they defined as more than or fewer than two admissions for disease exacerbation, accounting for only the most severe patients. Finally, the largest single study to date[95] studied 189 women who called a teratogen information service after exposure to AZA during pregnancy and compared them with 230 women who did not take any teratogenic medications during pregnancy. The rate of major malformations did not differ between groups with six neonates in each; for AZA, the rate was 3.5% and for the control group rate it was 3.0% (P = .775; OR 1.17; CI 0.37, 3.69).

Breastfeeding, initially discouraged, may now be compatible with AZA use. Small studies in IBD suggest that the overall exposure to the infant is low. Moretti and colleagues[96] reported four women breastfeeding on AZA. In two women, multiple breast milk samples did not have detectable levels of drug by high-performance liquid chromatography, and none of the four infants had any complications. Three other studies measured metabolite levels in the breastfeeding infant. Gardiner[97] reported four infants with undetectable metabolite levels despite mothers whose levels were in the therapeutic range. Sau[98] collected 31 samples from 10 breastfeeding women on AZA/6-MP. Only two samples had low levels of 6-MP in breast milk (1.2 and 7.6 ng/mL in one patient vs a serum level of 50 ng/mL). There were no detectable 6–thioguanine nucleotide or 6–methyl mercaptopurine levels in the 10 infants, nor were there signs of hematologic or clinical immunosuppression. Finally, an elegant study[99] of eight lactating women on AZA obtained milk and plasma samples at 30 and 60 minutes after drug administration and hourly for the following 5 hours. The variation in the bioavailability of the drug was reflected in a wide range of peak plasma values of 6-MP within the first 3 hours. A similar curve, but with an hour's delay and at significantly lower concentrations varying from 2-50 μg/L, was seen in maternal milk. Most 6-MP in breast milk was excreted within the first 4 hours after drug intake. On the basis of maximum concentration measured, the infant ingested 6-MP of less than 0.008 mg/kg bodyweight/24 h. The risks and benefits of breastfeeding must be considered carefully; however, at this time there does not appear to be an absolute contraindication to breastfeeding while on AZA/6-MP and mothers should be advised to wait 4 hours after dosing to feed.

Cyclosporine and tacrolimus

Cyclosporine is a pregnancy category C drug. A meta-analysis of 15 studies of pregnancy outcomes after cyclosporine therapy reported a total of 410 patients with data on major malformations.[100] The calculated OR of 3.83 for malformations did not achieve statistical significance (95% CI, 0.75–19.6). The rate of malformations was 4.1%, which is not different from the general population. The conclusion of the study was that cyclosporine did not appear to be a major human teratogen. In a study published in the obstetric literature,[101] a retrospective review of 38 pregnancies in 29 women between 1992 and 2002 was conducted. There were four spontaneous abortions and 10 first-trimester terminations for worsening liver function. The mean gestational age was 36.4 weeks, and there were no intrauterine or neonatal deaths. Five minor congenital anomalies were noted. The investigators concluded that planned pregnancy at least 2 years after liver transplantation with stable allograft function and continued immunosuppression had an excellent maternal and neonatal outcome.

There are several case reports of successful cyclosporine use during pregnancy to control UC and complete the pregnancy.[102–104] In the setting of severe, corticosteroid-refractory UC, cyclosporine may be a better option than colectomy given the substantial risk to the mother and fetus of surgery during this time.

Cyclosporine is excreted into breast milk in high concentrations. Therefore, the AAP considers cyclosporine contraindicated during breastfeeding because of the potential for immune suppression and neutropenia.

Tacrolimus is also a pregnancy category C drug. The earliest experience with this medication was in 1997, with a report of 27 pregnancies with exposure to tacrolimus.[105] Two infants died at weeks 23 and 24, but the mean gestational period was 36.6 weeks. There was a 36% incidence of transient perinatal hyperkalemia. One newborn had unilateral polycystic renal disease. Another study from Germany reported on 100 pregnancies in transplant recipients followed from 1992 to 1998.[106] There were a 68% live birth rate, 12% spontaneous abortion rate, and 3% stillbirth rate. Fifty-nine percent of the infants were premature. Malformations occurred in four neonates with no consistent defects. In a later single-center experience, 49 pregnancies in 37 women over 13 years were followed prospectively.[107] Thirty-six women survived the pregnancy, and two premature babies were seen. One infant died of Alagille syndrome; the rest survived, and 78% were of normal birth weight. No other congenital abnormalities were noted. A single case report of a patient with UC who had a successful pregnancy on maintenance tacrolimus was recently published.[108] No other data on IBD are published at this time. Tacrolimus is contraindicated in breastfeeding because of the high concentrations found in breast milk.

Thalidomide

Thalidomide, a pregnancy category X drug, has some anti–tumor necrosis factor (anti-TNF) effects and has been used successfully for the treatment of CD.[109] However, its teratogenicity has been extensively documented and includes limb defects, central nervous system effects, and abnormalities of the respiratory, cardiovascular, gastrointestinal, and genitourinary systems.[71] Thalidomide is contraindicated during pregnancy and in women of childbearing age who are not using two reliable methods of contraception for 1 month before starting therapy, during therapy, and for 1 month after stopping therapy.[110] There are no human data on breastfeeding, but it is not advised given the potential toxicity.

Biologic Therapy

Infliximab

Infliximab (INF), a pregnancy category B drug, is used for the management of CD[111] and UC.[112] INF is an IgG1 antibody, which does not cross the placenta in the first trimester, but very efficiently crosses in the second and third trimester.[113] Although this protects the infant from exposure during the crucial period of organogenesis, INF levels cross efficiently in the third trimester and are present in the infant for several months from birth.

There is a growing body of evidence that suggests INF is low risk in pregnancy. The two largest studies are from the TREAT Registry[114] and the INF Safety Database[115] maintained by Centocor (Malvern, PA). The TREAT Registry is a prospective registry of patients with CD.[114] Patients may or may not be treated with INF. Of the more than 6200 patients enrolled, 168 pregnancies were reported, 117 with INF exposure. The rates of miscarriage (10.0% vs 6.7%) and neonatal complications (6.9% vs 10.0%) were not significantly different between INF-treated and INF-naïve patients, respectively. The INF Safety Database is a retrospective data collection instrument.

Pregnancy outcome data are available for 96 women with direct exposure to INF.[115] This was primarily exposure in during conception and the first trimester. When patients found out they were pregnant, the treatment was often stopped. The 96 pregnancies resulted in 100 births. The expected versus observed outcomes among women exposed to INF were not different from those of the general population. A series of 10 women with maintenance INF use throughout pregnancy was also reported.[116] All 10 pregnancies ended in live births, with no reported congenital malformations. Another series[117] reported 22 patients with exposure to INF within 3 months of conception, continued until 20 weeks of gestation at which time the drug was stopped to minimize placental transfer. Several of the patients did have a flare of disease in the third trimester. There were three spontaneous abortions, one missed abortion, one stillbirth at 36 weeks (umbilical strangulation), two preterm births, three low birth weight infants, and no congenital anomalies.

INF crosses the placenta and is detectable in the infant for several months after birth. A case report[118] noted higher than detectable INF levels in an infant born to a mother on INF therapy every 4 weeks. The mother breast-fed and continued to receive INF but the infant's INF level dropped over 6 months, suggesting placental rather than breast milk transfer. The effect of high INF levels on the infant's developing immune system is not known, although at 7 months the infant had appropriate responses to vaccination. In a case series[119] of eight patients receiving INF during pregnancy, all eight patients delivered a healthy infant. The mothers were receiving INF 5 mg/kg every 8 weeks and the mean time between delivery and the last infusion was 66 days (range 2–120 days). The INF level at birth was always higher in the infant and cord blood than in the mother and it took anywhere from 2 to 7 months for the infant to have undetectable INF levels. These findings support the fact that IgG1 antibodies are very efficiently transported across the placenta in the third trimester, but the infant reticuloendothelial system is too immature to effectively clear the antibody rapidly. INF has not been detected in breast milk.[120,121]

So far, there has been no reported adverse event associated with elevated INF levels in the newborns. In our experience, infants exposed to INF in utero have an appropriate response to standard early vaccinations.[122] In adults receiving a similar agent, adalimumab, pneumococcal and influenza vaccinations were given safely and effectively.[123] However, live vaccinations, such as varicella and small pox, are contraindicated in immunosuppressed patients, such as those on anti-TNF therapy.[124] Traditionally, the first live virus encountered by an infant was at 1 year of age (varicella, measles-mumps-rubella) when INF levels would be undetectable. However, now, rotavirus live vaccine is given at 2 months of age. Although it is given orally and is significantly attenuated, its safety in this setting is not known and the mother and pediatrician should be cautioned against its use if INF or ADA levels may be present.

Adalimumab

Adalimumab (ADA), a pregnancy category B drug, is FDA approved for induction and maintenance of remission in CD.[125] Three case reports[126–128] document the successful use of ADA to treat CD during pregnancy, including one in which the patient received weekly dosing throughout pregnancy for a total of 38 doses.[128] OTIS (Organization for Teratology Information Specialists) reports 27 women enrolled in a prospective study of ADA in pregnancy and an additional 47 ADA exposed pregnant women in a registry (Chambers CD Johnson D, Jones KL. Pregnancy outcomes in women exposed to adalimumab: The OTIS autoimmune diseases in pregnancy project, personal communication; July 13, 2007). The rate of spontaneous abortion and stillbirth was similar to the diseased comparison and the general population. The rates of congenital malformation and preterm delivery are also within the expected range.

ADA, an IgG1 antibody, would be expected to cross the placenta in the third trimester as INF does. However, as ADA levels cannot be checked commercially, this has not been confirmed. ADA is considered compatible with breastfeeding although there are no human data.

Certolizumab pegol

Certolizumab pegol (CZP) is a PEGylated Fab' fragment of a humanized anti-TNFα monoclonal antibody. As it does not have an Fc portion, it should not be actively transported across the placenta as INF and ADA are. A study of pregnant rats[129] receiving a murinized IgG1 antibody of TNFα and a PEGylated FAB' fragment of this antibody, demonstrated much lower levels of drug in the infant and in breast milk with the Fab' fragment compared with the full antibody. These findings were confirmed in two patients with CD receiving CZP during pregnancy.[130] Both patients received the drug during the 2 weeks before delivery. The mothers' levels were high (19.60) but the infants' level (1.02) and cord blood level (1.65) were low on the day of birth. However, one concern may be that in theory the Fab' fragment (and the IgG1 antibodies) may cross the placenta passively in low levels in the first trimester during the period of organogenesis. A single case report in a patient with Crohn reported a successful pregnancy[131] on CZP. Further data are clearly needed on all the anti-TNF agents.

Timing of Anti–Tumor Necrosis Factor Therapy in Pregnancy

All three anti-TNFs should be continued through conception and the first and second trimester on schedule. In our practice, if the patient is in remission, we give the last dose of infliximab at week 30 gestation and then immediately after delivery. We give the last dose of adalimumab at approximately week 32 of gestation and then immediately after delivery. If the mother flares during this time period, the options include giving a dose of anti-TNF or using steroids to manage the patient until delivery. This decision is driven by how far the mother is from delivery. Although we would refrain from giving infliximab at week 39 of gestation, a mother who is flaring at week 34 on adalimumab would likely benefit from continuing dosing on schedule. Certolizumab, given its minimal transfer across the placenta, is continued on schedule until delivery. Rotavirus vaccine can be given to the infant if there is no detectable infliximab in its blood at time of vaccination or if they received certolizumab, as by 2 months little to no drug will be present. As adalimumab levels are not commercially available, we advise mothers not to have their child vaccinated against rotavirus.

Fish Oil Supplements

Many patients with IBD use fish oil supplements as an adjunct to standard medical therapy. Because this is a supplement and not a drug, it is not rated by the FDA. A randomized controlled trial of fish oil supplementation demonstrated a prolongation of pregnancy without detrimental effects on the growth of the fetus or on the course of labor.[132] Fish oil supplementation may also play a role in preventing miscarriage associated with the antiphospholipid antibody syndrome.[133] In women with IBD who may be at increased risk for preterm birth and miscarriage, fish oil supplementation is not harmful and may be of some benefit.

SUMMARY

The use of IBD medication during conception and pregnancy is generally low risk. For a drug to clearly be associated with congenital anomalies, the same defect must be seen repeatedly, a phenomenon not demonstrated with any IBD medication except methotrexate and thalidomide, both of which are contraindicated. The risk of an adverse fetal event must be weighed against the benefit to the health of the mother from continuing her medication and controlling her underlying disease.

Based on the available evidence, a woman with IBD contemplating pregnancy should be in optimal health and remission. Methotrexate and thalidomide should be discontinued 6 months before attempting conception. Aminosalicylates, AZA/6-MP, and anti-TNF agents are continued during conception and pregnancy. Two potential nuances to this policy: a patient on sulfasalazine may be switched to a mesalamine agent if tolerated to minimize antifolate effects and a stable patient on combination AZA/6-MP and an anti-TNF agent may consider discontinuing the AZA/6-MP before conception to minimize risk to the fetus. Although this may seem inconsistent, as data suggest continuing AZA/6-MP during pregnancy is low risk, at every opportunity we want to maintain the mother's health and minimize risk to the fetus. Discontinuing AZA/6-MP in a patient stable on INF has not been associated with an increase in adverse events.[134] Corticosteroids and antibiotics should be avoided in the first trimester to avoid the small risk of congenital malformations. However, if a patient is flaring, steroids may need to be used at any point in pregnancy. A patient naïve to AZA/6-MP should not get it for the first time during pregnancy as the risk of leucopenia and pancreatitis is unpredictable. Anti-TNFs can be started in a naïve patient during pregnancy. Use of INF and ADA should be minimized in the third trimester (we stop dosing of INF at week 30 and ADA at week 32 of gestation if tolerated) given the high rates of placental transfer. If an anti-TNF is to be given for the first time during pregnancy, CZP may be the ideal choice given the low rate of placental transfer.

REFERENCES

1. Andres PG, Friedman LS. Epidemiology and the natural course of inflammatory bowel disease. Gastroenterol Clin North Am 1999;28(2):255–81, vii.
2. Orholm M, Fonager K, Sorensen HT. Risk of ulcerative colitis and Crohn's disease among offspring of patients with chronic inflammatory bowel disease. Am J Gastroenterol 1999;94(11):3236–8.
3. Orholm M, Munkholm P, Langholz E, et al. Familial occurrence of inflammatory bowel disease. N Engl J Med 1991;324(2):84–8.
4. Yang H, McElree C, Roth MP, et al. Familial empirical risks for inflammatory bowel disease: differences between Jews and non-Jews. Gut 1993;34(4): 517–24.
5. Bennett RA, Rubin PH, Present DH. Frequency of inflammatory bowel disease in offspring of couples both presenting with inflammatory bowel disease. Gastroenterology 1991;100(6):1638–43.
6. Klement E, Reif S. Breastfeeding and risk of inflammatory bowel disease. Am J Clin Nutr 2005;82(2):486.
7. Fielding JF. Pregnancy and inflammatory bowel disease. Ir J Med Sci 1982; 151(6):194–202.
8. Mayberry JF, Weterman IT. European survey of fertility and pregnancy in women with Crohn's disease: a case control study by European collaborative group. Gut 1986;27(7):821–5.

9. Francella A, Dyan A, Bodian C, et al. The safety of 6-mercaptopurine for child-bearing patients with inflammatory bowel disease: a retrospective cohort study. Gastroenterology 2003;124(1):9–17.

10. Hudson M, Flett G, Sinclair TS, et al. Fertility and pregnancy in inflammatory bowel disease. Int J Gynaecol Obstet 1997;58(2):229–37.

11. Baird DD, Narendranathan M, Sandler RS. Increased risk of preterm birth for women with inflammatory bowel disease. Gastroenterology 1990;99(4): 987–94.

12. Willoughby CP, Truelove SC. Ulcerative colitis and pregnancy. Gut 1980;21(6): 469–74.

13. Ording Olsen K, Juul S, Berndtsson I, et al. Ulcerative colitis: female fecundity before diagnosis, during disease, and after surgery compared with a population sample. Gastroenterology 2002;122(1):15–9.

14. Wikland M, Jansson I, Asztely M, et al. Gynaecological problems related to anatomical changes after conventional proctocolectomy and ileostomy. Int J Colorectal Dis 1990;5(1):49–52.

15. Olsen KO, Juul S, Bulow S, et al. Female fecundity before and after operation for familial adenomatous polyposis. Br J Surg 2003;90(2):227–31.

16. Waljee A, Waljee J, Morris AM, et al. Threefold increased risk of infertility: a meta-analysis of infertility after ileal pouch anal anastomosis in ulcerative colitis. Gut 2006;55(11):1575–80.

17. Cornish JA, Tan E, Teare J, et al. The effect of restorative proctocolectomy on sexual function, urinary function, fertility, pregnancy and delivery: a systematic review. Dis Colon Rectum 2007;50(8):1128–38.

18. Timmer A, Bauer A, Dignass A, et al. Sexual function in persons with inflammatory bowel disease: a survey with matched controls. Clin Gastroenterol Hepatol 2007;5(1):87–94.

19. Van Horn C, Barrett P. Pregnancy, delivery, and postpartum experiences of fifty-four women with ostomies. J Wound Ostomy Continence Nurs 1997;24(3): 151–62.

20. Kane SV, Khatibi B, Reddy D. Use of immunosuppressants results in higher incidence of abnormal PAP smears in women with inflammatory bowel disease [abstract]. Gastroenterology 2006;130(4 Suppl 2):A2.

21. Venkatesan TBD, Ferrer V, Weber L, et al. Abnormal PAP smear, cervical dysplasia and immunomodulator therapy in women with inflammatory bowel disease [abstract]. Gastroenterology 2006;130(4 Suppl 2):A3.

22. Singh H, Demers AA, Nugent Z, et al. Risk of cervical abnormalities in women with inflammatory bowel disease: a population-based nested case-control study. Gastroenterology 2009;136(2):451–8.

23. Lees CW, Critchley J, Chee N, et al. Lack of association between cervical dysplasia and IBD: a large case-control study. Inflamm Bowel Dis 2009. [Epub ahead of print].

24. Fonager K, Sorensen HT, Olsen J, et al. Pregnancy outcome for women with Crohn's disease: a follow-up study based on linkage between national registries. Am J Gastroenterol 1998;93(12):2426–30.

25. Kornfeld D, Cnattingius S, Ekbom A. Pregnancy outcomes in women with inflammatory bowel disease–a population-based cohort study. Am J Obstet Gynecol 1997;177(4):942–6.

26. Norgard B, Fonager K, Sorensen HT, et al. Birth outcomes of women with ulcerative colitis: a nationwide Danish cohort study. Am J Gastroenterol 2000;95(11): 3165–70.

27. Dominitz JA, Young JC, Boyko EJ. Outcomes of infants born to mothers with inflammatory bowel disease: a population-based cohort study. Am J Gastroenterol 2002;97(3):641–8.
28. Norgard B, Puho E, Pedersen L, et al. Risk of congenital abnormalities in children born to women with ulcerative colitis: a population-based, case-control study. Am J Gastroenterol 2003;98(9):2006–10.
29. Mahadevan U, Sandborn WJ, Li DK, et al. Pregnancy outcomes in women with inflammatory bowel disease: a large community-based study from Northern California. Gastroenterology 2007;133(4):1106–12.
30. Cornish J, Tan E, Teare J, et al. A meta-analysis on the influence of inflammatory bowel disease on pregnancy. Gut 2007;56(6):830–7.
31. Larzilliere I, Beau P. Chronic inflammatory bowel disease and pregnancy. Case control study. Gastroenterol Clin Biol 1998;22(12):1056–60 [in French].
32. Nielsen OH, Andreasson B, Bondesen S, et al. Pregnancy in ulcerative colitis. Scand J Gastroenterol 1983;18(6):735–42.
33. Nielsen OH, Andreasson B, Bondesen S, et al. Pregnancy in Crohn's disease. Scand J Gastroenterol 1984;19(6):724–32.
34. Mogadam M, Korelitz BI, Ahmed SW, et al. The course of inflammatory bowel disease during pregnancy and postpartum. Am J Gastroenterol 1981;75(4): 265–9.
35. Morales M, Berney T, Jenny A, et al. Crohn's disease as a risk factor for the outcome of pregnancy. Hepatogastroenterology 2000;47(36):1595–8.
36. Kane S, Lemieux N. The role of breastfeeding in postpartum disease activity in women with inflammatory bowel disease. Am J Gastroenterol 2005;100(1): 102–5.
37. Agret F, Cosnes J, Hassani Z, et al. Impact of pregnancy on the clinical activity of Crohn's disease. Aliment Pharmacol Ther 2005;21(5):509–13.
38. Castiglione F, Pignata S, Morace F, et al. Effect of pregnancy on the clinical course of a cohort of women with inflammatory bowel disease. Ital J Gastroenterol 1996;28(4):199–204.
39. Riis L, Vind I, Politi P, et al. Does pregnancy change the disease course? A study in a European cohort of patients with inflammatory bowel disease. Am J Gastroenterol 2006;101(7):1539–45.
40. Nelson JL, Hughes KA, Smith AG, et al. Maternal-fetal disparity in HLA class II alloantigens and the pregnancy-induced amelioration of rheumatoid arthritis. N Engl J Med 1993;329(7):466–71.
41. Kane S, Kisiel J, Shih L, et al. HLA disparity determines disease activity through pregnancy in women with inflammatory bowel disease. Am J Gastroenterol 2004;99(8):1523–6.
42. Bush MC, Patel S, Lapinski RH, et al. Perinatal outcomes in inflammatory bowel disease. J Matern Fetal Neonatal Med 2004;15(4):237–41.
43. Fedorkow DM, Persaud D, Nimrod CA. Inflammatory bowel disease: a controlled study of late pregnancy outcome. Am J Obstet Gynecol 1989;160(4):998–1001.
44. Moser MA, Okun NB, Mayes DC, et al. Crohn's disease, pregnancy, and birth weight. Am J Gastroenterol 2000;95(4):1021–6.
45. Norgard B, Hundborg HH, Jacobsen BA, et al. Disease activity in pregnant women with Crohn's disease and birth outcomes: a regional Danish Cohort Study. Am J Gastroenterol 2007;102(9):1947–54.
46. Ilnyckyji A, Blanchard JF, Rawsthorne P, et al. Perianal Crohn's disease and pregnancy: role of the mode of delivery. Am J Gastroenterol 1999;94(11): 3274–8.

47. Brandt LJ, Estabrook SG, Reinus JF. Results of a survey to evaluate whether vaginal delivery and episiotomy lead to perineal involvement in women with Crohn's disease. Am J Gastroenterol 1995;90(11):1918–22.
48. Hahnloser D, Pemberton JH, Wolff BG, et al. Pregnancy and delivery before and after ileal pouch-anal anastomosis for inflammatory bowel disease: immediate and long-term consequences and outcomes. Dis Colon Rectum 2004;47(7):1127–35.
49. Craxi A, Pagliarello F. Possible embryotoxicity of sulfasalazine. Arch Intern Med 1980;140(12):1674.
50. Hoo JJ, Hadro TA, Von Behren P. Possible teratogenicity of sulfasalazine. N Engl J Med 1988;318(17):1128.
51. Newman NM, Correy JF. Possible teratogenicity of sulphasalazine. Med J Aust 1983;1(11):528–9.
52. Mogadam M, Dobbins WO 3rd, Korelitz BI, et al. Pregnancy in inflammatory bowel disease: effect of sulfasalazine and corticosteroids on fetal outcome. Gastroenterology 1981;80(1):72–6.
53. Norgard B, Czeizel AE, Rockenbauer M, et al. Population-based case control study of the safety of sulfasalazine use during pregnancy. Aliment Pharmacol Ther 2001;15(4):483–6.
54. Esbjorner E, Jarnerot G, Wranne L. Sulphasalazine and sulphapyridine serum levels in children to mothers treated with sulphasalazine during pregnancy and lactation. Acta Paediatr Scand 1987;76(1):137–42.
55. Habal FM, Hui G, Greenberg GR. Oral 5-aminosalicylic acid for inflammatory bowel disease in pregnancy: safety and clinical course. Gastroenterology 1993;105(4):1057–60.
56. Marteau P, Tennenbaum R, Elefant E, et al. Foetal outcome in women with inflammatory bowel disease treated during pregnancy with oral mesalazine microgranules. Aliment Pharmacol Ther 1998;12(11):1101–8.
57. Trallori G, d'Albasio G, Bardazzi G, et al. 5-Aminosalicylic acid in pregnancy: clinical report. Ital J Gastroenterol 1994;26(2):75–8.
58. Diav-Citrin O, Park YH, Veerasuntharam G, et al. The safety of mesalamine in human pregnancy: a prospective controlled cohort study. Gastroenterology 1998;114(1):23–8.
59. Norgard B, Fonager K, Pedersen L, et al. Birth outcome in women exposed to 5-aminosalicylic acid during pregnancy: a Danish cohort study. Gut 2003;52(2):243–7.
60. Nelis GF. Diarrhoea due to 5-aminosalicylic acid in breast milk. Lancet 1989;1(8634):383.
61. Burtin P, Taddio A, Ariburnu O, et al. Safety of metronidazole in pregnancy: a meta-analysis. Am J Obstet Gynecol 1995;172(2 Pt 1):525–9.
62. Caro-Paton T, Carvajal A, Martin de Diego I, et al. Is metronidazole teratogenic? A meta-analysis. Br J Clin Pharmacol 1997;44(2):179–82.
63. Piper JM, Mitchel EF, Ray WA. Prenatal use of metronidazole and birth defects: no association. Obstet Gynecol 1993;82(3):348–52.
64. Sorensen HT, Larsen H, Jensen ES, et al. Safety of metronidazole during pregnancy: a cohort study of risk of congenital abnormalities, preterm delivery and low birth weight in 124 women. J Antimicrob Chemother 1999;44(6):854–6.
65. Diav-Citrin O, Shechtman S, Gotteiner T, et al. Pregnancy outcome after gestational exposure to metronidazole: a prospective controlled cohort study. Teratology 2001;63(5):186–92.

66. Czeizel AE, Rockenbauer M. A population based case-control teratologic study of oral metronidazole treatment during pregnancy. Br J Obstet Gynaecol 1998; 105(3):322–7.

67. American Academy of Pediatrics. Committee on Drugs. Naloxone use in newborns. Pediatrics 1980;65(3):667–9.

68. Niebyl JR. Antibiotics and other anti-infective agents in pregnancy and lactation. Am J Perinatol 2003;20(8):405–14.

69. Loebstein R, Addis A, Ho E, et al. Pregnancy outcome following gestational exposure to fluoroquinolones: a multicenter prospective controlled study. Antimicrobial Agents Chemother 1998;42(6):1336–9.

70. Larsen H, Nielsen GL, Schonheyder HC, et al. Birth outcome following maternal use of fluoroquinolones. Int J Antimicrob Agents 2001;18(3):259–62.

71. Briggs. Drugs in pregnancy and lactation. 7th edition. Philadelphia: Lippincott Williams Wilkins; 2005.

72. Xifaxan. Package insert. 2005.

73. Czeizel AE, Rockenbauer M, Sorensen HT, et al. Augmentin treatment during pregnancy and the prevalence of congenital abnormalities: a population-based case-control teratologic study. Eur J Obstet Gynecol Reprod Biol 2001;97(2): 188–92.

74. Berkovitch M, Diav-Citrin O, Greenberg R, et al. First-trimester exposure to amoxycillin/clavulanic acid: a prospective, controlled study. Br J Clin Pharmacol 2004;58(3):298–302.

75. Rodriguez-Pinilla E, Martinez-Frias ML. Corticosteroids during pregnancy and oral clefts: a case-control study. Teratology 1998;58(1):2–5.

76. Carmichael SL, Shaw GM. Maternal corticosteroid use and risk of selected congenital anomalies. Am J Med Genet 1999;86(3):242–4.

77. Park-Wyllie L, Mazzotta P, Pastuszak A, et al. Birth defects after maternal exposure to corticosteroids: prospective cohort study and meta-analysis of epidemiological studies. Teratology 2000;62(6):385–92.

78. Gur C, Diav-Citrin O, Shechtman S, et al. Pregnancy outcome after first trimester exposure to corticosteroids: a prospective controlled study. Reprod Toxicol 2004;18(1):93–101.

79. Armenti VT, Moritz MJ, Cardonick EH, et al. Immunosuppression in pregnancy: choices for infant and maternal health. Drugs 2002;62(16):2361–75.

80. Beaulieu DB, Ananthakrishnan AN, Issa M, et al. Budesonide induction and maintenance therapy for Crohn's disease during pregnancy. Inflamm Bowel Dis 2009;15(1):25–8.

81. Gluck PA, Gluck JC. A review of pregnancy outcomes after exposure to orally inhaled or intranasal budesonide. Curr Med Res Opin 2005;21(7):1075–84.

82. Norjavaara E, de Verdier MG. Normal pregnancy outcomes in a population-based study including 2,968 pregnant women exposed to budesonide. J Allergy Clin Immunol 2003;111(4):736–42.

83. Patlas N, Golomb G, Yaffe P, et al. Transplacental effects of bisphosphonates on fetal skeletal ossification and mineralization in rats. Teratology 1999;60(2): 68–73.

84. Ornoy A, Wajnberg R, Diav-Citrin O. The outcome of pregnancy following pre-pregnancy or early pregnancy alendronate treatment. Reprod Toxicol 2006;22(4):578–9.

85. Del Campo M, Kosaki K, Bennett FC, et al. Developmental delay in fetal aminopterin/methotrexate syndrome. Teratology 1999;60(1):10–2.

86. American Academy of Pediatrics Committee on Drugs. The transfer of drugs and other chemicals into human milk. Pediatrics 2001;108:776–89.

87. Polifka JE, Friedman JM. Teratogen update: azathioprine and 6-mercaptopurine. Teratology 2002;65(5):240–61.

88. de Boer NK, Jarbandhan SV, de Graaf P, et al. Azathioprine use during pregnancy: unexpected intrauterine exposure to metabolites. Am J Gastroenterol 2006;101(6):1390–2.

89. Norgard B, Pedersen L, Fonager K, et al. Azathioprine, mercaptopurine and birth outcome: a population-based cohort study. Aliment Pharmacol Ther 2003;17(6):827–34.

90. Alstead EM, Ritchie JK, Lennard-Jones JE, et al. Safety of azathioprine in pregnancy in inflammatory bowel disease. Gastroenterology 1990;99(2):443–6.

91. Khan ZH, Mayberry JF, Spiers N, et al. Retrospective case series analysis of patients with inflammatory bowel disease on azathioprine. A district general hospital experience. Digestion 2000;62(4):249–54.

92. Moskovitz DN, Bodian C, Chapman ML, et al. The effect on the fetus of medications used to treat pregnant inflammatory bowel-disease patients. Am J Gastroenterol 2004;99(4):656–61.

93. Zlatanic J, Korelitz BI, Rajapakse R, et al. Complications of pregnancy and child development after cessation of treatment with 6-mercaptopurine for inflammatory bowel disease. J Clin Gastroenterol 2003;36(4):303–9.

94. Norgard B, Pedersen L, Christensen LA, et al. Therapeutic drug use in women with Crohn's disease and birth outcomes: a Danish nationwide cohort study. Am J Gastroenterol 2007;102(7):1406–13.

95. Goldstein LH, Dolinsky G, Greenberg R, et al. Pregnancy outcome of women exposed to azathioprine during pregnancy. Birth Defects Res A Clin Mol Teratol 2007;79(10):696–701.

96. Moretti ME, Verjee Z, Ito S, et al. Breast-feeding during maternal use of azathioprine. Ann Pharmacother 2006;40(12):2269–72.

97. Gardiner SJ, Gearry RB, Roberts RL, et al. Exposure to thiopurine drugs through breast milk is low based on metabolite concentrations in mother-infant pairs. Br J Clin Pharmacol 2006;62(4):453–6.

98. Sau A, Clarke S, Bass J, et al. Azathioprine and breastfeeding: is it safe? BJOG 2007;114(4):498–501.

99. Christensen LA, Dahlerup JF, Nielsen MJ, et al. Azathioprine treatment during lactation. Aliment Pharmacol Ther 2008;28(10):1209–13.

100. Bar Oz B, Hackman R, Einarson T, et al. Pregnancy outcome after cyclosporine therapy during pregnancy: a meta-analysis. Transplantation 2001;71(8):1051–5.

101. Nagy S, Bush MC, Berkowitz R, et al. Pregnancy outcome in liver transplant recipients. Obstet Gynecol 2003;102(1):121–8.

102. Angelberger S, Reinisch W, Dejaco C. Prevention of abortion by ciclosporin treatment of fulminant ulcerative colitis during pregnancy. Gut 2006;55(9):1364–5.

103. Bertschinger P, Himmelmann A, Risti B, et al. Cyclosporine treatment of severe ulcerative colitis during pregnancy. Am J Gastroenterol 1995;90(2):330.

104. Reindl W, Schmid RM, Huber W. Cyclosporin A treatment of steroid-refractory ulcerative colitis during pregnancy: report of two cases. Gut 2007;56(7):1019.

105. Jain A, Venkataramanan R, Fung JJ, et al. Pregnancy after liver transplantation under tacrolimus. Transplantation 1997;64(4):559–65.

106. Kainz A, Harabacz I, Cowlrick IS, et al. Analysis of 100 pregnancy outcomes in women treated systemically with tacrolimus. Transpl Int 2000;13(Suppl 1): S299–300.
107. Jain AB, Reyes J, Marcos A, et al. Pregnancy after liver transplantation with tacrolimus immunosuppression: a single center's experience update at 13 years. Transplantation 2003;76(5):827–32.
108. Baumgart DC, Sturm A, Wiedenmann B, et al. Uneventful pregnancy and neonatal outcome with tacrolimus in refractory ulcerative colitis. Gut 2005; 54(12):1822–3.
109. Ehrenpreis ED, Kane SV, Cohen LB, et al. Thalidomide therapy for patients with refractory Crohn's disease: an open-label trial. Gastroenterology 1999;117(6): 1271–7.
110. Celgene-Corporation. Thalomid. Product Information. 2000.
111. Hanauer SB, Feagan BG, Lichtenstein GR, et al. Maintenance infliximab for Crohn's disease: the ACCENT I randomised trial. Lancet 2002;359(9317): 1541–9.
112. Rutgeerts P, Sandborn WJ, Feagan BG, et al. Infliximab for induction and maintenance therapy for ulcerative colitis. N Engl J Med 2005;353(23):2462–76.
113. Simister NE. Placental transport of immunoglobulin G. Vaccine 2003;21(24): 3365–9.
114. Lichtenstein G, Cohen RD, Feagan BG, et al. Safety of infliximab in Crohn's disease: data from the 5000- patient TREAT Registry [abstract]. Gastroenterology 2004;126(Suppl 4):A54.
115. Katz JA, Antoni C, Keenan GF, et al. Outcome of pregnancy in women receiving infliximab for the treatment of Crohn's disease and rheumatoid arthritis. Am J Gastroenterol 2004;99(12):2385–92.
116. Mahadevan U, Kane S, Sandborn WJ, et al. Intentional infliximab use during pregnancy for induction or maintenance of remission in Crohn's disease. Aliment Pharmacol Ther 2005;21(6):733–8.
117. Schnitzler F, Fidder H, Ferrante M, et al. Intentional treatment with infliximab during pregnancy in women with inflammatory bowel disease [abstract]. Gastroenterology 2007;132(4 Suppl 2):958.
118. Vasiliauskas EA, Church JA, Silverman N, et al. Case report: evidence for transplacental transfer of maternally administered infliximab to the newborn. Clin Gastroenterol Hepatol 2006;4(10):1255–8.
119. Mahadevan U, Terdiman J, Church J, et al. Infliximab levels in infants born to women with inflammatory bowel disease [abstract]. Gastroenterol 2007;132(4 Suppl 2):A144.
120. Kane S, Ford J, Cohen R, et al. Absence of infliximab in infants and breast milk from nursing mothers receiving therapy for Crohn's disease before and after delivery. J Clin Gastroenterol 2009;43(7):613–6.
121. Peltier M, James D, Ford J, et al. Infliximab levels in breast-milk of a nursing Crohn's patient [abstract]. Am J Gastroenterol 2001;96(9 Suppl 1):P258.
122. Mahadevan UKS, Church J, Vasiliauskas E, et al. The effect of maternal peripartum infliximab use on neonatal immune response [abstract]. Gastroenterology 2008;134(4 suppl 1):A69.
123. Kaine JL, Kivitz AJ, Birbara C, et al. Immune responses following administration of influenza and pneumococcal vaccines to patients with rheumatoid arthritis receiving adalimumab. J Rheumatol 2007;34(2):272–9.
124. Sands BE, Cuffari C, Katz J, et al. Guidelines for immunizations in patients with inflammatory bowel disease. Inflamm Bowel Dis 2004;10(5):677–92.

125. Hanaver SB, Sandborn WJ, Rutgeerts P, et al. Human anti-tumor necrosis factor monoclonal antibody (adalimumab) in Crohn's disease: the CLASSIC-I trial. Gastroenterology 2006;130:323–33 [quiz 591].

126. Coburn LA, Wise PE, Schwartz DA. The successful use of adalimumab to treat active Crohn's disease of an ileoanal pouch during pregnancy. Dig Dis Sci 2006; 51(11):2045–7.

127. Mishkin DS, Van Deinse W, Becker JM, et al. Successful use of adalimumab (Humira) for Crohn's disease in pregnancy. Inflamm Bowel Dis 2006;12(8): 827–8.

128. Vesga L, Terdiman JP, Mahadevan U. Adalimumab use in pregnancy. Gut 2005; 54(6):890.

129. Nesbitt ABD, Stephens S, Foulkes R. Placental transfer and accumulation in milk of the anti-TNF antibody TN3 in rats: immunoglobulin G1 versus PEGylated Fab' [abstract]. Am J Gastroenterol 2006;101:1119.

130. Mahadevan USC, Abreu M. Certolizumab use in pregnancy: low levels detected in cord blood [abstract]. Gastroenterology 2009;136(5):960.

131. Oussalah A, Bigard MA, Peyrin-Biroulet L. Certolizumab use in pregnancy. Gut 2009;58(4):608.

132. Olsen SF, Sorensen JD, Secher NJ, et al. Randomised controlled trial of effect of fish-oil supplementation on pregnancy duration. Lancet 1992;339(8800):1003–7.

133. Rossi E, Costa M. Fish oil derivatives as a prophylaxis of recurrent miscarriage associated with antiphospholipid antibodies (APL): a pilot study. Lupus 1993; 2(5):319–23.

134. Van Assche G, Magdelaine-Beuzelin C, D'Haens G, et al. Withdrawal of immunosuppression in Crohn's disease treated with scheduled infliximab maintenance: a randomized trial. Gastroenterology 2008;134(7):1861–8.

Pouchitis and Pouch Dysfunction

Hao Wu, MB[a], Bo Shen, MD[b],*

KEYWORDS

- Classification • Complications • Ileal pouch
- Inflammatory bowel disease
- Pouchitis • CAP restorative proctocolectomy

Approximately 30% of patients with ulcerative colitis (UC) eventually require colectomy at some point in their disease course, despite advances in medical therapy.[1] Restorative proctocolectomy with ileal pouch-anal anastomosis (IPAA) has become the surgical treatment of choice for most patients with UC who fail medical therapy or develop dysplasia, and for most patients with familial adenomatous polyposis (FAP). The main advantage of IPAA surgery includes re-establishment of gastrointestinal continuity and improvement of health-related quality of life. However, the trade-off of the procedure is its high risk for the development of inflammatory and noninflammatory complications, with cumulative pouch failure rates ranging from 4% to 10%.[2–6] The most common causes for pouch failure are pelvic sepsis,[7,8] followed by Crohn disease (CD) of the pouch and chronic pouchitis.[9]

Pouchitis is one of the most challenging disorders in IPAA. This article updates the information on diagnosis and treatment of pouchitis.

INCIDENCE AND PREVALENCE OF POUCHITIS

Pouchitis significantly affects patients' quality of life and long-term surgical outcome.[10] Reported cumulative frequencies of pouchitis 10 to 11 years after IPAA surgery range from 23% to 46%.[11–14] It is estimated that approximately 50% of patients who have undergone IPAA surgery for UC develop at least 1 episode of pouchitis.[15] The estimated incidence within the first 12 months after ileostomy closure was as high as 40%, as reported in a clinical trial.[16] In patients with pouchitis, 70% had the initial episode during the first 12 months after ileostomy closure.[17] As the incidence of

This article originally appeared in *Gastroenterology Clinics of North America*, Volume 38, Issue 4.
This work is partially supported by a grant from BMRP, Eli and Edyth Broad Foundation.
a Department of Gastroenterology, Zhongshan Hospital, Fudan University, Shanghai, China
b Digestive Disease Institute-Desk A31, Cleveland Clinic, 9500 Euclid Avenue, Cleveland, OH 44195, USA
* Corresponding author.
E-mail address: shenb@ccf.org (B. Shen).

inflammatory bowel disease (IBD), including UC, seems to be increasing, the authors expect a growing number of patients with pouchitis or other pouch disorders in clinical practice.

ETIOLOGY AND PATHOGENESIS OF POUCHITIS

Pouchitis occurs almost exclusively in patients with underlying UC, not in patients with FAP who undergo the same surgical procedure.[18,19] It is generally believed that pouchitis results from alternations in luminal microflora (ie, dysbiosis), leading to abnormal mucosal immune response in genetically susceptible hosts. Attempts have been made to identify true pathogenic microbes. In a subset of patients with pouchitis, pathogenic factors may be identified. A recent study showed that 18% of patients seen in a specialty pouchitis clinic tested positive for *Clostridium difficile* toxins A or B.[20] Cytomegalovirus (CMV)[21,22] and fungi (such as *Candida albicans*)[23] have also been implicated in pouchitis, particularly in patients with chronic antibiotic-refractory pouchitis.

Although microbiological investigation of the bacterial communities in the gut failed to demonstrate consistently the existence of pathogens in pouchitis, a large body of evidence suggests that alteration in the bacteria community, ie, dysbiosis, of the human gut likely plays a key role in the initiation and development of pouchitis. In a culture-based study of fecal specimens in patients with UC pouches or FAP pouches, viable sulfate-reducing bacteria were exclusively detected in pouches of UC patients, but not in patients with FAP. Sulfate-reducing bacteria were detected in higher numbers in active pouchitis than in those without a history of pouchitis, past episode(s) of pouchitis, or on antibiotic therapy, and in patients with FAP.[24] This particular group of bacteria was sensitive to antibiotic treatment.[24] Gosselink and colleagues[25] analyzed bacteria content at the episode of pouchitis before and during treatment with ciprofloxacin or metronidazole, and during pouchitis-free periods, and found that, in the absence of inflammation, the pouch microbiota was characterized by the presence of *Lactobacilli* and large numbers of anaerobes. During pouchitis episodes, there was a decreased number of anaerobes, an increased number of aerobic bacteria, lower numbers of *Lactobacilli*, and higher numbers of *Clostridium perfringens*. In addition, hemolytic strains of *Escherichia coli* were observed. Administration of metronidazole was shown to eradicate anaerobic microbiota including *C perfringens*, whereas treatment with ciprofloxacin inhibited the growth of *C perfringens* and that of coliforms, including hemolytic strains of *E coli*.

Advances in molecular microbiology with 16S ribosomal RNA techniques have provided a cornerstone of microbial taxonomy and made the assay of bacterial composition in the gut community possible.[26] In a case study, mucosa-associated bacteria of the pouch were assayed using tissue biopsy samples at the time of colectomy, pouch construction, ileostomy closure, and postoperative routine pouch examination at 1, 3, and 12 months after ileostomy closure.[26] The pouch microbiota were similar to the normal colon microbiota except for the presence of clones with sequences resembling those of the *C perfringens* group and *Turicibacter*. The bacterial composition differed between the 2 patients studied and the microbiota changed with time, suggesting that the composition is not stable during the first year of ileostomy closure.[26] Komanduri and colleagues[27] studied pouch biopsy specimens from 5 patients with active pouchitis and 15 patients with normal pouches, using a fingerprinting technique. The study showed mucosa-associated microbiota patterns unique to each individual. Moreover, specific bacterial amplicons were unique to active pouchitis mucosa: clostridial cluster XIVa, Enterobacteriaceae, and *Streptococci* were associated with control pouches. The persistence of *Fusobacter* and enteric species associated with the disease state was also shown.

Alterations in innate and adaptive mucosal immunity in the pouch and pouchitis have been reported.[28–33] An increased bacterial permeability was associated with duration of having a pouch with mucosal adaptive changes in an ex vivo study.[28] UC patients with backwash ileitis were shown to have impaired barrier function in the future course of the IPAA.[34] Toll-like receptors (TLR) serve an important immune and nonimmune function in human intestinal epithelial cells (IEC) by binding microbial signature molecules and triggering innate and adaptive immune responses on stimulation.[35] TLRs comprise a defense line against invading pathogens challenging the IEC layer. TLRs can trigger the secretion of antibacterial peptides, and also link innate and adaptive immune responses of the intestinal mucosa by attracting immune cells from the lamina propria. An aberrant TLR expression pattern has been found in IBD.[36] An immunohistochemical study showed that TLR2 expression is up-regulated in pouchitis and TLR4 expression is increased in the normal pouch and in pouchitis compared with the normal ileum.[37] Alterations in mRNA levels of TLR3 and TLR5 were present.[38] TLR3 expression was decreased significantly, whereas TLR5 expression was increased significantly in normal pouch mucosa compared with normal ileal mucosa.[38] A combined carriership of the TLR9-1237C and CD14-260T allele seemed to be associated with development of chronic pouchitis.[39]

Antimicrobial peptides produced from Paneth cells and other gut epithelial cells are an important component of innate immunity in the intestinal tract.[40–43] Paneth cells synthesize and secrete several antimicrobial peptides, including lysozyme, secretory phospholipase 2, and human α-defensins 5 and 6 (HD5 and HD6).[42–45] The copy number of HD5 mRNA was significantly decreased in the inflamed or noninflamed pouch compared with the normal terminal ileum.[46] Tissue mRNA copies of HD5 produced by Paneth cells and β (hBD-1, 2, 3)-defensins produced by gut epithelial cells were increased in UC and FAP pouches immediately after surgery, compared with ileum of controls. Initially, α- and β-defensin mRNAs were higher in UC pouches than in FAP pouches. However, the defensin expression declined in UC and FAP pouch groups and increased again slightly in pouchitis in patients with UC. FAP pouches without pouchitis had strong expression of hBD-1, whereas all other defensins remained at low levels.[47]

As in IBD, adaptive immune mechanisms for pouchitis have been extensively studied. For example, proliferation of immature plasma cells was increased in pouchitis.[32–34,48] Proinflammatory cytokines, such as tumor necrosing factor-α, are released mostly in the inflamed mucosa by macrophages and monocytes, leading to tissue injury, and are considered to be involved as a secondary pathophysiologic mechanism in pouchitis.[33] The production of inflammatory mediators is increased including proinflammatory cytokines,[47,49–52] cell adhesion molecules,[53] platelet-activating factor,[54] lipoxygenase products of arachidonic acids,[55,56] vascular endothelial growth factor,[56] proinflammatory neuropeptides, and other mediators.[50,57–59] In general, UC pouches expressed higher levels of inflammatory cytokines than FAP pouches.[60] Abnormalities in immunoregulatory cytokines such as IL-2, interferon-γ,[47,61] IL-4,[47,61] and IL-10[47] are also observed in pouchitis. Imbalance between proinflammatory and immunoregulatory cytokines has been described in patients with pouchitis.[52] However, it is likely that those abnormalities in mucosal adaptive immunity reflect activation of nonspecific inflammatory cascade.[50]

The natural history of pouchitis may mimic that of UC, starting from an acute disease process of bacterial etiology to chronic disease of persistent inflammation. There are similarities in clinical presentations and immunologic abnormalities between chronic pouchitis and UC. The presence of fecal stasis in the pouch, exposure to fecal contents, and an increased microbial load of the pouch epithelia may result in inflammatory changes leading to morphologic alterations in the ileal pouch mucosa mimicking the colon epithelia in UC, namely colonic metaplasia.[54,62] Colonic metaplasia, characterized by villous blunting, crypt cell hyperplasia, and colon epithelium-specific antigens such as human tropomyosin 5, may be associated with UC-like clinical presentations.[63] Colonic metaplasia seems to be associated with dysbiosis, particularly the presence of sulfate-reducing bacteria.[64] It has been reported that mucosal butyrate oxidation in pouchitis is similar to the findings in UC.[65] An alteration in mucin glycoproteins occurs in pouchitis similar to that seen in UC.[66] It is possible that the altered glycoproteins are more susceptible to enzymatic degradation by bacteria, making the mucus barrier less effective.[67]

RISK FACTORS FOR POUCHITIS

Factors associated with pouchitis have been studied extensively as part of the investigation of the etiology and pathogenesis of pouchitis. In addition, the identification of risk factors may have a direct impact on disease prevention and prognostication. Immunogenetic studies showed that genetic polymorphisms, such as those of the IL-1 receptor antagonist[68] and NOD2/CARD15,[69] may increase the risk for pouchitis. Other reported risk factors include extensive UC,[70,71] the presence of backwash ileitis,[17,70] precolectomy thrombocytosis,[72] the presence of concurrent primary sclerosing cholangitis (PSC)[17,73,74] or arthralgia/arthropathy,[75] seropositive perinuclear antineutrophil cytoplasmic antibodies (pANCA)[14,76,77] or anti-CBir1 flagellin,[14] being a nonsmoker,[14,71,75] and the use of nonsteroidal anti-inflammatory drugs (NSAID).[71,74] Acute antibiotic-responsive pouchitis and chronic antibiotic-refractory pouchitis may represent different disease processes associated with different etiopathogenetic pathways. As such, acute and chronic pouchitis may be associated with different risk factors.[71] In a recent study of 238 patients with different phenotypes of pouchitis, antibiotic-responsive pouchitis developed in 37 pANCA-positive patients (22%) versus 6 pANCA-negative patients (9%), and in 12 anti-CBir1–positive patients (26%) versus 31 anti-CBir1–negative patients (16%) during a median of 47 months of follow-up.[14] In one report, patients with backwash ileitis or PSC were associated with chronic pouchitis, but not with acute pouchitis.[17] Smoking was associated with acute pouchitis,[14] whereas extraintestinal manifestations,[14] preoperative thrombocytosis, a long duration of IPAA,[14] and postoperative surgery-related complications[78] were reported to be associated with chronic pouchitis. Smoking seems to be protective against the development of chronic pouchitis.[79] These findings suggest that chronic pouchitis and UC may share similar pathogenetic pathways, as smoking has also been shown to be protective against progression of UC.[80] Patients with chronic antibiotic-refractory pouchitis, not acute pouchitis, were associated with concurrent autoimmune disorders.[81]

Concurrent PSC is associated with an increased risk for backwash ileitis in patient with UC. Furthermore, the prevalence of PSC among patients with UC needing proctocolectomy was higher than in patients with UC in general.[74] Although PSC seems to be a risk factor for pouchitis,[73,74] particularly chronic pouchitis,[82,83] orthotopic liver transplantation together with post-transplant use of immunosuppressive agents seems not to have a detrimental impact on the disease course of pouchitis.[84,85]

There have been discrepancies in the literature in reported risk factors associated with pouchitis. With regard to inconsistency in the reported risk factors, there were intrainstitutional and interinstitutional variations. These variations could largely be due to the difference in study design, sample size, diagnostic criteria used for pouchitis, referral pattern, and statistical methods.

DIAGNOSIS OF POUCHITIS

Diagnosis of pouchitis is not always straightforward, because there are no specific symptoms and signs. Patients with pouchitis have a wide range of clinical presentations, ranging from increased stool frequency, urgency, incontinence, night-time seepage, to abdominal perianal discomfort. These symptoms, however, can be present in other inflammatory and noninflammatory disorders of the pouch, such as cuffitis, CD of the pouch, and irritable pouch syndrome. Therefore, the diagnosis of pouchitis should not be solely dependent on symptom assessment. In addition, severity of symptoms does not necessarily correlate with the degree of endoscopic or histologic inflammation of the pouch.[86,87] To complicate the matter even more, the diagnosis of pouch disorders can resemble hitting a moving target, as the disease process may not be static. For example, a patient may have typical pouchitis at 1 point, and may present CD of the pouch several months later. Therefore, a combined assessment of symptoms, endoscopic, and histologic features is advocated for the diagnosis and differential diagnosis of pouchitis.[86,88] Pouch endoscopy provides the most valuable information on the severity and extent of mucosal inflammation, backwash ileitis, CD of the pouch or cuffitis, and the presence of other abnormalities such as polyps, strictures, sinuses, and fistula openings (**Fig. 1**). Although histology has a limited role in grading the degree of pouch inflammation, it can provide valuable information on some special features, such as granulomas, viral inclusion bodies (for CMV infection), pyloric gland metaplasia (a sign of chronic mucosal inflammation), and dysplasia. A diagnostic and treatment algorithm is proposed (**Fig. 2**).

Laboratory testing is often necessary as a part of the evaluation of patients with pouch disorders, particular patients with chronic pouchitis. In patients with persistent symptoms of pouchitis, celiac serology, salicylate screening, and microbiological assays for *C difficile* and CMV may be performed.[89] As most patients undergo repeated or chronic antibiotic exposure, *C difficile* infection has been a growing problem.[20] Fecal assays of lactoferrin and calprotectin have been evaluated for the diagnosis and differential diagnosis of pouchitis. Quantitative[90] and qualitative[91] assays of lactoferrin have been used to distinguish pouchitis from normal pouches or irritable pouch syndrome. Fecal lactoferrin may be used as an inexpensive

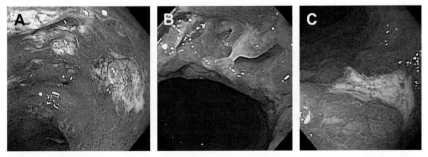

Fig. 1. Endoscopy of inflammatory disorders of the pouch. (*A*) Pouchitis, inflammation of the pouch body; (*B*) cuffitis, inflammation of the cuff; (*C*) Crohn disease of the pouch, ulcers at the neoterminal ileum.

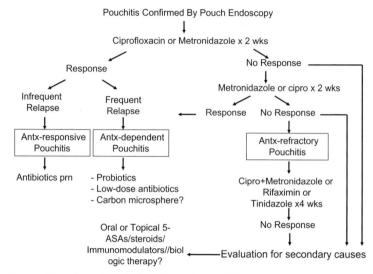

Fig. 2. Diagnostic and treatment algorithm of pouchitis.

screening test for pouchitis.[91,92] Fecal calprotectin assay had a sensitivity of 90% and a specificity of 76.5% for the diagnosis of pouchitis in a recent study.[93] However, the diagnostic accuracy of these studies was assessed based on the comparison of patients with pouchitis and patients with healthy pouches, whereas other inflammatory conditions such as cuffitis and CD of the pouch were not included in the prior studies. Other laboratory tests, such as assays of fecal dimeric M2-pyruvate kinase[94] and tissue proinflammatory cytokine gene scripts,[95] may also be useful in distinguishing pouchitis from noninflammatory conditions of the pouch. However, laboratory tests should not replace pouch endoscopy as the first-line evaluation for the diagnosis and differential diagnosis of pouchitis.

DIFFERENTIAL DIAGNOSIS OF POUCHITIS

There are overlaps in clinical presentations between a variety of inflammatory and noninflammatory disorders of ileal pouches (see **Fig. 1**). Cuffitis is considered a variant form of UC in the rectal cuff, particularly in patients with IPAA without mucosectomy. Patients with cuffitis often present with bloody bowel movements, which seldom occur in conventional pouchitis. When IPAA is constructed, there are 2 techniques to be used for the pouch-anal anastomosis, hand-sewn versus staple techniques: the hand-sewn IPAA with mucosectomy of the anal transition zone (ATZ) mucosa (or rectal cuff mucosa) or a stapled IPAA at the level of the anorectal ring without mucosectomy of the ATZ. To remove the rectal mucosa as completely as possible, a mucosectomy with hand-sewn anastomosis is necessary. This technique normally takes longer and has a high risk for postoperative functional problems related to seepage and incontinence due to anal canal manipulation. In contrast, the stapled anastomosis is easy to perform and is less likely to result in functional and septic complications. The preservation of ATZ is meant to optimize anal canal sensation, eliminate sphincter stretching, and preserve normal postoperative resting and squeeze pressures.[5,7,8] However, to allow transanal insertion of the stapler head, it is usually necessary to leave a 1- to

2-cm strip of rectal cuff/ATZ mucosa that is at risk for developing symptomatic inflammation (cuffitis) or even dysplasia.

Another common inflammatory disorder of the pouch is CD. It has been speculated that IPAA surgery with change of bowel anatomy, anastomoses, and fecal stasis creates a "CD-friendly" environment. CD of the pouch can occur after IPAA intentionally performed in a selected group of patients with Crohn colitis with no small intestinal or perianal diseases[96]; CD is also inadvertently found in proctocolectomy specimens of patients with a preoperative diagnosis of UC or indeterminate colitis. De novo CD of the pouch, by far the most common form of CD, may develop weeks to years after IPAA for UC or indeterminate colitis. Clinical phenotypes of CD of the pouch can be inflammatory, fibrostenotic, or fistulizing. There are symptoms and signs that would suggest a diagnosis of CD, particularly fibrostenotic and fistulizing CD. It is critical to differentiate NSAID-induced ileitis/pouchitis from CD ileitis, backwash ileitis from diffuse pouchitis. Making a diagnosis of CD of the pouch often needs a combined assessment of symptoms, endoscopy, histology, radiography, and sometimes examination under anesthesia.

Irritable pouch syndrome is a functional disorder in patients with IPAA.[97] The disease entity has a significant negative impact on health-related quality of life. There are great overlaps in clinical presentation between irritable pouch syndrome and pouchitis. Contributing factors for the pathophysiology of irritable pouch syndrome include visceral hypersensitivity, enterochromaffin cell hyperplasia,[98] and proximal small bowel bacterial overgrowth. Currently, irritable pouch syndrome is a diagnosis of exclusion. Pouch endoscopy is the diagnostic modality of choice for to distinguish between pouchitis and irritable pouch syndrome.

Patients with surgical complications (such as pouch sinus and pouch ischemia) can present symptoms resembling those of pouchitis. Again, pouch endoscopy is considered the first-line diagnostic modality.

CLASSIFICATION OF POUCHITIS

The natural history of pouchitis is poorly defined. Patients with initial episodes of pouchitis almost uniformly respond to antibiotic therapy. However, relapse of pouchitis is common. Among patients with acute pouchitis, 39% had a single acute episode that responded to antibiotic therapy; the remaining 61% developed at least 1 recurrence.[99] Approximately 5% to 19% of patients with acute pouchitis develop refractory or rapidly relapsing forms of the disease.[100–102] Pouchitis likely represents a disease spectrum from an acute, antibiotic-responsive type to a chronic, antibiotic-refractory entity. Based on the cause, disease duration, and activity, and response to medical therapy, pouchitis can be categorized into: (1) idiopathic versus secondary, with causes such as NSAID use and C difficile or CMV infection; (3) acute versus chronic, with a cut-off time of 4 weeks of persistent symptoms; (4) infrequent episodes versus relapsing versus continuous; and (5) responsive versus refractory to antibiotic therapy.[103]

Classification based on the response to antibiotic therapy is useful in clinical practice.[104] Analogous to the classification of UC according to the response to or dependency on corticosteroids, pouchitis can be classified into antibiotic-responsive, antibiotic-dependent, and antibiotic-refractory pouchitis (**Table 1**).[75] Pouchitis can be diffuse or patchy. Based on the distribution of inflammation, pouchitis can be categorized into diffuse pouchitis, pouchitis with backwash ileitis, pouchitis with concurrent cuffitis, and segmental pouchitis. It is now clear that pouchitis can be seen as

Table 1
Classification of pouchitis

Classification Based on Disease Course	Classification Based on Response to Antibiotic Therapy	Classification Based on Etiology
Acute pouchitis	Antibiotic-responsive pouchitis	Idiopathic pouchitis (with unidentified pathogens or triggering factors)
Acute relapsing pouchitis Chronic pouchitis	Antibiotic-dependent pouchitis Antibiotic-refractory pouchitis	Secondary pouchitis - *Clostridium difficile*–associated pouchitis - Cytomegalovirus-associated pouchitis - NSAID-induced pouchitis - Ischemic pouchitis - Autoimmune pouchitis

a heterogeneous group, with different clinical phenotypes, that may be associated with different risk factors, pathogenetic pathways, natural courses, and outcomes.

PROPHYLAXIS OF POUCHITIS

Some of the risk factors for pouchitis are modifiable, such as avoidance of the use of broad-spectrum antibiotics or NSAIDs. It has been speculated that small bowel bacterial overload may be common, as there is no valve mechanism between the pouch and distal small bowel, and pouch contents can easily reflux back to the segment of small bowel. A diet with a low quantify of poorly absorbed short-chain carbohydrates may reduce stool frequency in patients with or without pouchitis.[105]

Given that approximately 40% of patients develop pouchitis within the first 12 months after ileostomy closure,[16] and that most patients who develop acute pouchitis do so within the first year after IPAA,[17,106] it is reasonable to consider primary or secondary prophylaxis therapy, particularly in patients at risk.[107] Efficacy and safety of several probiotic agents have been evaluated. In a randomized trial of VSL#3 (containing viable lyophilized bacteria of 4 strains of *Lactobacillus*, 3 *Bifidobacterium* species, and *Streptococcus salivarius* subsp *thermophillus*) for the primary prophylaxis of the initial episode of pouchitis, 2 of 20 patients (10%) in the study group and 8 of 20 patients (40%) in the placebo group developed pouchitis within 12 months after IPAA.[16] *Lactobacillus rhamnosus* GG has also shown some efficacy in delaying the first episodes of pouchitis.[9,108] Although the efficacy of probiotic or prebiotic agents in the primary prophylaxis remains to be further investigated, patients with risk factors for pouchitis may try these agents.

In addition to primary prophylaxis, probiotic or antibiotic agents have been used as a maintenance therapy for secondary prophylaxis in patients with relapsing pouchitis or antibiotic-dependent pouchitis (see later discussion).

MANAGEMENT OF POUCHITIS

It is speculated that in most patients with pouchitis, the disease process is triggered and maintained by bacterial causes from dysbiosis of commensal bacteria. However, there are types of pouchitis that have identifiable pathogenic factors, such as

C difficile,[20] *Candida albicans*, and CMV infection, NSAID use, and pouch ischemia. Pathogen-targeted therapy is often effective.

There might be a new disease category named "autoimmune pouchopathy."[81] The patients often present with symptoms similar to "bacteria-associated" pouchitis, such as increased stool frequency, cramps, and urgency. On endoscopy examination, mucosal inflammation can be present in the pouch as well as a long segment of afferent limb. Although there are currently no established diagnostic criteria, the diagnosis of autoimmune pouchopathy may be suspected if a patient has antibiotic-refractory pouchitis, concurrent autoimmune disorders (such as rheumatoid arthritis and Hashimoto thyroiditis), and serum autoantibodies. For patients with autoimmune pouchopathy, treatment with oral budesonide or a low dose of immunomodulator may be attempted.

The therapeutic effect of probiotics parallels the restoration of mucosal immune response to altered microflora in the pouch.[2,9,108–110] For example, probiotic-treated patients were shown to have a significant increase in the percentage of regulatory T cells.[111] Changes in mucosa-associated bacteria in pouchitis were also reflected by therapeutic administration of probiotic agents. Kuhbacher and colleagues[23] conducted a double-blind, placebo-controlled trial to study the impact of a probiotic agent containing viable lyophilized bacteria, comprising *Lactobacilli*, *Bifidobacteria*, and *Streptococci*, on the dominant mucosa-associated bacteria from patients with chronic pouchitis in remission induced by antibiotics. The mucosal microbiota was mainly detected within the epithelium and nearly all bacteria were affiliated with the Enterobacteriaceae group. Compared with the placebo group, an increase in Enterobacteriaceae within the mucosa during the probiotic therapy was observed. Investigation of the molecular species was performed with the construction of taxonomic group–specific clone libraries. Using Proteobacteria/Enterobacteriaceae group–specific primers, slight differences in terms of phylotypic composition were observed between the placebo and probiotic groups. *Enterobacter* species and *E coli* were mainly identified. *Lactobacillus* and *Bifidobacterium* clone libraries generated from the probiotic group displayed a diverse spectrum of species in comparison with the 2 other experimental groups (pretreatment remission group and placebo group). Analysis of the mucosa-associated microbiota using an electrophoretic fingerprinting technique showed that the probiotic therapy increased the bacterial diversity in comparison with the patients in the pretreatment remission and placebo administration groups.

Probiotics have been used as a maintenance therapy for patients with antibiotic-dependent pouchitis or relapsing pouchitis. A randomized trial of VSL#3 at a dose of 6 g/d was conducted for the maintenance and secondary prophylaxis of relapse of pouchitis, after remission was induced by oral ciprofloxacin (1000 mg/d) plus rifaximin (2000 mg/d). During the 9-month trial of 40 patients with relapsing pouchitis, 15% in the probiotic group relapsed versus 100% in the placebo group.[109] A separate randomized trial of VSL#3 in patients with antibiotic-dependent pouchitis showed that 17 of 20 patients (85%) in the VSL#3 group maintained clinical remission, compared with remission in 1 of 16 patients (6%) in the placebo group.[110] A meta-analysis of 5 randomized, placebo-controlled clinical trials was performed. Pooling of the results from these trials yielded an odds ratio of 0.04 in the treatment group in comparison with the placebo group. The benefit of probiotics in the management of pouchitis after IPAA operation was confirmed by the meta-analysis.[107] In addition, high-dose probiotics have been used for treating pouchitis. In a study of the probiotic agent, VSL#3, 3600 billion bacteria/d in treating mild pouchitis, 16 of 23 patients (69%) were in remission after treatment.[112]

Routine use of probiotics for induction and maintenance therapy has generated some controversy. However, some postmarket open-labeled studies reported a much lower response rate. These outstanding results have been challenged by 2 recent postmarket open-labeled trials. In a study of 31 patients with antibiotic-dependent pouchitis treated with VSL#3 for maintenance therapy after 2 weeks of treatment with ciprofloxacin, 25 patients (81%) had stopped the agent at 8 months, mainly because of the lack of efficacy or development of adverse effects.[113] Similar results were reported in a separate open-labeled trial.[114]

Management strategies vary based on different types of pouchitis (see **Fig. 2**).[9] Because most pouchitis is caused by bacteria, antibiotic therapy is the mainstream therapy. For antibiotic-responsive pouchitis, the first-line therapy includes a 14-day course of metronidazole (15–20 mg/kg/d) or ciprofloxacin (1000 mg/d).[115,116] A randomized trial of ciprofloxacin and metronidazole showed that patients treated with ciprofloxacin experienced significantly greater reductions in disease activity scores and fewer adverse effects than those treated with metronidazole.[116] A small randomized trial of oral rifaximin 1200 mg/d versus placebo showed only a marginal therapeutic benefit for active pouchitis.[117] Diffuse pouchitis can be associated with backwash ileitis, particularly in patients with concurrent PSC. Combination therapy with ciprofloxacin and metronidazole for 28 days was shown to be effective in treating backwash ileitis in a recent open-labeled trial.[118] Other agents were reported in open-labeled trials, including tetracycline, clarithromycin, amoxicillin/clavulanic acid, doxy-cycline, budesonide enemas, alicaforsen enemas (an antisense inhibitor of intercellular adhesion molecule-1), leukocytapheresis,[119] AST-120 (a highly adsorptive, porous, carbon microsphere),[120] and dietary supplement of short-chain carbohydrates.

The gut-specific nonabsorbable antibiotic, rifaximin, may be a candidate for maintenance therapy in patients who need long-term antibiotics. In our recent study, 51 patients began maintenance therapy with rifaximin (median dose 200 mg/d); 33 (65%) maintained remission for 3 months. Of these 33 patients, 26 (79%) successfully continued maintenance for 6 months after beginning maintenance, 19 (58%) successfully continued for 12 months, and 2 (6%) successfully continued for 24 months.[121]

Treatment of chronic antibiotic-refractory pouchitis is often challenging. In fact, this phenotype of pouchitis is one of the most common causes for pouch failure. It is important to investigate contributing causes related to failure of antibiotic therapy. Secondary causes of refractory disease include use of NSAIDs, concurrent C diffi-cile,[20] CMV,[21,22] or fungal[23] infection, celiac disease and other autoimmune disorders, cuffitis, and CD of the pouch. Chronic pouchitis can be associated with single or multiple small or large inflammatory polyps. Large (>1 cm) pouch polyps can occasionally cause bleeding and can be dysplastic. Endoscopic polypectomy is feasible, which may be helpful in controlling patients' symptoms, in conjunction with medical therapy.[122] For patients without obvious causes, treatment options include a prolonged course of combined antibiotic therapy, mesalamine, corticosteroids, immunosuppressive agents, or even biologic therapy. In open-labeled trials, combined agents of ciprofloxacin (1000 mg/d) with rifaximin (2000 mg/d),[123,124] metronidazole (1000 mg/d),[125] or tinidazole (1000–1500 mg/d) for 4 weeks were reported to be effective.[126] However, maintenance of remission in this group of patients after the induction therapy with the dual antibiotic therapy remains challenging.[127]

Anti-inflammatory agents, immunomodulators, and biologic therapy have been used to treat pouchitis. These agents include bismuth carbomer enemas, short-chain fatty acid enemas, glutamine enemas, mesalamine enemas, 6-mercaptopurine, and infliximab. In an open-labeled study of 20 patients with chronic refractory pouchitis, oral budesonide 9 mg/d for 8 weeks induced remission in 15 (75%).[128] Biologic agents have been used in chronic pouchitis. Infliximab was studied for treating 10 patients with chronic refractory pouchitis complicated by ileitis, using wireless capsule endoscopy. Clinical remission was achieved in 9 patients and endoscopic (with video capsule endoscopy and pouch endoscopy) remission.[129]

In summary, management of pouchitis and other pouch disorders can be difficult. One of the contributing factors for the complexity is the surgical component, which may not be familiar to practicing gastroenterologists. A multidisciplinary approach involving gastroenterologists and colorectal surgeons, together with a team of gastrointestinal pathologists and gastrointestinal radiologists, has been advocated. Few institutions have even established subspecialty pouchitis clinics.[10,130] The practice model has been feasible and effective in treating complicated pouch disorders in a tertiary-care setting.

SUMMARY

Pouchitis is the most common long-term complication of IPAA, which represents a spectrum of disease processes with different clinical phenotypes, risk factors, pathogenetic pathways, natural history, and prognosis. Pouch endoscopy is the most valuable tool for diagnosis and differential diagnosis. Although most patients with pouchitis respond favorably to antibiotic therapy, antibiotic dependency and refractory disease have posed therapeutic challenges. Secondary causes of pouchitis, such as *C difficile* infection, should be evaluated.

REFERENCES

1. Dhillon S, Loftus EV Jr, Tremaine WJ, et al. The natural history of surgery for ulcerative colitis in a population-based cohort from Olmsted County, Minnesota [abstract]. Am J Gastroenterol 2005;100:A819.
2. Sandborn WJ. Pouchitis following ileal pouch-anal anastomosis: definition, pathogenesis, and treatment. Gastroenterology 1994;107:1856–60.
3. Winther KV, Jess T, Langholz E, et al. Survival and cause-specific mortality in ulcerative colitis - follow-up of a population-based cohort in Copenhagen County. Gastroenterology 2003;125:1576–82.
4. Tulchinsky H, Hawley PR, Nicholls J. Long-term failure after restorative proctocolectomy for ulcerative colitis. Ann Surg 2003;238:229–34.
5. Belliveau P, Trudel J, Vasilevsky CA, et al. Ileoanal anastomosis with reservoirs: complications and long-term results. Can J Surg 1999;42:345–52.
6. Hueting WE, Buskens E, van der Tweel I, et al. Results and complications after ileal pouch anal anastomosis: a meta-analysis of 43 observational studies comprising 9,317 patients. Dig Surg 2005;22:69–79.
7. Sagap I, Remzi FH, Hammel JP, et al. Factors associated with failure in managing pelvic sepsis after ileal pouch-anal anastomosis (IPAA) – a multivariate analysis. Surgery 2006;140:691–703 [discussion: 703–4].
8. Prudhomme M, Dehni N, Dozois RR, et al. Causes and outcomes of pouch excision after restorative proctocolectomy. Br J Surg 2006;93:82–6.
9. Nicholls RJ. Review article: ulcerative colitis-surgical indications and treatment. Aliment Pharmacol Ther 2002;16:25–8.
10. Shen B, Fazio VW, Lashner BA, et al. Comprehensive evaluation of inflammatory and non-inflammatory sequelae of ileal pouch-anal anastomosis. Am J Gastroenterol 2005;100:93–101.

11. Penna C, Dozois R, Tremaine W, et al. Pouchitis after ileal pouch-anal anastomosis for ulcerative colitis occurs with increased frequency in patients with associated primary sclerosing cholangitis. Gut 1996;38:234–9.
12. Fazio VW, Ziv Y, Church JM, et al. Ileal pouch-anal anastomosis complications and function in 1005 patients. Ann Surg 1995;222:120–7.
13. Ferrante M, Declerck S, De Hertogh G, et al. Outcome after proctocolectomy with ileal pouch-anal anastomosis for ulcerative colitis. Inflamm Bowel Dis 2008;14:20–8.
14. Fleshner P, Ippoliti A, Dubinsky M, et al. Both preoperative perinuclear antineutrophil cytoplasmic antibody and anti-CBir1 expression in ulcerative colitis patients influence pouchitis development after ileal pouch-anal anastomosis. Clin Gastroenterol Hepatol 2008;6:561–8.
15. Stocchi L, Pemberton JH. Pouch and pouchitis. Gastroenterol Clin North Am 2001;30:223–41.
16. Gionchetti P, Rizzello F, Helwig U, et al. Prophylaxis of pouchitis onset with probiotic therapy: a double-blind placebo controlled trial. Gastroenterology 2003; 124:1202–9.
17. Abdelrazeq AS, Kandiyil N, Botterill ID, et al. Predictors for acute and chronic pouchitis following restorative proctocolectomy for ulcerative colitis. Colorectal Dis 2008;10:805–13.
18. Penna C, Tiret E, Kartheuser A, et al. Function of ileal J pouch-anal anastomosis in patients with familial adenomatous polyposis. Br J Surg 1993;80:765–7.
19. Tjandra JJ, Fazio VW, Church JM, et al. Similar functional results after restorative proctocolectomy in patients with familial adenomatous polyposis and mucosal ulcerative colitis. Am J Surg 1993;165:322–5.
20. Shen B, Jiang Z-D, Fazio VW, et al. *Clostridium difficile* infection in patients with ileal pouch-anal anastomosis. Clin Gastroenterol Hepatol 2008;6:782–8.
21. Munoz-Juarez M, Pemberton JH, Sandborn WJ, et al. Misdiagnosis of specific cytomegalovirus infection of ileoanal pouch as a refractory idiopathic chronic pouchitis. Report of two cases. Dis Colon Rectum 1999;42:117–20.
22. Mooka D, Furth EE, MacDermott RP, et al. Pouchitis associated with primary cytomegalovirus infection. Am J Gastroenterol 1998;93:264–6.
23. Kühbacher T, Ott SJ, Helwig U, et al. Bacterial and fungal microbiota in relation to probiotic therapy (VSL#3) in pouchitis. Gut 2006;55:833–41.
24. Ohge H, Furne JK, Springfield J, et al. Association between fecal hydrogen sulfide production and pouchitis. Dis Colon Rectum 2005;48:469–75.
25. Gosselink MP, Schouten WR, van Lieshout LM, et al. Eradication of pathogenic bacteria and restoration of normal pouch flora: comparison of metronidazole and ciprofloxacin in the treatment of pouchitis. Dis Colon Rectum 2004;47: 1519–25.
26. Falk A, Olsson C, Ahrne S, et al. Ileal pelvic pouch microbiota from two former ulcerative colitis patients, analysed by DNA-based methods, were unstable over time and showed the presence of *Clostridium perfringens*. Scand J Gastroenterol 2007;42:973–85.
27. Komanduri S, Gillevet PM, Sikaroodi M, et al. Dysbiosis in pouchitis: evidence of unique microfloral patterns in pouch inflammation. Clin Gastroenterol Hepatol 2007;5:352–60.
28. Kroesen AJ, Leistenschneider P, Lehmann K, et al. Increased bacterial permeation in long-lasting ileoanal pouches. Inflamm Bowel Dis 2006;12:736–44.
29. DeSilva HJ, Jones M, Prince C, et al. Lymphocyte and macrophage subpopulations in pelvic ileal reservoirs. Gut 1991;32:1160–5.

30. Hirata I, Berrebi G, Austin LL, et al. Immunohistological characterization of intraepithelial and lamina propria lymphocytes in control ileum and colon and inflammatory bowel disease. Dig Dis Sci 1986;31:593–603.
31. Stallmach A, Schafer F, Hoffman S, et al. Increased state of activation of CD4 positive T cells and elevated interferon gamma production in pouchitis. Gut 1998;43:499–505.
32. Thomas PD, Forbes A, Nicholls RJ, et al. Altered expression of the lymphocyte activation markers CD30 and CD27 in patients with pouchitis. Scand J Gastroenterol 2001;36:258–64.
33. Goldberg PA, Herbst F, Beckett CG, et al. Leukocyte typing, cytokine expression and epithelial turnover in the ileal pouch in patients with ulcerative colitis and familial adenomatous polyposis. Gut 1996;38:549–53.
34. Kroesen AJ, Dullat S, Schulzke JD, et al. Permanently increased mucosal permeability in patients with backwash ileitis after ileoanal pouch for ulcerative colitis. Scand J Gastroenterol 2008;43:704–11.
35. Akira S, Takeda A. Toll like receptors signalling. Nat Rev Immunol 2004;4(7): 499–511.
36. Cario E, Podolsky DK. Differential alteration in intestinal epithelial cell expression of toll-like receptor 3 (TLR3) and TLR4 in inflammatory bowel disease. Infect Immun 2000;68(12):7010–7.
37. Toiyama T, Araki T, Yoshiyama S, et al. The expression patterns of toll-like receptors in the ileal pouch mucosa of postoperative ulcerative colitis patients. Surg Today 2006;36:287–90.
38. Heuschen G, Leowardi C, Hinz U, et al. Differential expression of toll-like receptor 3 and 5 in ileal pouch mucosa of ulcerative colitis patients. Int J Colorectal Dis 2007;22:293–301.
39. Lammers KM, Ouburg S, Morre SA, et al. Combined carriership of TLR9 -1237C and CD14 -260T alleles enhances the risk for developing chronic relapsing pouchitis. World J Gastroenterol 2005;11:7323–9.
40. Ayabe T, Satchell DP, Wilson CL, et al. Secretion of microbicidal alpha-defensins by intestinal Paneth cells in response to bacteria. Nat Immunol 2000;1:113–8.
41. Salzman NH, Ghosh D, Huttner KM, et al. Protection against enteric salmonellosis in transgenic mice expressing a human intestinal defensin. Nature 2003; 422:522–6.
42. Ouellette A, Bevins CL. Paneth cell defensins and innate immunity of the small bowel. Inflamm Bowel Dis 2001;7:43–50.
43. Porter EM, Bevins CL, Ghosh D, et al. The multifaceted Paneth cell. Cell Mol Life Sci 2002;59:156–70.
44. Ghosh D, Porter EM, Shen B, et al. Paneth cell trypsin is the processing enzyme for human defensin-5. Nat Immunol 2002;3:583–90.
45. Porter E, van Dam E, Valore E, et al. Broad spectrum antimicrobial activity of human intestinal defensin 5. Infect Immun 1997;65:2396–401.
46. Wehkamp J, Salzman NH, Porter E, et al. Decreased Paneth cell defensins and antimicrobial activity in ileal Crohn's disease. Proc Natl Acad Sci U S A 2005; 102:18129–34.
47. Kiehne K, Brunke G, Wegner F, et al. Defensin expression in chronic pouchitis in patients with ulcerative colitis or familial adenomatous polyposis coli. World J Gastroenterol 2006;12:1056–62.
48. Hirata N, Oshitani N, Kamata N, et al. Proliferation of immature plasma cells in pouchitis mucosa in patients with ulcerative colitis. Inflamm Bowel Dis 2008; 14:1084–90.

49. Patel RT, Bain I, Youngs D, et al. Cytokine production in pouchitis is similar to that in ulcerative colitis. Dis Colon Rectum 1995;38:831–7.

50. Schmidt C, Giese T, Ludwig B, et al. Increased cytokine transcripts in pouchitis reflect the degree of inflammation but not the underlying entity. Int J Colorectal Dis 2006;21:419–26.

51. Gionchetti P, Campieri M, Belluzzi A, et al. Mucosal concentrations of interleukin-1β, interleukin-6, interleukin-8, and tumor necrosis factor-α in pelvic ileal pouches. Dig Dis Sci 1994;39:1525–31.

52. Bulois P, Tremaine WJ, Maunoury V, et al. Pouchitis is associated with mucosal imbalance between interleukin-8 and interleukin-10. Inflamm Bowel Dis 2000;6:157–64.

53. Patel RT, Pall AA, Adu D, et al. Circulating soluble adhesion molecules in inflammatory bowel disease. Eur J Gastroenterol Hepatol 1995;7:1037–41.

54. Chaussade S, Denizot Y, Valleur P, et al. Presence of PAF-acether in stool of patients with pouch ileoanal anastomosis and pouchitis. Gastroenterology 1991;100:1509–14.

55. Gertner DJ, Rampton DS, Madden MV, et al. Increased leukotriene B4 release from ileal pouch mucosa in ulcerative colitis compared with familial adenomatous polyposis. Gut 1994;35:1429–32.

56. Romano M, Cuomo A, Tuccillo C, et al. Vascular endothelial growth factor and cyclooxygenase-2 are overexpressed in ileal pouch-anal anastomosis. Dis Colon Rectum 2007;50:650–9.

57. Stucchi AF, Shebani KO, Leeman SE, et al. A neurokinin 1 receptor antagonist reduces an ongoing ileal pouch inflammation and the response to a subsequent inflammatory stimulus. Am J Physiol Gastrointest Liver Physiol 2003;285:G1259–67.

58. Stallmach A, Chan CC, Ecker K-W, et al. Comparable expression of matrix metalloproteinases 1 and 2 in pouchitis and ulcerative colitis. Gut 2000;47:415–22.

59. Ulisse S, Gionchetti P, Alo S, et al. Expression of cytokine, inducible nitric oxide synthase, matrix metalloproteinases in pouchitis: effects of probiotic therapy. Am J Gastroenterol 2001;96:2691–6.

60. Leal RF, Coy CS, Ayrizono ML, et al. Differential expression of pro-inflammatory cytokines and a pro-apoptotic protein in pelvic ileal pouches for ulcerative colitis and familial adenomatous polyposis. Tech Coloproctol 2008;12:33–8.

61. Thomas PD, Forbes A, Nicholls RJ, et al. Increased mucosal IFN-γ production in pouchitis despite normal functional responses of isolated CD4 cells [abstract]. Gut 1999;44(Suppl 4):32A.

62. Shepherd NA, Healey CJ, Warren BF, et al. Distribution of mucosal morphology and an assessment of colonic phenotype change in the pelvic ileal reservoir. Gut 1993;34:101–5.

63. Biancone L, Palmieri G, Lombardi A, et al. Tropomyosin expression in the ileal pouch: a relationship with the development of pouchitis in ulcerative colitis. Am J Gastroenterol 2003;98:2719–26.

64. Coffey JC, Rowan F, Burke J, et al. Pathogenesis of and unifying hypothesis for idiopathic pouchitis. Am J Gastroenterol 2009;104:1013–23.

65. De Preter V, Bulteel V, Suenaert P, et al. Pouchitis, similar to active ulcerative colitis, is associated with impaired butyrate oxidation by intestinal mucosa. Inflamm Bowel Dis 2009;15:335–40.

66. Tysk C, Riedesel H, Lindberg E, et al. Colonic glycoproteins in monozygote twins with inflammatory bowel disease. Gastroenterology 1991;100:1509–14.

67. Merrett MN, Soper N, Mortensen N, et al. Intestinal permeability in the ileal pouch. Gut 1996;39:226–30.
68. Carter K, Di Giovine FS, Cox A, et al. The interleukin 1 receptor antagonist gene allele 2 as a predictor of pouchitis following colectomy and IPAA in ulcerative colitis. Gastroenterology 2001;121:805–11.
69. Meier C, Hegazi RA, Aisenberg J, et al. Innate immune receptor genetic polymorphisms in pouchitis: is NOD2/CARD15 a susceptibility factor? Inflamm Bowel Dis 2005;11:965–71.
70. Schmidt CM, Lazenby AJ, Hendrickson RJ, et al. Pre-operative terminal ileal and colonic resection histopathology predicts risk of pouchitis in patients after ileoanal pull-through procedure. Ann Surg 1998;227:654–62.
71. Achkar JP, Al-Haddad M, Lashner B, et al. Differentiating risk factors for acute and chronic pouchitis. Clin Gastroenterol Hepatol 2005;3:60–6.
72. Okon A, Dubinsky M, Vasilauskas EA, et al. Elevated platelet count before ileal pouch–anal anastomosis for ulcerative colitis is associated with the development of chronic pouchitis. Am Surg 2005;71:821–6.
73. Hata K, Watanabe T, Shinozaki M, et al. Patients with extraintestinal manifestations have a higher risk of developing pouchitis in ulcerative colitis – multivariate analysis. Scand J Gastroenterol 2003;38:1055–8.
74. Lepistö A, Kärkkäinen P, Järvinen HJ. Prevalence of primary sclerosing cholangitis in ulcerative colitis patients undergoing proctocolectomy and ileal pouch-anal anastomosis. Inflamm Bowel Dis 2008;14:775–9.
75. Shen B, Fazio VW, Remzi FH, et al. Risk factors for diseases of ileal pouch-anal anastomosis in patients with ulcerative colitis. Clin Gastroenterol Hepatol 2006; 4:81–9.
76. Fleshner PR, Vasiliauskas EA, Kam LY, et al. High level perinuclear antineutrophil cytoplasmic antibody (pANCA) in ulcerative colitis patients before colectomy predicts the development of chronic pouchitis after ileal pouch-anal anastomosis. Gut 2001;49:671–7.
77. Kuisma J, Jarvinen H, Kahri A, et al. Factors associated with disease activity of pouchitis after surgery for ulcerative colitis. Scand J Gastroenterol 2004;39: 544–8.
78. Hoda KM, Collins JF, Knigge KL, et al. Predictors of pouchitis after ileal pouch-anal anastomosis: a retrospective review. Dis Colon Rectum 2008;51:554–60.
79. Fleshner P, Ippoliti A, Dubinsky M, et al. A prospective multivariate analysis of clinical factors associated with pouchitis after ileal pouch-anal anastomosis. Clin Gastroenterol Hepatol 2007;5:952–8.
80. Boyko EJ, Koepsell TD, Perera DR, et al. Risk of ulcerative colitis among former and current cigarette smokers. N Engl J Med 1987;316:707–10.
81. Shen B, Remzi FH, Bennett AE, et al. Association between immune-associated disorders and adverse outcomes of ileal pouch-anal anastomosis. Am J Gastroenterol 2009;104:655–64.
82. Mathis KL, Dozois EJ, Larson DW, et al. Ileal pouch-anal anastomosis and liver transplantation for ulcerative colitis complicated by primary sclerosing cholangitis. Br J Surg 2008;95:882–6.
83. Cho CS, Dayton MT, Thompson JS, et al. Proctocolectomy-ileal pouch-anal anastomosis for ulcerative colitis after liver transplantation for primary sclerosing cholangitis: a multi-institutional analysis. J Gastrointest Surg 2008;12:1221–6.
84. Zins BJ, Sandborn WJ, Penna CR, et al. Pouchitis disease course after orthotopic liver transplantation in patients with primary sclerosing cholangitis and an ileal pouch-anal anastomosis. Am J Gastroenterol 1995;90:2177–80.

85. Freeman K, Shao Z, Remzi FH, et al. Orthotopic liver transplantation for primary sclerosing cholangitis in patients with ulcerative colitis: impact on occurrence of chronic pouchitis. Clin Gastroenterol Hepatol 2008;6:62–8.

86. Shen B, Achkar J-P, Lashner BA, et al. Endoscopic and histologic evaluations together with symptom assessment are required to diagnose pouchitis. Gastroenterology 2001;121:261–7.

87. Moskowitz RL, Shepherd NA, Nicholls RJ. An assessment of inflammation in the reservoir after restorative proctocolectomy with ileoanal ileal reservoir. Int J Colorectal Dis 1986;1:167–74.

88. Sandborn WJ, Tremaine WJ, Batts KP, et al. Pouchitis after ileal pouch-anal anastomosis: a pouchitis disease activity index. Mayo Clin Proc 1994;69:409–15.

89. Shen B, Fazio VW, Bennett AE, et al. Effect of withdrawal of non-steroidal anti-inflammatory drug use in patients with the ileal pouch. Dig Dis Sci 2007;52:3321–8.

90. Parsi MA, Shen B, Achkar JP, et al. Fecal lactoferrin for diagnosis of symptomatic patients with ileal pouch-anal anastomosis. Gastroenterology 2004;126:1280–6.

91. Lim M, Gonsalves S, Thekkinkattil D, et al. The assessment of a rapid noninvasive immunochromatographic assay test for fecal lactoferrin in patients with suspected inflammation of the ileal pouch. Dis Colon Rectum 2008;51:96–9.

92. Parsi MA, Ellis JJ, Lashner BA. Cost-effectiveness of quantitative fecal lactoferrin assay for diagnosis of symptomatic patients with ileal pouch-anal anastomosis. J Clin Gastroenterol 2008;42:799–805.

93. Johnson MW, Maestranzi S, Duffy AM, et al. Faecal calprotectin: a noninvasive diagnostic tool and marker of severity in pouchitis. Eur J Gastroenterol Hepatol 2008;20:174–9.

94. Johnson MW, Maestranzi S, Duffy AM, et al. Faecal M2-pyruvate kinase: a novel, noninvasive marker of ileal pouch inflammation. Eur J Gastroenterol Hepatol 2009;21:544–60.

95. Schmidt C, Häuser W, Giese T, et al. Irritable pouch syndrome is associated with depressiveness and can be differentiated from pouchitis by quantification of mucosal levels of proinflammatory gene transcripts. Inflamm Bowel Dis 2007;13:1502–8.

96. Panis Y, Poupard B, Nemeth J, et al. Ileal pouch-anal anastomosis for Crohn's disease. Lancet 1996;347:854–7.

97. Shen B, Achkar J-P, Lashner BA, et al. Irritable pouch syndrome: a new category of diagnosis for symptomatic patients with ileal pouch-anal anastomosis. Am J Gastroenterol 2002;97:972–7.

98. Shen B, Liu W, Remzi FH, et al. Enterochromaffin cell hyperplasia in irritable pouch syndrome. Am J Gastroenterol 2008;103:2293–300.

99. Lohmuller JL, Pemberton HJ, Dozois RR, et al. Pouchitis and extraintestinal manifestations of inflammatory bowel disease after ileal pouch-anal anastomosis. Ann Surg 1990;211:622–9.

100. Mowschenson PM, Critchlow JF, Peppercorn MA. Ileoanal pouch operation: long-term outcome with or without diverting ileostomy. Arch Surg 2000;135:463–5.

101. Hurst RD, Chung TP, Rubin M, et al. Implications of acute pouchitis on the long-term functional results after restorative proctocolectomy. Inflamm Bowel Dis 1998;4:280–4.

102. Madiba TE, Bartolo DC. Pouchitis following restorative proctocolectomy for ulcerative colitis: incidence and therapeutic outcome. J R Coll Surg Edinb 2001;46:334–7.

103. Sandborn WJ. Pouchitis: risk factors, frequency, natural history, classification and public health prospective. In: McLeod RS, Martin F, Sutherland LR, et al, editors. Trends in inflammatory bowel disease 1996. Lancaster (UK): Kluwer Academic Publishers; 1997. p. 51–63.

104. Shen B. Diagnosis and management of patients with pouchitis. Drugs 2003;65: 453–61.

105. Croagh C, Shepherd SJ, Berryman M, et al. Pilot study on the effect of reducing dietary FODMAP intake on bowel function in patients without a colon. Inflamm Bowel Dis 2007;13:1522–8.

106. Stahlberg D, Gullberg K, Liljeqvist L, et al. Pouchitis following pelvic pouch operation for ulcerative colitis. Incidence, cumulative risk, and risk factors. Dis Colon Rectum 1996;39:1012–8.

107. Elahi B, Nikfar S, Derakhshani S, et al. On the benefit of probiotics in the management of pouchitis in patients underwent ileal pouch anal anastomosis: a meta-analysis of controlled clinical trials. Dig Dis Sci 2008;53:1278–84.

108. Gosselink MP, Schouten WR, van Lieshout LMC, et al. Delay of the first onset of pouchitis by oral intake of the probiotic strain *Lactobacillus rhamnosus* GG. Dis Colon Rectum 2004;47:876–84.

109. Gionchetti P, Rizzello F, Venturi A, et al. Oral bacteriotherapy as maintenance treatment in patients with chronic pouchitis: a double-blind, placebo-controlled trial. Gastroenterology 2000;119:305–9.

110. Mimura T, Rizzello F, Helwig U, et al. Once daily high dose probiotic therapy (VSL#3) for maintaining remission in recurrent or refractory pouchitis. Gut 2004;53:108–14.

111. Pronio A, Montesani C, Butteroni C, et al. Probiotic administration in patients with ileal pouch-anal anastomosis for ulcerative colitis is associated with expansion of mucosal regulatory cells. Inflamm Bowel Dis 2008;14:662–8.

112. Gionchetti P, Rizzello F, Morselli C, et al. High-dose probiotics for the treatment of active pouchitis. Dis Colon Rectum 2007;50:2075–82 [discussion: 2082–4].

113. Shen B, Brzezinski A, Fazio VW, et al. Maintenance therapy with a probiotic in antibiotic-dependent pouchitis – experience in clinical practice. Aliment Pharmacol Ther 2005;22:721–8.

114. McLaughlin SD, Johnson MW, Clark SK, et al. VSL#3 for chronic pouchitis; experience in UK clinical practice [abstract]. Gastroenterology 2008;134(Suppl 1): A711.

115. Madden MV, McIntyre AS, Nicholls RJ. Double-blinded crossover trial of metronidazole versus placebo in chronic unremitting pouchitis. Dig Dis Sci 1994;39: 1193–6.

116. Shen B, Achkar JP, Lashner BA, et al. A randomized trial of ciprofloxacin and metronidazole in treating acute pouchitis. Inflamm Bowel Dis 2001;7:301–5.

117. Isaacs KL, Sandler RS, Abreu M, et al. Crohn's and Colitis Foundation of America Clinical Alliance. Rifaximin for the treatment of active pouchitis: a randomized, double-blind, placebo-controlled pilot study. Inflamm Bowel Dis 2007;13:1250–5.

118. McLaughlin SD, Clark SK, Bell AJ, et al. An open study of antibiotics for the treatment of pre-pouch ileitis following restorative proctocolectomy with ileal pouch-anal anastomosis. Aliment Pharmacol Ther 2008 Oct 3. [Epub ahead of print].

119. Araki Y, Mitsuyama K, Nagae T, et al. Leukocytapheresis for the treatment of active pouchitis: a pilot study. J Gastroenterol 2008;43:571–5.
120. Shen B, Pardi DS, Bennett AE, et al. The efficacy and tolerability of AST-120 (spherical carbon adsorbent) in active pouchitis. Am J Gastroenterol 2009; 104:1468–74.
121. Shen B, Remzi FH, Lopez AR, et al. Rifaximin for maintenance therapy in antibiotic-dependent pouchitis [abstract]. BMC Gastroenterol 2008;8:26.
122. Schaus BJ, Fazio VW, Remzi FH, et al. Large polyps in the ileal pouch in patients with underlying ulcerative colitis. Dis Colon Rectum 2007;50:832–8.
123. Gionchetti P, Rizzello F, Venturi A, et al. Antibiotic combination therapy in patients with chronic treatment-resistant pouchitis. Aliment Pharmacol Ther 1999;13:713–8.
124. Abdelrazeq AS, Kelly SM, Lund JN, et al. Rifaximin-ciprofloxacin combination therapy is effective in chronic active refractory pouchitis. Colorectal Dis 2005; 7:182–6.
125. Mimura T, Rizzello R, Helwig U, et al. Four-week open-label trial of metronidazole and ciprofloxacin for the treatment of recurrent or refractory pouchitis. Aliment Pharmacol Ther 2002;16:909–17.
126. Shen B, Fazio VW, Remzi FH, et al. Combined ciprofloxacin and tinidazole in the treatment of chronic refractory pouchitis. Dis Colon Rectum 2007;50:498–508.
127. Viscido A, Kohn A, Papi C, et al. Management of refractory fistulizing pouchitis with infliximab. Eur Rev Med Pharmacol Sci 2004;8:239–46.
128. Gionchetti P, Rizzello F, Poggioli G, et al. Oral budesonide in the treatment of chronic refractory pouchitis. Aliment Pharmacol Ther 2007;25:1231–6.
129. Calabrese C, Gionchetti P, Rizzello F, et al. Short-term treatment with infliximab in chronic refractory pouchitis and ileitis. Aliment Pharmacol Ther 2008;27: 759–64.
130. Tulchinsky H, Dotan I, Alper A, et al. Comprehensive pouch clinic concept for follow-up of patients after ileal pouch anal anastomosis: report of 3 years' experience in a tertiary referral center. Inflamm Bowel Dis 2008;14:1125–32.

Safety Profile of IBD: Lymphoma Risks

Meenakshi Bewtra, MD, MPH[a],*, James D. Lewis, MD, MSCE[a,b]

KEYWORDS

- Inflammatory bowel disease • Thiopurine analogs
- TNF-antagonists • Lymphoma
- Hepatosplenic T cell lymphoma

An increasingly daunting challenge in the care of patients with inflammatory bowel disease (IBD) is managing the risks associated with medical therapies. One of the most worrisome issues for patients is the risk of cancer associated with their medical therapy. In this article, the cancer risks of commonly used IBD medications are described, with an emphasis on hematologic malignancy risks. Lymphoma, particularly non-Hodgkin lymphoma (NHL), has been associated with other immune-mediated diseases (eg, rheumatoid arthritis [RA] and lupus) and with states of immunosuppression, whether as a consequence of the underlying disease (eg, acquired immune deficiency syndrome [AIDS]) or the treatment (eg, organ transplantation). The increasing use of immunosuppressant therapies in the treatment of IBD has raised this question to an even higher level of importance for patients and physicians.

DOES IBD INCREASE THE RISK OF LYMPHOMA INDEPENDENT OF MEDICAL THERAPIES?

Before considering whether certain medical therapies increase the risk of malignancy, one must first determine whether the baseline risk of cancer among patients with IBD is elevated by virtue of their disease. Other immune-mediated diseases, such as RA, are associated with an increased risk of lymphoma that seems to be independent of the medical therapy.[1,2] One could hypothesize that IBD patients have a similarly elevated risk of lymphoma due to chronic inflammation from their underlying IBD.

Several studies have sought to evaluate this underlying risk, with conflicting results (**Table 1**).[3–9,11–18] In evaluating these studies, 2 important features should be considered. First, it is important to assess the source of the IBD patients being studied. Population-based studies evaluate all IBD patients in a region. In contrast, tertiary-referral–based studies evaluate IBD patients referred to specialty centers.

This article originally appeared in *Gastroenterology Clinics of North America*, Volume 38, Issue 4.
[a] Division of Gastroenterology, Department of Medicine, University of Pennsylvania, 3400 Spruce Street, Philadelphia, PA 19104, USA
[b] Center for Clinical Epidemiology and Biostatistics, University of Pennsylvania, Philadelphia, PA 19104, USA
* Corresponding author.
E-mail address: meenakshi.bewtra@uphs.upenn.edu (M. Bewtra).

Med Clin N Am 94 (2010) 93–113
doi:10.1016/j.mcna.2009.08.015
0025-7125/09/$ – see front matter © 2010 Elsevier Inc. All rights reserved.

Table 1
Risk of lymphoma in hospital- and population-based studies

Study	Type of Study	N	Cases of Lymphoma CD	Cases of Lymphoma UC	SIR, RR or OR in CD Patients (95% CI)	SIR, RR or OR in UC Patients (95% CI)
Greenstein et al[3]	H	1227 CD; 734 UC	3	3	4.69 (P<.05)	8.82 (P<.005)
Ekbom et al[4]	P	1655 CD; 3121 UC	1	8	0.4 (0.0–2.4)	1.2 (0.5–2.4)
Persson et al[5]	P	1251 CD	a	N/A	1.4 (0.4–3.5)	—
Kerlen et al[6]	P	1573 UC	N/A	3	N/A	1.2 (0.3–3.5)
Mellemkjaer et al[7]	P	2645 CD	4	N/A	1.5 (0.4–3.7)	N/A
Loftus et al[8]	P	216 CD; 238 UC	1	0	2.4 (0.1–13.1)	0 (0–6.4)
Palli et al[9]	P	231 CD; 689 UC	2[a]	2 NHL 4 HD	2.5 (0.28–9.0)[a]	1.8 (0.20–6.5) 9.3 (2.50–23.82)
Farrell et al[10]	H	267 CD; 515 UC	1	3	31.2 (2.0–85)[b]	31.2 (2.0–85)[b]
Bernstein et al[11]	P	2857 CD; 2672 UC	9 NHL 0 HD	7 NHL 0 HD	2.40 (1.17–4.97)	1.03 (0.47–2.24)
Lewis et al[12]	P	7988 CD; 12,185 UC	7	11	1.59 (0.63–3.29)	1.20 (0.59–2.15)
Winther et al[13]	P	1160 UC	N/A	2	—	0.51 (0.06–1.82)
Askling et al[14]	P	20,120 CD; 27,559 UC	65	87	1.3 (1.0–1.6)	1.0 (0.8–1.3)
Goldacre et al[15]	P	5127 CD; 6990 UC	6	14	1.01 (0.37–2.20)	1.19 (0.64–2.01)
Hemminki et al[16]	P	27,606 UC	—	75	—	1.52 (1.20–1.91)
von Roon et al[17]	M	36,576 CD	—	—	1.42 (1.16–1.73)	—

Abbreviations: NHL, Non-Hodgkin lymphoma; HD, Hodgkin disease; H, hospital-based study; P, population-based study; M, meta-analysis.
[a] Included 1 case of HD, 1 case of myeloma; no cases of NHL.
[b] Reported SIR for IBD, not specifically for CD/UC.

These patients may be under closer surveillance by their physicians, leading to over-reporting or earlier diagnosis of malignancies. They may also have other coexisting diseases in addition to their IBD, thus inflating any underlying association with lymphoma. Patients in tertiary referral centers may also have had a longer duration of disease, more severe disease, and may be more likely to have received immuno-suppressive therapies. For example, in the study by Farrell and colleagues,[10] which showed a significantly elevated risk of lymphoma in IBD, all 4 cases occurred in patients on immunosuppressive therapy, often on multiple immunosuppressants. In RA, it has been shown that the risk of lymphoma is greater in those with more severe arthritis, independent of the medical therapy.[1,2,19–27] Such studies have not been performed in IBD. However, referral-based studies have tended to observe a higher relative risk of lymphoma among IBD patients than population-based studies (see **Table 1**). One interesting comparison came from a single study from Olmsted County and the Mayo clinic.[8] In their population-based study of 454 IBD patients identified in Olmstead County between 1940 and 1993, they found only a single case of NHL in 6662 patient-years, resulting in a crude risk of 0.002 in IBD patients in Olmstead County and an incidence rate of 15 cases per 100,000 person-years. In an effort to clarify the clinical features and outcomes of IBD patients, all patients with IBD and lymphoma seen at the Mayo Clinic between 1976 and 1997 were also studied. Among approximately 15,000 patients seen at the Mayo Clinic during this time, 61 had a lymphoma, resulting in a crude risk of lymphoma in these tertiary-referral patients of 0.004, twice that seen in the population-based study. Although these are only rough calculations, these divergent findings from a single study illustrate two critical points. First, there was a higher risk of lymphoma in the tertiary-based study than in the population-based study. Second, although there was an elevated risk, the absolute risk remained low.

Another important aspect in evaluating these studies is the ability to control for concomitant medication use. Because patients with the most severe disease are also more likely to be treated with more potent immunosuppression, it is difficult to separate these factors. Furthermore, most population-based studies do not have the ability to control for medication use. In a meta-analysis of cancer risk in Crohn disease (CD) patients, the pooled relative risk of developing lymphoma was 1.42 (95% CI 1.16–1.73).[17] However, when evaluating the two studies within the meta-analysis in which patients were specifically only on corticosteroids, the pooled relative risk of developing lymphoma in 9462 patients was 2.01 (95% 1.17–3.46).[17]

Although the estimated relative risk of lymphoma in ulcerative colitis (UC) and CD may differ from study to study, most population-based studies suggest minimal, if any, increased risk of lymphoma compared with the general population.[17] Further-more, in the general population, lymphoma is rare. For example, in the United States, the annual incidence is approximately 22 per 100,000 people per year.[28] As a result, in the IBD population as a whole, the absolute risk of lymphoma is low.

IMMUNOSUPPRESSION AND LYMPHOMA RISK

Defective host immune function increases the risk of lymphoma, as shown by the increased risk of lymphoma in patients with human immunodeficiency virus (HIV) and AIDS populations. Elevated risks for lymphoma have been found in HIV-positive patients with even modest levels of immunosuppression, before the onset of AIDS.[29] Furthermore, the risk of lymphoma has been found to be inversely related to the CD4 count in several studies, lending additional credence to the concept that a deficient immune system enhances oncogenesis.[29–31]

The post-transplant population has broadened the link between immunosuppression and malignancy to incorporate medications as causal mechanisms. By reducing components of the host immune system, and therefore undermining the immunologic surveillance of tumor cells, it is believed that chronic use of immunosuppressive medications can prevent early elimination of malignant cells.[32,33] This has specifically been implicated in the prevalence of Epstein-Barr virus (EBV)–positive lymphomas in immunocompromised patients.[34–37] EBV is a human herpesvirus that infects more than 90% of the population, with the primary infection usually occurring in childhood. After this primary infection, which can range from asymptomatic forms to overt mononucleosis, EBV-infected B-lymphocytes exist in a life-long asymptomatic latent infection that is typically controlled by cell-mediated host immunosurveillance including natural killer cells, and CD4+ and CD8+ T cells.[38] Immunocompromised states, including congenital syndromes and medically induced immunosuppression, remove the host's control and allow the emergence of lymphoproliferative disorders associated with EBV infections.[39] Data from the transplant population also support the hypothesis that the risk of lymphoma is directly correlated with the degree of immunosuppression, and that lymphoma can develop shortly after the onset of immunosuppressive therapy.[40] Many of these tumors completely regress when the immunosuppressive therapy is reduced or stopped.[26,36,39,41–44]

CLASSES OF MEDICATIONS IN IBD AND THEIR LYMPHOMA RISK
5-Aminosalicylate Medications

To date, there has been no association between the 5-aminosalicylate (5-ASA) class of medications and lymphoma in IBD. 5-ASA is a major metabolite of salicylazosulfapyridine (SASP). In rodent models and in vitro studies, SASP, 5-ASA, and sulfapyridine (SP) have not been demonstrated to exhibit mutagenicity or DNA reactivity, nor were they found to be genotoxic.

Corticosteroids

Corticosteroids, specifically oral prednisone, have been a mainstay in the therapy for IBD. Despite having numerous well-known side effects, corticosteroids have not been associated with an increased risk of lymphoma. Corticosteroids have long been a standard medication in first-line and salvage therapy for NHL.[45–48] Of theoretical interest, however, is the possibility of masking evolving malignancies by the use of corticosteroids in IBD. In addition, because of the widespread immunosuppressant effects of corticosteroids, combination therapy with other immunosuppressive medications could theoretically potentiate the risk of immunosuppression-related lymphoma.

Cyclosporine

Cyclosporine (CsA) is a calcineurin inhibitor that blocks production of interleukin 2 by activated CD4-positive T cells. Although not directly mutagenic, it may impair the hosts' immunosurveillance for transformed cells and has been implicated in EBV-positive lymphoproliferative disorders.[35,41,49] The number of IBD patients treated with CsA is too small to precisely estimate the risk of rare events such as malignancies associated with this medication. However, there is greater experience in the fields of dermatology and organ transplantation. A worldwide study of more than 5000 organ transplant patients found that 0.5% of men (10 men in total) and fewer than 0.1% of women (1 female patient) developed lymphoma, with differing latency periods from time of drug therapy to malignancy diagnosis for different transplant indications.[50]

This translated into an approximately 28-times higher risk of lymphoma in patients treated with CsA.[50] A 5-year prospective cohort study of 1252 patients with psoriasis treated with CsA found no trend toward an increased incidence of malignancies over time within the cohort.[51] Two patients developed lymphoma in the study, translating into a standardized incidence ratio (SIR) of 2.0 (0.2–7.2), similar to a previously reported incidence in moderate to severe psoriasis patients not exposed to CsA.[51,52] However, the investigators conceded that this cohort was not large enough to adequately assess this risk.

In the IBD literature, there is a paucity of data on lymphomas associated with CsA therapy. A hospital-based study followed 782 patients for 8 years at a single institution.[10] Of those patients, 238 received immunosuppressive therapy. Four cases of NHL were reported, all of which occurred in patients on immunosuppression. One of these patients had received 5 months of methotrexate (MTX) therapy followed by 12 months of CsA and ultimately underwent a colectomy. At surgery, the patient was found to have a lymph node with pathology consistent with large cell diffuse B-cell type lymphoma. No other evidence of lymphoma was found and the patient required no treatment.[10] Two additional case reports in IBD patients with CsA exposure have been published. The first was a case report of rectal lymphoma reported in a patient with a 13-year history of UC who had been treated with CsA for 4 years.[53] Therapy with CsA was discontinued and the patient was treated medically with good response. Another case report involved a UC patient who was found to have B-cell lymphoma after ileal pouch-anal anastomosis (IPAA) surgery in the pouch and diffusely in the lymph nodes.[54] The patient had only a 4-year duration of IBD before surgery, and had been treated with a combination of 4 immunosuppressant therapies including CsA, 6-MP, and infliximab.[54]

As noted previously, the hypothesis that immunosuppression directly increases the risk of lymphoma is supported by observations of lymphoma regression with discontinuation of immunosuppression therapy. In the setting of organ transplantation and treatment of dermatologic disorders, complete remission of lymphomas associated with CsA treatment has occurred after dose reduction or discontinuation of the drug.[50]

Methotrexate

MTX is a structural analogue of folic acid that inhibits the activity of dihydrofolate reductase, the enzyme responsible for converting folic acid to folate cofactors. This inhibition, in turn, inhibits DNA synthesis. MTX is cytotoxic and can induce immunosuppression and leucopenia. It has been implicated in impairing cellular immune control of tumor proliferation, and specifically immune control of EBV-induced B-cell proliferation. Animal studies examining this primary carcinogenic effect of MTX have shown a trend toward increased rates of malignant lymphomas in Swiss mice and Syrian hamsters, although numbers were small and no significant difference was detected.[55] In a second animal study, buccal pouches of hamsters injected with MTX showed increased rates of chemically induced carcinomas.[56]

MTX has been used for several decades to treat psoriasis and RA, and most studies of MTX-associated lymphoproliferative disease come from these specialties. In examining these rates, it is important to appreciate that there seems to be an increased risk of lymphoma at baseline in patients with connective-tissue disorders as a result of the disease itself. The theory is that prolonged stimulation of lymphoid tissue by the underlying disease inflammation induces lymphoma development, and it is believed that this explains the 2- to 3-fold increased risk of lymphoma in RA patients who are not receiving any immunosuppressive therapy.[10,19–27] However, a similar increased rate of malignancy at baseline in psoriasis patients has been questioned.[57]

Numerous case reports of lymphoproliferative disorders occurring in patients with RA and psoriasis treated with MTX have been published,[36,37,42–44,57–62] including several cases of EBV-positive lymphomas.[26,36,37,42,44,60,62] However, several cohort and case-control studies have not shown an elevated risk of lymphoma in patients with RA and psoriasis treated with MTX compared with those not treated with MTX. In psoriasis, in a multicenter prospective cohort study that included 28,554 person-years of follow-up, the incidence of lymphoma in patients with psoriasis who were not exposed to MTX was comparable to the general population (incidence rate ratio [IRR] 0.85, 95% CI 0.27–1.67).[63] However, the investigators of this study did find an elevated risk of lymphoma in patients with psoriasis who were treated with MTX for 3 or more years (IRR 3.74, 95% CI 1.61–7.36).[63] In contrast, a matched case-control study of 26 patients with severe psoriasis and noncutaneous cancer and 104 matched psoriasis controls nested within a cohort of 1380 patients found a relative risk of non-cutaneous cancer of 0.95 (95% CI 0.4–2.2).[64] The only 2 cases of leukemia or lymphoma occurred in patients with psoriasis who were not treated with MTX.[64] The RA literature also supports no increased risk of lymphoma associated with MTX. A large study of 18,572 patients with RA compared overall rates and MTX-associated rates of lymphoma to those expected from the survey, epidemiology and end results (SEER) cancer database.[24] The rate of lymphoma for patients with RA who were treated with MTX specifically was nonsignificantly increased compared with expected rates in the United States (SIR 1.7, 95% CI 0.9–3.2).[24] In this same study, patients who had not been exposed to MTX or anti-TNF therapies had no increased incidence of lymphoma (SIR 1.0, 95% CI 0.4–2.5).[24] Two studies compared MTX-treated RA with their nonexposed RA counterparts. In a comparison of patients associated with MTX, those not associated with MTX, and those with sporadic lymphoproliferative disease compiled from several studies, RA patients exposed to MTX had a shorter time between their RA and lymphoproliferative disorder diagnosis, but no other significant differences were found.[26] In a nested case-control study of 23,810 patients with RA from Canada, a nonsignificant adjusted relative risk of developing lymphoma was found for patients with exposure to MTX (risk ratio [RR] = 1.23, 95% CI 0.99–1.40).[65] These studies suggest that among patients with RA and psoriasis, if there is any increased risk of lymphoma associated with MTX therapy, the increase is likely small, although long-term therapy may be associated with a higher risk.

In the IBD literature there is limited data evaluating the risk of lymphoproliferative disease associated with MTX use. In a single-center study of 782 IBD patients, 238 of whom were receiving immunosuppression, 4 cases of NHL were seen, all of which occurred in immunosuppressed IBD patients.[10] Two of the 4 cases had exposure to MTX: 1 patient had been on MTX for 4 years, the other had received MTX for 5 months followed by 12 months of CsA. These data translated into a statistically significant overall risk of NHL in the population (SIR 31.2, 95% CI 2.0–85) and substantially increased odds of NHL in immunosuppressed IBD patients.[10] However, issues of power and selection bias, given the hospital base of this study, confound interpretation of these results.

6-Mercaptopurine/Azathioprine

Azathioprine (AZA) is a prodrug that yields 6-mercaptopurine (6-MP). The final active metabolite of these compounds is believed to be 6-thioguanine (6TG), which becomes incorporated into ribonucleotides and causes an antiproliferative effect on mitotically active lymphocytes. It is also believed that 6-MP and AZA may directly inhibit cyto-toxic T cell and natural killer cell function, yielding defective cell-mediated immune surveillance and allowing the development of lymphoproliferative disorders, including EBV-infected lymphocytes, to proliferate out of check.

Transplant and RA literature have pointed to an increased incidence of lymphoma in patients treated with the thiopurine analogues. An early large collaborative study of 3823 renal transplant patients reported a nearly 60-fold increased risk of NHL in patients exposed to AZA.[66] Fifteen of the NHLs affected the brain and presented as space-occupying lesions, an observation noted in prior transplantation literature.[66,67] A more recent multicenter study of 6500 transplant patients found a lower, but still significantly elevated, risk of post-transplant lymphoproliferative disorder (PTLD) in those with AZA exposure.[68] However, in many of these studies, patients were concomitantly receiving multiple immunosuppressive medications or receiving dosages much higher than those given in nontransplant populations. Several studies of patients with RA have also shown increased risks of NHL in patients exposed to AZA or 6-MP with estimates ranging from a 3- to 13-fold increased risk of reticuloen-dothelial cancers.[27,67,69] A large nested case-control study found no increased risk of lymphoma associated with AZA after adjustment for concomitant medications.[65] When evaluating the rheumatologic studies, issues of baseline risk of cancer in this patient population and increased dosages of AZA used in some of these studies must be taken into account.

Several cohort studies have also been performed examining the risk of lymphoma in IBD patients treated with thiopurine analogues (**Table 2**). A study from Mount Sinai in the late 1980s evaluated their experience with 6-MP in their IBD patients in the previous 18-year period.[70] Twelve neoplasms were seen during this period, including 1 diffuse lymphoma of the brain in a 53-year-old patient with long-standing CD who had been treated with 6-MP for approximately 9 months.[70] Connell and colleagues[71] conducted a prospective study of 755 patients with IBD treated with 2 mg/kg AZA for a median of 12.5 months between the years of 1962 and 1991. They found no excess cancer in the patients treated with AZA and no cases of NHL.[71] A study from France surveyed 157 CD patients treated with AZA/6-MP for at least 6 months.[72] A large percentage (27%) of these patients stopped taking their medication during the 20-year follow-up period. Four malignancies were seen in the follow-up period including 1 case of CNS lymphoma that occurred in a 37-year-old patient who had been on AZA for 17 months.[72] A study of 6-MP in 90 patients with chronic refractory UC found 6 malignancies (including 3 colonic neoplasms) in 368 cumulative patient-years, but no cases of NHL.[73] In a single-center study of 550 patients taking 6-MP for an average of 5 years, 2 cases of NHL developed, including 1 cerebral and 1 abdominal.[74]

Farrell and colleagues reported a dramatically increased incidence of lymphoma in IBD patients treated with immunosuppressive medications. In their tertiary care center–based retrospective study of 238 IBD patients, they reported 4 cases of NHL, 2 of which were on AZA. Their overall reported SIR for NHL in patients receiving AZA was 37.5 (95% CI 3.5–138). However, in a population-based study using the General Practice Research Database (GPRD) from the United Kingdom evaluating 1465 IBD patients treated with the thiopurine analogues, only 1 case of Hodgkin lymphoma was found in a patient with UC who had received 1 prescription for AZA 10 months earlier.[12] This resulted in a nonsignificant SIR of 1.57 (95% CI 0.04–8.75) that remained nonsignificant even after sensitivity analyses were performed.[12] A 15-year review from the Mayo Clinic identified all IBD patients who developed lymphoma and then divided the patient population into 2 8-year intervals (1985–1992, 1993–2000) corresponding to the introduction of thiopurine analogue therapy in 1993.[75] They identified 18 patients with lymphoma, 6 within the first interval and 12 occurring in the second interval. Fifty percent of the lymphomas occurring between

Table 2
Studies investigating incidence of lymphoma in IBD patients treated with AZA or 6-MP

Study	Type of Study	Drug Therapy	Number of Patients Studied	Mean Duration of Therapy (Months)	Number of Cases of Lymphoma	SIR, RR or OR (95% CI)
Kinlen[67]	H	AZA, 6-MP	321 IBD	N/R	2	12.5 (1.2–46.0)
Present et al[70]	H	6-MP	276 CD 120 UC	38.3 CD 24.2 UC	0 CD 1 UC[a]	N/R
Connell et al[71]	H	AZA	450 CD 282 UC 23 indeterminate colitis	12.5 (median)	0	0
Bouhnik et al[72]	H	AZA, 6-MP	157 CD	25	1[a]	N/R
George et al[73]	H	6-MP	90 UC	42	0	0
Korelitz et al[74]	H	6-MP	380 CD 170 UC	60	2 CD[a] 0 UC	4.9 (0.9–14.5)
Farrell et al[10]	H	AZA	238 IBD	21.6	2	37.5 (3.5–138)
Lewis et al[12]	P	AZA/6-MP	837 CD 628 UC	24	0 CD 1 UC	1.6 (0.0006–9.0)
Dayharsh et al[75]	P	AZA/6-MP	1200 IBD	42 (median)	6[b]	N/R
Fraser et al[76]	H	AZA	271 CD 355 UC	27	0 CD 3 UC	4.6 (0.9–13.7)
Glazier et al[77]	H	6-MP	160 CD 125 UC	27	1 CD 0 UC	N/R
Kandiel et al[78]	M	Pooled analysis	3891 IBD	N/R	11	4.18 (2.07–7.51)

Abbreviations: H, hospital-based study; P, population-based study; M, meta-analysis; N/R, not reported.
[a] Included 1 case of CNS lymphoma.
[b] Reported 18 total lymphomas, 6 of which occurred in patients with AZA/6-MP exposure.

1993 and 2000 occurred in patients treated with thiopurine analogues; and of these 6 patients, 5 were EBV-positive. This figure was in comparison to only one EBV-positive lymphoma occurring during the first period. The investigators also noted that 5 of the 6 lymphomas arising in the AZA/6-MP–treated patients were extranodal lymphoma, in comparison with 5 of the 12 lymphomas in the unexposed patients. In addition, 5 of the 6 lymphomas in the AZA/6-MP–treated patients were diffuse large B-cell type in comparison with only 4 of the 12 lymphomas in the unexposed patients. Although the investigators did not evaluate dosages or duration of treatment during their study, they did estimate that from 1993 to 2000 they treated approximately 1200 patients with AZA or 6-MP, giving an estimated risk of developing EBV-positive lymphoma of 0.5%.[75] Two retrospective chart reviews from 2 different hospital-based studies observed no significantly increased risk of NHL in AZA/6-MP treated patients.[76,77] Fraser and colleagues[76] evaluated 626 patients and found 3 cases of NHL, a rate that was not significantly different from IBD patients not receiving thiopurine analogue therapy. A 10-year single-center experience of 285 IBD patients found a single case of large B-cell colonic lymphoma in a 44-year-old patient with a history of Crohn colitis.[77]

A meta-analysis was performed using 6 studies evaluating the risk of NHL in IBD patients treated with AZA or 6-MP.[78] When pooling the data from the 6 studies, the investigators observed a significant increased risk of lymphoma in IBD patients treated with thiopurine analogues compared with the expected rates in the general population (SIR 4.18 95% CI 2.07–7.51). There was significant heterogeneity among the studies but excluding any 1 study did not appreciably affect their results, with statistically significant SIRs ranging from 2.90 to 5.21. When evaluating studies that directly compared IBD patients treated with thiopurine analogues with those who were not treated with thiopurine analogues, the investigators found a lower, but still significantly elevated, relative risk of NHL in IBD patients treated with thiopurine analogues.[78]

Most of these studies have been single-center or hospital-based, raising the issues of ascertainment and referral bias. In addition, there is potential bias in studies from tertiary care centers if the cases of lymphoma that prompted the investigators to undertake the study were included in the study cohort. It is also unclear whether the increased incidence of lymphoma in patients receiving AZA or 6-MP is due to the immunomodulators or is a consequence of the more aggressive or refractory nature of disease in patients who tend to receive these medications.

Overall, treatment with thiopurines seems likely to be associated with an increased risk of lymphoma, particularly EBV-associated lymphoproliferative disorder. The magnitude of this risk is likely on the order of a 3- to 5-fold relative risk. Several unanswered questions remain, such as whether the risk persists after the medication is discontinued, and whether combination therapy with other immunosuppressants potentiates the risk.

Anti-TNF Therapy

Three anti-TNF agents, infliximab, adalimumab, and certolizumab, have been approved for the treatment of IBD. In addition, etanercept is approved for the treatment of RA and psoriasis in the United States. Shortly after the approval of the first three anti-TNF agents, questions were raised regarding whether these agents may increase the risk of lymphoma.

Infliximab

Infliximab, previously known as cA2, is a chimeric monoclonal antibody directed against human tumor necrosis factor (TNF). It consists of a linkage of variable regions of mouse antihuman TNF monoclonal antibody to human IgG1 with k light chains. Mouse studies have shown that infliximab binds to and neutralizes soluble TNF in vitro and protects against the effects of TNF in vivo.[79] Infliximab has also been shown to bind to the transmembrane form of TNF with a high specificity, affecting down-regulation of several inflammatory mediators.[79,80] Like many of the immunosuppressive medications, infliximab was initially used extensively for RA. Initial clinical trials did not observe an increased incidence of lymphoma in RA patients treated with infliximab, although these studies were not designed to specifically address this question and were underpowered for this outcome.[81,82] More recent population-based prospective observational studies have suggested a possible increased risk of lymphoma among RA patients treated with anti-TNF agents. Investigators from the National Data Bank for Rheumatologic Disease compared outcomes in 18,572 RA patients to the SEER cancer database matched for age and gender.[24] The investigators found an overall SIR for lymphoma with biologic use of 2.9 (95% CI 1.7–4.9). For infliximab specifically (with or without etanercept), the SIR for lymphoma was 2.6 (1.4–4.5); and for infliximab alone, the SIR was 2.2 (1.0–4.9).[24] This must be viewed against the expected increased risk of lymphoma among RA patients in general, albeit such an increased risk was not observed in this study population among patients who had not received MTX or TNF therapy. In a large multicenter registry of 757 RA patients treated with either etanercept or infliximab and 800 RA patents who were treated conventionally, the investigators identified a nearly 5-fold increased rate of lymphoma in the anti-TNF–treated patients compared with the patients treated conventionally (RR = 4.9, 95% CI 0.9–26.2).[83] A recent meta-analysis of randomized controlled trials of anti-TNF therapy in RA patients calculated a pooled odds ratio (OR) for total malignancies of 3.3 (95% CI 1.2–9.1).[84] Although a separate, specific analysis for lymphoma risk was not made, a total of 10 lymphomas were observed in the anti-TNF–treated patients, whereas no lymphomas were observed in the control arms. Six of these 10 lymphomas were not included in the analysis because they occurred in follow-up after the trials ended.[84] Even after updating their estimates to include 2 additional RA studies, the OR for overall malignancy remained significant (OR 2.4, 95% CI 1.2–4.8).[85] The results of these studies must be interpreted with caution. First, the limited number of observations and, in some cases, short follow-up, limit interpretation, as demonstrated by the wide and often overlapping confidence intervals. Studies evaluating lymphoma risk in RA are also complicated by the uncertainty of the true cause. Given the known association between RA and lymphoma, and RA disease severity and lymphoma, it is impossible to determine whether these elevated risks are due to the anti-TNF therapy, the underlying disease severity, or a combination of both.

Infliximab received US Food and Drug Administration (FDA) approval for CD in October 1998 and licensing in the European Union in September 1999; it received FDA approval for UC in September 2005. At the time of FDA approval, there were 2 small open-labeled studies and another 2 randomized placebo-controlled trials (**Table 3**). Neither of the randomized controlled trials at that time had reported any lymphomas;[86,87] however, given the small number of patients, the FDA felt there was not even evidence to exclude a relationship between infliximab and lymphoma development.[100] Subsequently, an extension of 1 of the studies did find a single case of lymphoma in a patient with a 6-year history of AZA and a single infusion of infliximab.[88]

After commercial release of infliximab, an increasing number of lymphoma cases were reported. Three single-center and 2 multicenter retrospective studies found no cases of lymphoma reported at their respective institutions.[89,90,93,94,101] Three additional prospective randomized trials, including ACT 1 and ACT 2, also reported no

Table 3
Studies investigating incidence of lymphoma in IBD patients treated with infliximab

Study	Study Design	Patient Number	Cases of Lymphoma	Median Follow-up
Targan et al[86]	Randomized controlled trial	83	0	12 wk
Present et al[87]	Randomized controlled trial	94	0	N/R
Rutgeerts et al[88]	Randomized controlled trial	73	1	48 wk
Cohen et al[89]	Single-center cohort	129	0	54 wk
Farrell et al[90]	Multiple-center cohort	100	0	24 wk
Ardizzone et al[91]	Single-center cohort	63	0	10 wk
Hanauer et al[92]	Randomized controlled trial	573	1[a]	54 wk
Wenzl et al[93]	Multiple-center cohort	153	0	29 mo (mean)
Seiderer et al[94]	Single-center cohort	100	0	26 mo
Sands et al[95]	Randomized control trial	282	0	54 wk
Colombel et al[96]	Single-center cohort	500	2[b]	17 mo
Ljung et al[97]	Population-based cohort	217	3	N/R
Rutgeerts et al[98]	Randomized controlled trial	243w (ACT 1) 241w (ACT 2)	0 0	54 wk 30 wk
Caspersen et al[99]	Population-based cohort	651	0	29.1 mo

Abbreviation: N/R, not reported.
[a] The same patient as reported by Rutgeerts and colleagues.[88]
[b] One case of NHL and 1 case of Hodgkin lymphoma.

lymphomas in their evaluation of the clinical efficacy of infliximab.[95,98] A recent retrospective population-based cohort study using the Danish Crohn and Colitis Database found no lymphomas in 651 patients observed from 1999 to 2005.[99] However, the ACCENT 1 trial, a large multicenter randomized controlled trial to evaluate infliximab as a maintenance medication in CD, did report a single case of lymphoma.[92] A subsequent large population-based cohort study from Sweden found 3 cases of lymphoma developing, all of which occurred in CD patients and 2 of which were fatal.[97] More than half of the patients in this study were receiving concomitant thiopurine analogue therapy.[97] The Mayo Clinic reported their experience of 500 consecutive patients treated with infliximab at their institution and reported 1 case of NHL and 1 case of Hodgkin lymphoma.[96] Both patients had had several infusions of infliximab and both had exposure to thiopurine analogue therapy, although in 1 case it was only for 5 months.[96]

In 2002, a study was performed using the FDA's MedWatch postmarketing adverse event surveillance system to evaluate the incidence of lymphoproliferative disorders in patients with RA and CD who were treated with either etanercept or infliximab.[102] They found a total of 26 cases of lymphoproliferative disorders reported, 8 of which occurred in patients treated with infliximab. Five of these were NHL and the remaining 3 were Hodgkin lymphoma.[102] The findings raised concerns for the FDA, especially the short temporal relationship between initiation of medication and development of lymphoma (median 8 weeks).[102] Several "possible" or "probable" infliximab-associated lymphoma cases were also reported, and in March 2003, the Arthritis Advisory Committee of the FDA calculated an 8-fold increased rate of lymphoma in CD patients treated with infliximab in clinical trials compared with age-, gender- and race-matched populations.[103] In October 2004, the risk of malignancy, including lymphoma, was added to the infliximab package insert as a potential adverse reaction to the drug, stating a rate of 0.10 cases per 100 patient-years of follow-up or an approximately 4-fold increased risk over that of the general population.[104]

In contrast to these findings are the observational outcomes from the Crohn therapy, resource, evaluation and assessment tool (TREAT) registry, a long-term registry set up to assess the safety of infliximab. As of August 2005, it has been reported that the registry contains more than 6000 CD patients, of whom approximately half have had exposure to infliximab, comprising almost 15,000 patient-years of follow-up. The incidence of lymphoma has been reported to be 0.06 per 100 patient-years, with a nonsignificant risk of infliximab-related lymphoma (relative risk 1.3, 95% CI 0.4–5.0). This registry is subject to selection and ascertainment bias.

It is difficult to fully evaluate the lymphoma risk of infliximab in IBD patients. Infliximab is often used with other immunosuppressants, and is used in sicker patients with worse disease severity. The low event rate of lymphoma compounds the difficulty of precisely ascertaining the magnitude of risk. However, given the low, but possibly elevated, predisposition for lymphoma in chronically ill IBD patients, the known elevated lymphoma risk in other immunosuppressed populations, and the immunosuppressive effects of anti-TNF medications, it is possible that there is a small increased risk associated with infliximab therapy alone in IBD patients that is compounded by the disease and likely the concomitant use of other immunosuppressives. Therefore, it seems prudent, given the biologic basis, to warn patients taking infliximab of this potential, and to carefully monitor them.

Adalimumab

Adalimumab is a recombinant human immunoglobulin IgG1 monoclonal antibody that binds with high affinity and specificity to human soluble TNF. Adalimumab was approved in 2002 for RA. In preregulation studies in RA, 10 cases of lymphoma in 2468 patients with a median follow-up of 2 years was observed, with an SIR of 5.4 (95% CI 2.6–10) compared with the general population.[105–107] A postmarketing surveillance study analyzed more than 10,050 patients, representing 12,506 patient-years of adalimumab exposure in RA patients, including safety data from randomized controlled trials, open-label trials, and postmarketing spontaneous reports as of 2005, and found an SIR of 3.19 (95% CI 1.78–5.26), consistent with the observed increased incidence of lymphoma in the general RA population.[108]

In early 2007, adalimumab was approved in the United States and Europe as a treatment of adults with moderate to severely active CD who had an inadequate response to conventional therapy or lost response to, or were intolerant to, infliximab. The CLASSIC-1 and CHARM trials established efficacy of adalimumab for induction and maintenance of remission.[109,110] No lymphomas were noted in either the 4-week induction or 56-week maintenance follow-up, nor were lymphomas seen in a 4-week multicenter trial of adalimumab for patients previously treated with infliximab.[111] Despite the lack of reported lymphoma in IBD patients treated with adalimumab, given the more extensive data in the RA population, current FDA guidelines report an approximate 3-fold higher risk of lymphoma in adalimumab-treated patients compared with the general population, based on a combination of controlled and uncontrolled open-label portions of clinical trials including 6539 patients and more than 16,000 patient-years of therapy.[112]

Certolizumab pegol

Certolizumab pegol (CDP870), referred to as certolizumab, is a polyethylene glycolated Fab' fragment of humanized anti-TNF-α monoclonal antibody. The polyethylene glycolation increases the half-life of the antibody fragment, thereby reducing the frequency of the subcutaneous dosing. Certolizumab was approved for CD in 2008 based on several studies showing clinical efficacy in CD patients with moderate to severe active disease who were intolerant to or lost response to infliximab.[113–115] In these studies, only 1 case of lymphoma has been reported in a patient treated in the placebo arm who was also on 6-MP.[114] Currently, there is no FDA warning for lymphoproliferative diseases associated with certolizumab.

Pooled data on the risk of cancer with anti-TNF therapy for IBD

A recent meta-analysis of 21 placebo-controlled trials of these 3 anti-TNF agents and several other anti-TNF agents that have not proven efficacious for treatment of IBD did not identify an increased risk of cancer among patients treated with anti-TNF therapy.[116] However, these were small studies, and there were only a total of 16 malignancies between the treatment groups. The investigators did not report separate assessment of the risk of lymphoma.[116]

HEPATOSPLENIC T CELL LYMPHOMA

Hepatosplenic T cell lymphoma (HSTCL) is an uncommon extranodal T cell lymphoma that primarily affects young men in the second and third decade of life (median age 32). These malignancies are not EBV-related and were first described in 1990 as a distinct entity among post-transplant lymphoproliferative diseases in the World Health Organization (WHO) classification. Patients typically present with hepatosplenomegaly without lymphadenopathy. The typical course is aggressive, despite combination chemotherapy, with the median survival less than 1 year.[117]

A large percentage of reported cases of HSTCL arise in immunocompromised patients, mainly after solid organ transplantation (15%–25%).[118,119] Most have been reported after renal transplantation, although this may be due to the larger number of renal transplantations performed compared with other solid transplants. At least 6 cases of HSTCL have been reported in IBD patients receiving thiopurine analogue therapy alone.[119–123] As of July 2008, the FDA's adverse event reporting system (AERS) database had received reports of 17 cases of HSTCL involving anti-TNF therapy.[123] Most of these patients were treated with concomitant thiopurine analogue therapy and corticosteroids. Nearly all patients were men, and the outcome in all known cases was death.

The black-box warning for infliximab now includes information cautioning about the risk of HSTCL in adolescent and young adult patients with CD. Although a concern, it is impossible to determine whether infliximab has a primary or even causative role in the pathogenesis of the reported cases of HSTCL. Several potential confounders exist, including underlying disease severity, duration of disease, and the concomitant use of immunosuppression such as thiopurine analogue therapy. Like other malignancies, the low event rate limits the ability to generate precise estimates of absolute and relative risks.

WEIGHING RISKS AND BENEFITS

Weighed against the risk of lymphoma is the real disease that affects these young adults with disabling and, at times, lethal outcomes.[124] Several decision models have evaluated the risk of immunosuppressant use in CD patients. These models have illustrated that the substantial clinical improvement, decrease in surgeries, and incremental increase in quality-adjusted life years gained by treatment with infliximab outweighed the risks in most populations of IBD patients.[125,126] For older patients in whom the baseline risk of lymphoma is higher, the risk-benefit tradeoff is less clear.[126]

Additional studies have illustrated that patients with CD are willing to accept much higher than anticipated levels of life-threatening risks of death in exchange for medication efficacy in their disease.[127] Although not directly measuring the risk of HSTCL, these findings demonstrate a strong opinion on the part of IBD patients regarding their willingness to accept risks in exchange for medication efficacy.

A major limitation of most studies to date is lack of clarity on whether any increased risk of lymphoma persists after a therapy is discontinued. There is reason to believe that the risk is lower once the medication is discontinued and the immunosuppression resolves. However, other mechanisms of oncogenesis, such as injury to DNA, could result in elevated risk of neoplasia even after the therapy is discontinued. If the risk of lymphoma resolves, or is at least substantially lower once a therapy is discontinued, this may affect patient risk-taking thresholds. Specifically, once a medication is proven beneficial for a given patient, the risk-benefit balance is much more favorable than the same assessment made before initiating therapy. In contrast, if the medication is not efficacious for the patient, and discontinuation of the medication results in return to the baseline risk of lymphoma, the patient has only been at increased risk for development of lymphoma for a limited time period. Future studies are critically needed to address this question of persistence of lymphoma risk after discontinuation of the currently available medical therapies for IBD.

A related, and particularly challenging, issue in planning medical therapy for patients with IBD is whether or not to employ combination therapy or monotherapy with immunosuppressive medications. Given that increasing levels of immunosuppression seem to increase the risk of lymphoma and the risk of opportunistic infections, there is reason to favor monotherapy.[128] In addition, a clinical trial examining withdrawal of thiopurine therapy among patients treated with combination thiopurines and anti-TNF agents demonstrated no difference in relapse rates for a period of 2 years.[129] In contrast, evidence from the SONIC trial showed that in patients newly initiating therapy, a combination of a thiopurine analogue plus infliximab was superior to either alone, arguing in favor of combination therapy, at least initially.[130] Thus, an open and frank dialog with patients contemplating treatment with thiopurines or anti-TNF agents is imperative. In the future, studies clarifying the relative risk of lymphoma with anti-TNF agents in combination with thiopurines compared with the 2 classes of agents used individually will help to clarify this clinical dilemma.

SUMMARY

The risk of lymphoma in the treatment of IBD is a complicated issue. Most population-based studies show little if any increased risk of lymphoma among patients with IBD. Several studies from tertiary care centers have suggested higher lymphoma rates, which may be confounded by increased disease severity in these populations, referral bias, or a complication of medical therapy. IBD patients treated with thiopurines seem to have a 3- to 5-fold increased risk of lymphoma compared with patients not receiving these therapies and compared with patients without IBD. There are fewer data on MTX, but if there is any increased risk of lymphoma with MTX, data from other diseases suggest that this increased risk is lower than that observed with thiopurines. The data on anti-TNF therapies are even more complicated, because most patients treated with anti-TNF agents have been previously, or are concurrently, treated with thiopurines or MTX, and are also likely to have the most severe disease. Given the evidence that more profound immunosuppression is associated with further increased risk of lymphoma in other disease states, it is logical that the same may apply to patients with IBD. However, definitive data are lacking at the present. HSTCL has been observed among multiple IBD patients treated with combined immunosuppression. However, the absolute magnitude of this risk is remains low. The potential risks of all therapies must be weighed against the real benefits these therapies can offer. Availability of thiopurines, MTX, and anti-TNF has dramatically changed the management of these diseases and improves the quality of life for patients with IBD. Future studies will continue to provide the necessary data to determine the optimal approach with the available therapies and optimally balance the risks and benefits for individual patients.

REFERENCES

1. Baecklund E, Ekbom A, Sparen P, et al. Disease activity and risk of lymphoma in patients with rheumatoid arthritis: nested case-control study. BMJ 1998;317:180–1.
2. Baecklund E, Iliadou A, Askling J, et al. Association of chronic inflammation, not its treatment, with increased lymphoma risk in rheumatoid arthritis. Arthritis Rheum 2006;54:692–701.
3. Greenstein AJ, Gennuso R, Sachar DB, et al. Extraintestinal cancers in inflammatory bowel disease. Cancer 1985;56:2914–21.
4. Ekbom A, Helmick C, Zack M, et al. Extracolonic malignancies in inflammatory bowel disease. Cancer 1991;67:2015–9.
5. Persson PG, Karlen P, Bernell O, et al. Crohn's disease and cancer: a population-based cohort study. Gastroenterology 1994;107:1675–9.
6. Karlen P, Lofberg R, Brostrom O, et al. Increased risk of cancer in ulcerative colitis: a population-based cohort study. Am J Gastroenterol 1999;94:1047–52.
7. Mellemkjaer L, Johansen C, Gridley G, et al. Crohn's disease and cancer risk (Denmark). Cancer Causes Control 2000;11:145–50.
8. Loftus EV Jr, Tremaine WJ, Habermann TM, et al. Risk of lymphoma in inflammatory bowel disease. Am J Gastroenterol 2000;95:2308–12.
9. Palli D, Trallori G, Bagnoli S, et al. Hodgkin's disease risk is increased in patients with ulcerative colitis. Gastroenterology 2000;119:647–53.
10. Farrell RJ, Ang Y, Kileen P, et al. Increased incidence of non-Hodgkin's lymphoma in inflammatory bowel disease patients on immunosuppressive therapy but overall risk is low. Gut 2000;47:514–9.
11. Bernstein CN, Blanchard JF, Kliewer E, et al. Cancer risk in patients with inflammatory bowel disease: a population-based study. Cancer 2001;91:854–62.
12. Lewis JD, Bilker WB, Brensinger C, et al. Inflammatory bowel disease is not associated with an increased risk of lymphoma. Gastroenterology 2001;121:1080–7.
13. Winther KV, Jess T, Langholz E, et al. Long-term risk of cancer in ulcerative colitis: a population-based cohort study from Copenhagen County. Clin Gastroenterol Hepatol 2004;2:1088–95.
14. Askling J, Brandt L, Lapidus A, et al. Risk of haematopoietic cancer in patients with inflammatory bowel disease. Gut 2005;54:617–22.
15. Goldacre MJ, Wotton CJ, Yeates D, et al. Cancer in patients with ulcerative colitis, Crohn's disease and coeliac disease: record linkage study. Eur J Gastroenterol Hepatol 2008;20:297–304.
16. Hemminki K, Li X, Sundquist J, et al. Cancer risks in ulcerative colitis patients. Int J Cancer 2008;123:1417–21.
17. von Roon AC, Reese G, Teare J, et al. The risk of cancer in patients with Crohn's disease. Dis Colon Rectum 2007;50:839–55.
18. Ekstrom Smedby K, Vajdic CM, Falster M, et al. Autoimmune disorders and risk of non-Hodgkin lymphoma subtypes: a pooled analysis within the InterLymph Consortium. Blood 2008;111:4029–38.

19. Hakulinen T, Isomaki H, Knekt P. Rheumatoid arthritis and cancer studies based on linking nationwide registries in Finland. Am J Med 1985;78:29–32.
20. Prior P. Cancer and rheumatoid arthritis: epidemiologic considerations. Am J Med 1985;78:15–21.
21. Symmons DP. Neoplasms of the immune system in rheumatoid arthritis. Am J Med 1985;78:22–8.
22. Isomaki HA, Hakulinen T, Joutsenlahti U. Excess risk of lymphomas, leukemia and myeloma in patients with rheumatoid arthritis. J Chronic Dis 1978;31:691–6.
23. Gridley G, McLaughlin JK, Ekbom A, et al. Incidence of cancer among patients with rheumatoid arthritis. J Natl Cancer Inst 1993;85:307–11.
24. Wolfe F, Michaud K. Lymphoma in rheumatoid arthritis: the effect of methotrexate and anti-tumor necrosis factor therapy in 18,572 patients. Arthritis Rheum 2004;50:1740–51.
25. Santana V, Rose NR. Neoplastic lymphoproliferation in autoimmune disease: an updated review. Clin Immunol Immunopathol 1992;63:205–13.
26. Hoshida Y, Xu JX, Fujita S, et al. Lymphoproliferative disorders in rheumatoid arthritis: clinicopathological analysis of 76 cases in relation to methotrexate medication. J Rheumatol 2007;34:322–31.
27. Silman AJ, Petrie J, Hazleman B, et al. Lymphoproliferative cancer and other malignancy in patients with rheumatoid arthritis treated with azathioprine: a 20 year follow up study. Ann Rheum Dis 1988;47:988–92.
28. Available at: http://seer.cancer.gov/index.html. Accessed June 13, 2009.
29. Engels EA, Biggar RJ, Hall HI, et al. Cancer risk in people infected with human immunodeficiency virus in the United States. Int J Cancer 2008;123:187–94.
30. Mbulaiteye SM, Biggar RJ, Goedert JJ, et al. Immune deficiency and risk for malignancy among persons with AIDS. J Acquir Immune Defic Syndr 2003;32:527–33.
31. Biggar RJ, Chaturvedi AK, Goedert JJ, et al. HIV/AIDS Cancer Match Study. AIDS-related cancer and severity of immunosuppression in persons with AIDS. J Natl Cancer Inst 2007;99:962–72.
32. Alamartine E, Sabido O, Berthoux F. In-vitro effects of cyclosporin A, FK506, 6-mercaptopurine, and prednisolone on lymphokine-activated killer cells. Nephrol Dial Transplant 1994;9:1456–61.
33. Tamura F, Masuhara A, Sakaida I, et al. FK506 promotes liver regeneration by suppressing natural killer cell activity. J Gastroenterol Hepatol 1998;13:703–8.
34. Pietersma F, Piriou E, van Baarle D. Immune surveillance of EBV-infected B cells and the development of non-Hodgkin lymphomas in immunocompromised patients. Leuk Lymphoma 2008;49:1028–41.
35. Nalesnik MA, Jaffe R, Starzl TE, et al. The pathology of posttransplant lymphoproliferative disorders occurring in the setting of cyclosporine A-prednisone immunosuppression. Am J Pathol 1988;133:173–92.
36. Kamel OW, van de Rijn M, Weiss LM, et al. Brief report: reversible lymphomas associated with Epstein-Barr virus occurring during methotrexate therapy for rheumatoid arthritis and dermatomyositis. N Engl J Med 1993;328:1317–21.
37. Paul C, Le Tourneau A, Cayuela JM, et al. Epstein-Barr virus-associated lymphoproliferative disease during methotrexate therapy for psoriasis. Arch Dermatol 1997;133:867–71.
38. Losco A, Gianelli U, Cassani B, et al. Epstein-Barr virus-associated lymphoma in Crohn's disease. Inflamm Bowel Dis 2004;10:425–9.
39. Salloum E, Cooper DL, Howe G, et al. Spontaneous regression of lymphoproliferative disorders in patients treated with methotrexate for rheumatoid arthritis and other rheumatic diseases. J Clin Oncol 1996;14:1943–9.

40. Buell JF, Gross TG, Woodle ES. Malignancy after transplantation. Transplantation 2005;80:S254–64.
41. Starzl TE, Nalesnik MA, Porter KA, et al. Reversibility of lymphomas and lymphoproliferative lesions developing under cyclosporin-steroid therapy. Lancet 1984; 1:583–7.
42. Liote F, Pertuiset E, Cochand-Priollet B, et al. Methotrexate related B lymphoproliferative disease in a patient with rheumatoid arthritis. Role of Epstein-Barr virus infection. J Rheumatol 1995;22:1174–8.
43. Viraben R, Brousse P, Lamant L. Reversible cutaneous lymphoma occurring during methotrexate therapy. Br J Dermatol 1996;135:116–8.
44. Bachman TR, Sawitzke AD, Perkins SL, et al. Methotrexate-associated lymphoma in patients with rheumatoid arthritis: report of two cases. Arthritis Rheum 1996;39:325–9.
45. Ladetto M, De Marco F, Benedetti F, et al. Prospective, multicenter randomized GITMO/IIL trial comparing intensive (R-HDS) versus conventional (CHOP-R) chemoimmunotherapy in high-risk follicular lymphoma at diagnosis: the superior disease control of R-HDS does not translate into an overall survival advantage. Blood 2008;111:4004–13.
46. Kalinka-Warzocha E, Wajs J, Lech-Maranda E, et al. Randomized comparison of cladribine alone or in combination with cyclophosphamide, and cyclophosphamide, vincristine and prednisone in previously untreated low-grade B-cell non-Hodgkin lymphoma patients: final report of the Polish Lymphoma Research Group. Cancer 2008;113:367–75.
47. Hochster H, Weller E, Gascoyne RD, et al. Maintenance rituximab after cyclophosphamide, vincristine, and prednisone prolongs progression-free survival in advanced indolent lymphoma: results of the randomized phase III ECOG1496 study. J Clin Oncol 2009;27:1607–14.
48. Lazar AD, Shpilberg O, Shaklai M, et al. Salvage chemotherapy with dexamethasone, etoposide, ifosfamide and cisplatin (DVIP) for relapsing and refractory non-Hodgkin's lymphoma. Isr Med Assoc J 2009;11:16–22.
49. Zijlmans JM, van Rijthoven AW, Kluin PM, et al. Epstein-Barr virus-associated lymphoma in a patient with rheumatoid arthritis treated with cyclosporine. N Engl J Med 1992;326:1363.
50. Cockburn IT, Krupp P. The risk of neoplasms in patients treated with cyclosporine A. J Autoimmun 1989;2:723–31.
51. Paul CF, Ho VC, McGeown C, et al. Risk of malignancies in psoriasis patients treated with cyclosporine: a 5 y cohort study. J Invest Dermatol 2003;120: 211–6.
52. Hannuksela-Svahn A, Pukkala E, Laara E, et al. Psoriasis, its treatment, and cancer in a cohort of Finnish patients. J Invest Dermatol 2000;114:587–90.
53. Shibahara T, Miyazaki K, Sato D, et al. Rectal malignant lymphoma complicating ulcerative colitis treated with long-term cyclosporine A. J Gastroenterol Hepatol 2006;21:336–8.
54. Schwartz LK, Kim MK, Coleman M, et al. Case report: lymphoma arising in an ileal pouch anal anastomosis after immunomodulatory therapy for inflammatory bowel disease. Clin Gastroenterol Hepatol 2006;4:1030–4.
55. Rustia M, Shubik P. Life-span carcinogenicity tests with 4-amino-N10-methyl-pteroylglutamic acid (methotrexate) in Swiss mice and Syrian golden hamsters. Toxicol Appl Pharmacol 1973;26:329–38.
56. Shklar G, Cataldo E, Fitzgerald AL. The effect of methotrexate on chemical carcinogenesis of hamster buccal pouch. Cancer Res 1966;26:2218–24.

57. Khopkar U, Bhor U. Hodgkin's lymphoma in a patient of psoriasis treated with long-term, low-dose methotrexate therapy. Indian J Dermatol Venereol Leprol 2008;74:379–82.
58. Ellman MH, Hurwitz H, Thomas C, et al. Lymphoma developing in a patient with rheumatoid arthritis taking low dose weekly methotrexate. J Rheumatol 1991;18: 1741–3.
59. Kingsmore SF, Hall BD, Allen NB, et al. Association of methotrexate, rheumatoid arthritis and lymphoma: report of 2 cases and literature review. J Rheumatol 1992;19:1462–5.
60. Thomason RW, Craig FE, Banks PM, et al. Epstein-Barr virus and lymphoproliferation in methotrexate-treated rheumatoid arthritis. Mod Pathol 1996;9:261–6.
61. Ebeo CT, Girish MR, Byrd RP, et al. Methotrexate-induced pulmonary lymphoma. Chest 2003;123:2150–3.
62. Suzuki M, Hirano S, Ito H, et al. Pulmonary lymphoma developed during long-term methotrexate therapy for psoriasis. Respirology 2007;12:774–6.
63. Stern RS. Lymphoma risk in psoriasis: results of the PUVA follow-up study. Arch Dermatol 2006;142:1132–5.
64. Stern RS, Zierler S, Parrish JA. Methotrexate used for psoriasis and the risk of noncutaneous or cutaneous malignancy. Cancer 1982;50:869–72.
65. Bernatsky S, Clarke AE, Suissa S. Hematologic malignant neoplasms after drug exposure in rheumatoid arthritis. Arch Intern Med 2008;168:378–81.
66. Kinlen LJ, Sheil AG, Peto J, et al. Collaborative United Kingdom-Australasian study of cancer in patients treated with immunosuppressive drugs. Br Med J 1979;2:1461–6.
67. Kinlen LJ. Incidence of cancer in rheumatoid arthritis and other disorders after immunosuppressive treatment. Am J Med 1985;78:44–9.
68. Pourfarziani V, Taheri S, Lessan-Pezeshki M, et al. Lymphoma after living donor kidney transplantation: an Iranian multicenter experience. Int Urol Nephrol 2008; 40:1089–94.
69. Asten P, Barrett J, Symmons D. Risk of developing certain malignancies is related to duration of immunosuppressive drug exposure in patients with rheumatic diseases. J Rheumatol 1999;26:1705–14.
70. Present DH, Meltzer SJ, Krumholz MP, et al. 6-Mercaptopurine in the management of inflammatory bowel disease: short- and long-term toxicity. Ann Intern Med 1989;111:641–9.
71. Connell WR, Kamm MA, Dickson M, et al. Long-term neoplasia risk after azathioprine treatment in inflammatory bowel disease. Lancet 1994;343:1249–52.
72. Bouhnik Y, Lemann M, Mary JY, et al. Long-term follow-up of patients with Crohn's disease treated with azathioprine or 6-mercaptopurine. Lancet 1996; 347:215–9.
73. George J, Present DH, Pou R, et al. The long-term outcome of ulcerative colitis treated with 6-mercaptopurine. Am J Gastroenterol 1996;91:1711–4.
74. Korelitz BI, Mirsky FJ, Fleisher MR, et al. Malignant neoplasms subsequent to treatment of inflammatory bowel disease with 6-mercaptopurine. Am J Gastroenterol 1999;94:3248–53.
75. Dayharsh GA, Loftus EV Jr, Sandborn WJ, et al. Epstein-Barr virus-positive lymphoma in patients with inflammatory bowel disease treated with azathioprine or 6-mercaptopurine. Gastroenterology 2002;122:72–7.
76. Fraser AG, Orchard TR, Robinson EM, et al. Long-term risk of malignancy after treatment of inflammatory bowel disease with azathioprine. Aliment Pharmacol Ther 2002;16:1225–32.

77. Glazier KD, Palance AL, Griffel LH, et al. The ten-year single-center experience with 6-mercaptopurine in the treatment of inflammatory bowel disease. J Clin Gastroenterol 2005;39:21–6.
78. Kandiel A, Fraser AG, Korelitz BI, et al. Increased risk of lymphoma among inflammatory bowel disease patients treated with azathioprine and 6-mercaptopurine. Gut 2005;54:1121–5.
79. Bewtra M, Lichtenstein GR. Infliximab use in Crohn's disease. Expert Opin Biol Ther 2005;5:589–99.
80. Sandborn WJ, Hanauer SB. Antitumor necrosis factor therapy for inflammatory bowel disease: a review of agents, pharmacology, clinical results, and safety. Inflamm Bowel Dis 1999;5:119–33.
81. Maini R, St. Clair EW, Breedveld F, et al. Infliximab (chimeric anti-tumour necrosis factor alpha monoclonal antibody) versus placebo in rheumatoid arthritis patients receiving concomitant methotrexate: a randomised phase III trial. ATTRACT Study Group. Lancet 1999;354:1932–9.
82. Markham A, Lamb HM. Infliximab: a review of its use in the management of rheumatoid arthritis. Drugs 2000;59:1341–59.
83. Geborek P, Bladstrom A, Turesson C, et al. Tumour necrosis factor blockers do not increase overall tumour risk in patients with rheumatoid arthritis, but may be associated with an increased risk of lymphomas. Ann Rheum Dis 2005;64:699–703.
84. Bongartz T, Sutton AJ, Sweeting MJ, et al. Anti-TNF antibody therapy in rheumatoid arthritis and the risk of serious infections and malignancies: systematic review and meta-analysis of rare harmful effects in randomized controlled trials. JAMA 2006;295:2275–85.
85. Matteson EL, Bongartz T. Investigation, explanation, and apology for incomplete and erroneous disclosures. JAMA 2006;296:2205.
86. Targan SR, Hanauer SB, van Deventer SJ, et al. A short-term study of chimeric monoclonal antibody cA2 to tumor necrosis factor alpha for Crohn's disease. Crohn's Disease cA2 Study Group. N Engl J Med 1997;337:1029–35.
87. Present DH, Rutgeerts P, Targan S, et al. Infliximab for the treatment of fistulas in patients with Crohn's disease. N Engl J Med 1999;340:1398–405.
88. Rutgeerts P, D'Haens G, Targan S, et al. Efficacy and safety of retreatment with anti-tumor necrosis factor antibody (infliximab) to maintain remission in Crohn's disease. Gastroenterology 1999;117:761–9.
89. Cohen RD, Tsang JF, Hanauer SB. Infliximab in Crohn's disease: first anniversary clinical experience. Am J Gastroenterol 2000;95:3469–77.
90. Farrell RJ, Shah SA, Lodhavia PJ, et al. Clinical experience with infliximab therapy in 100 patients with Crohn's disease. Am J Gastroenterol 2000;95:3490–7.
91. Ardizzone S, Colombo E, Maconi G, et al. Infliximab in treatment of Crohn's disease: the Milan experience. Dig Liver Dis 2002;34:411–8.
92. Hanauer SB, Feagan BG, Lichtenstein GR, et al. Maintenance infliximab for Crohn's disease: the ACCENT I randomised trial. Lancet 2002;359:1541–9.
93. Wenzl HH, Reinisch W, Jahnel J, et al. Austrian infliximab experience in Crohn's disease: a nationwide cooperative study with long-term follow-up. Eur J Gastroenterol Hepatol 2004;16:767–73.
94. Seiderer J, Goke B, Ochsenkuhn T. Safety aspects of infliximab in inflammatory bowel disease patients. A retrospective cohort study in 100 patients of a German university hospital. Digestion 2004;70:3–9.
95. Sands BE, Anderson FH, Bernstein CN, et al. Infliximab maintenance therapy for fistulizing Crohn's disease. N Engl J Med 2004;350:876–85.

96. Colombel JF, Loftus EV Jr, Tremaine WJ, et al. The safety profile of infliximab in patients with Crohn's disease: the mayo clinic experience in 500 patients. Gastroenterology 2004;126:19–31.

97. Ljung T, Karlen P, Schmidt D, et al. Infliximab in inflammatory bowel disease: clinical outcome in a population based cohort from Stockholm County. Gut 2004;53:849–53.

98. Rutgeerts P, Sandborn WJ, Feagan BG, et al. Infliximab for induction and maintenance therapy for ulcerative colitis. N Engl J Med 2005;353:2462–76.

99. Caspersen S, Elkjaer M, Riis L, et al. Infliximab for inflammatory bowel disease in Denmark 1999-2005: clinical outcome and follow-up evaluation of malignancy and mortality. Clin Gastroenterol Hepatol 2008;6:1212–7, quiz 1176.

100. Kornbluth A. Infliximab approved for use in Crohn's disease: a report on the FDA GI Advisory Committee conference. Inflamm Bowel Dis 1998;4:328–9.

101. Ricart E, Panaccione R, Loftus EV, et al. Infliximab for Crohn's disease in clinical practice at the mayo clinic: the first 100 patients. Am J Gastroenterol 2001;96: 722–9.

102. Brown SL, Greene MH, Gershon SK, et al. Tumor necrosis factor antagonist therapy and lymphoma development: twenty-six cases reported to the food and drug administration. Arthritis Rheum 2002;46:3151–8.

103. FDA board document. Update on the TNF-alpha blocking agents; 2003. Available at: http://proxy.library.upenn.edu:2669/ohrms/dockets/ac/03/briefing/3930b1.htm. 2003. Accessed June 13, 2009.

104. Centocor. Remicade (infliximab) for IV injection. Prescribing information. Available at: http://www.remicade.com/remicade/global/hcp/hcp_pi.html. Accessed June 13, 2009.

105. Khanna D, McMahon M, Furst DE. Safety of tumour necrosis factor-alpha antagonists. Drug Saf 2004;27:307–24.

106. Mikuls TR, Weaver AL. Lessons learned in the use of tumor necrosis factor-alpha inhibitors in the treatment of rheumatoid arthritis. Curr Rheumatol Rep 2003;5: 270–7.

107. Scheinfeld N. A comprehensive review and evaluation of the side effects of the tumor necrosis factor alpha blockers etanercept, infliximab and adalimumab. J Dermatolog Treat 2004;15:280–94.

108. Schiff MH, Burmester GR, Kent JD, et al. Safety analyses of adalimumab (HUMIRA) in global clinical trials and US postmarketing surveillance of patients with rheumatoid arthritis. Ann Rheum Dis 2006;65:889–94.

109. Hanauer SB, Sandborn WJ, Rutgeerts P, et al. Human anti-tumor necrosis factor monoclonal antibody (adalimumab) in Crohn's disease: the CLASSIC-I trial. Gastroenterology 2006;130:323–33, quiz 591.

110. Colombel JF, Sandborn WJ, Rutgeerts P, et al. Adalimumab for maintenance of clinical response and remission in patients with Crohn's disease: the CHARM trial. Gastroenterology 2007;132:52–65.

111. Sandborn WJ, Rutgeerts P, Enns R, et al. Adalimumab induction therapy for Crohn disease previously treated with infliximab: a randomized trial. Ann Intern Med 2007;146:829–38.

112. Humira injection prescribing information and medication guide Jan 2008. Available at: http://proxy.library.upenn.edu:2669/Safety/MedWatch/SafetyInformation/Safety-RelatedDrugLabelingChanges/ucm106686.htm. Accessed June 13, 2009.

113. Schreiber S, Rutgeerts P, Fedorak RN, et al. A randomized, placebo-controlled trial of certolizumab pegol (CDP870) for treatment of Crohn's disease. Gastroenterology 2005;129:807–18.

114. Sandborn WJ, Feagan BG, Stoinov S, et al. Certolizumab pegol for the treatment of Crohn's disease. N Engl J Med 2007;357:228–38.
115. Schreiber S, Khaliq-Kareemi M, Lawrance IC, et al. Maintenance therapy with certolizumab pegol for Crohn's disease. N Engl J Med 2007;357:239–50.
116. Peyrin-Biroulet L, Deltenre P, de Suray N, et al. Efficacy and safety of tumor necrosis factor antagonists in Crohn's disease: meta-analysis of placebo-controlled trials. Clin Gastroenterol Hepatol 2008;6:644–53.
117. Khan WA, Yu L, Eisenbrey AB, et al. Hepatosplenic gamma/delta T-cell lymphoma in immunocompromised patients. report of two cases and review of literature. Am J Clin Pathol 2001;116:41–50.
118. Steurer M, Stauder R, Grunewald K, et al. Hepatosplenic gammadelta-T-cell lymphoma with leukemic course after renal transplantation. Hum Pathol 2002;33:253–8.
119. Navarro JT, Ribera JM, Mate JL, et al. Hepatosplenic T-gammadelta lymphoma in a patient with Crohn's disease treated with azathioprine. Leuk Lymphoma 2003;44:531–3.
120. Mackey AC, Green L, Liang LC, et al. Hepatosplenic T cell lymphoma associated with infliximab use in young patients treated for inflammatory bowel disease. J Pediatr Gastroenterol Nutr 2007;44:265–7.
121. Mittal S, Milner BJ, Johnston PW, et al. A case of hepatosplenic gamma-delta T-cell lymphoma with a transient response to fludarabine and alemtuzumab. Eur J Haematol 2006;76:531–4.
122. Thayu M, Markowitz JE, Mamula P, et al. Hepatosplenic T-cell lymphoma in an adolescent patient after immunomodulator and biologic therapy for Crohn disease. J Pediatr Gastroenterol Nutr 2005;40:220–2.
123. Shale M, Kanfer E, Panaccione R, et al. Hepatosplenic T cell lymphoma in inflammatory bowel disease. Gut 2008;57:1639–41.
124. Lewis JD, Gelfand JM, Troxel AB, et al. Immunosuppressant medications and mortality in inflammatory bowel disease. Am J Gastroenterol 2008;103:1428–35, quiz 1436.
125. Siegel CA, Hur C, Korzenik JR, et al. Risks and benefits of infliximab for the treatment of Crohn's disease. Clin Gastroenterol Hepatol 2006;4:1017–24, quiz 976.
126. Lewis JD, Schwartz JS, Lichtenstein GR. Azathioprine for maintenance of remission in Crohn's disease: benefits outweigh the risk of lymphoma. Gastroenterology 2000;118:1018–24.
127. Johnson FR, Ozdemir S, Mansfield C, et al. Crohn's disease patients' risk-benefit preferences: serious adverse event risks versus treatment efficacy. Gastroenterology 2007;133:769–79.
128. Toruner M, Loftus EV Jr, Harmsen WS, et al. Risk factors for opportunistic infections in patients with inflammatory bowel disease. Gastroenterology 2008;134:929–36.
129. Van Assche G, Magdelaine-Beuzelin C, D'Haens G, et al. Withdrawal of immunosuppression in Crohn's disease treated with scheduled infliximab maintenance: a randomized trial. Gastroenterology 2008;134:1861–8.
130. Sandborn WJ, Rutgeerts PJ, Reinisch W, et al. One year data from the Sonic study: a randomized, double-blind trial comparing infliximab and infliximab plus azathioprine to azathioprine in patients with Crohn's disease naive to immunomodulators and biologic therapy [abstract]. Gastroenterology 2009;136:A116.

Safety Profile of IBD Therapeutics: Infectious Risks

Waqqas Afif, MD, Edward V. Loftus Jr, MD*

KEYWORDS

- Inflammatory bowel disease • Infection • Corticosteroids
- Immunomodulator • Anti–tumor necrosis factor

The treatment of inflammatory bowel disease (IBD) has changed dramatically over the last decade. With increasing evidence that a "top-down" approach may alter the natural history of disease, a more aggressive treatment approach, including the use of combination immunomodulator and biologic therapy, is being advocated.[1,2] Immunomodulator therapy includes the use of azathioprine (AZA), 6-mercaptopurine (6-MP), and methotrexate (MTX). Biologic therapy includes the use of anti–tumor necrosis factor (TNF)-α agents, and more recently the use of a humanized monoclonal antibody against the cellular adhesion molecule α_4 integrin.

With the increasing use of immunomodulator and biologic therapy in the treatment of IBD, it is vitally important that the safety profile of these agents be carefully reviewed, particularly in terms of infectious risks. Corticosteroids (CS), which have been a mainstay of IBD treatment for many years, have increasingly been shown to be a major risk factor for the development of infectious complications.[3] A recent case-control study demonstrated that the use of CS, thiopurines (AZA/6-MP), and anti–TNF-α agents were each individually associated with a threefold increased risk of developing opportunistic infections and that the combination of these agents dramatically increased the risk.[4]

It is with this backdrop that this article reviews the infectious risks of IBD therapeutic agents. Throughout this article, serious infections are defined as those that lead to prolonged hospitalizations, are fatal or life threatening, result in significant disability, or are opportunistic in nature.[5] Opportunistic infections include viral infections (eg, cytomegalovirus, Epstein-Barr virus, herpes simplex virus, and varicella zoster); bacterial infections (tuberculosis [TB] and streptococcal); and fungal infections (histoplasmosis, aspergillosis, candidiasis, and blastomycosis).[4]

This article originally appeared in *Gastroenterology Clinics of North America,* Volume 38, Issue 4.
Doctor Loftus has received research support from Abbott Laboratories, Schering-Plough, and UCB. Doctor Loftus has consulted for UCB and Abbott Laboratories (fees to Mayo Clinic).
Division of Gastroenterology and Hepatology, Mayo Clinic, 200 First Street SW, Rochester, MN 55905, USA
* Corresponding author.
E-mail address: loftus.edward@mayo.edu (E.V. Loftus).

Med Clin N Am 94 (2010) 115–133
doi:10.1016/j.mcna.2009.08.016
0025-7125/09/$ – see front matter © 2010 Elsevier Inc. All rights reserved.

medical.theclinics.com

The first section of this article assesses the risk of serious infections with IBD therapeutic medications and the second section focuses on specific infectious diseases and particular circumstances.

PHARMACOEPIDEMIOLOGY

There are several challenges in determining the infectious risk of any given therapy.[6] Briefly, the determination of whether a particular adverse event is related to a specific treatment is difficult if the event in question occurs infrequently. Serious and opportunistic infections in patients with IBD fall into this category. In addition, in patients with IBD, the underlying disease process can complicate interpretation because the disease itself may increase the risk of developing an adverse event.

The strongest evidence that an adverse event is related to a particular therapy is best demonstrated through randomized controlled trials.[6] These randomized controlled trials are not powered to assess adverse events, however, especially those that occur rarely or over a longer period of time. Large observational cohort data or registry data can help to detect infrequent events, but they are neither randomized nor controlled and can be subject to bias. Case-control studies are an effective tool to study the risk of adverse events, but the identification of proper controls can be difficult and time-consuming.

CORTICOSTEROIDS

Population-based studies have shown that 42% of patients with Crohn disease are on CS within the first 3 years of diagnosis, and that 39% to 56% are on CS at some point during the course of their disease.[7–11] The absolute infectious risk of CS in IBD is difficult to quantify, but there is significant evidence that they increase the risk of infection.

A meta-analysis of 71 controlled trials assessed the association between CS and subsequent infections.[12] The overall risk of infectious complications was 12.7% in the CS group and 8% in the controlled group (relative risk [RR], 1.6; 95% confidence interval [CI], 1.3–1.9). In those receiving CS, there was a significantly increased risk of death (RR, 2.6; 95% CI, 1.2–5.3). The risk of infections in the intestinal disease subgroup was lower but still significant (RR, 1.4; 95% CI, 1.1–1.7). The rate was not increased in those patients receiving less than 10 mg/day of prednisone or those who had a cumulative dose of less than 700 mg.[12]

Increased risks of serious infection and mortality secondary to CS use were demonstrated specifically in patients with Crohn disease through the Crohn Therapy, Resource, Evaluation, and Assessment Tool (TREAT) registry.[3] This registry was initially created to monitor the toxicity of therapy with infliximab, and is an ongoing, prospective, observational, multicenter registry of North American patients with Crohn disease. There are approximately 6000 patients in the registry, half of whom are on other therapies aside from infliximab. Analysis of the TREAT registry demonstrated that in multivariate logistical analysis, CS were associated with an increased mortality risk (odds ratio [OR], 2.10; 95% CI, 1.15–3.83). Out of the 2142 patients on CS, 2.85% developed serious infections compared with 1.09% of patients not on CS. Serious infection risk was independently associated with CS use (OR, 2.21; 95% CI, 1.46–3.34), but not with infliximab treatment. Although this estimate of increased risk seems quite robust, it is important to note that this registry had a dropout rate of 20%, and that the reporting of adverse events was based primarily on the review of gastroenterologists' medical records, raising concerns about the completeness of safety data.[6]

Several studies have characterized the risk of CS in specific clinical circumstances. The European Cooperative Crohn Disease Study demonstrated that 3 out of the 43 patients who presented with an abdominal (phlegmonous) mass and were treated with CS died from sepsis.[13] A retrospective case-control study examined the effect of CS on intra-abdominal and pelvic abscess formation. Systemic CS therapy was associated with an increased rate of intra-abdominal and pelvic abscesses in patients with perforating disease (OR, 9.03; 95% CI, 2.40–33.98) and in patients with nonpenetrating disease (OR, 9.31; 95% CI, 1.03–83.91).[14] There was a trend toward an increased rate of abscess formation in patients receiving more than 20 mg per day of prednisone (OR, 2.81; 95% CI, 0.99–7.99).

Combined, all of these findings demonstrate the increased infectious risk with CS use and support the recommendation that patients who require frequent CS to control their disease should be considered for steroid-sparing therapy with immunomodulators or biologic agents.[15]

Budesonide

Budesonide, a highly potent 17-α substitute glucocorticoid with a reduced bioavailability caused by rapid first-pass hepatic metabolism, has been used in the induction of remission in patients with mild to moderate ileal or proximal colonic Crohn disease.[16] A meta-analysis to assess the safety of budesonide in patients with Crohn disease showed that the CS-related adverse event profile, including infectious complications, was similar to that of placebo.[16] Unfortunately, budesonide has a limited role in the treatment of Crohn disease because it is significantly less effective than conventional CS for inducing remission in patients with active inflammatory disease.[16]

IMMUNOMODULATOR THERAPY
AZA and 6-MP

Immunomodulator therapy with thiopurine agents (AZA and 6-MP) has been shown to be effective in the induction and maintenance of remission in patients with Crohn disease and ulcerative colitis (UC).[17–19] Although effective, they can cause multiple adverse events that can lead to drug discontinuation.

Treatment with AZA in patients with rheumatoid arthritis (RA) has been shown to increase the risk of serious infections. In a nested case-control study of a cohort of more than 23,000 patients between 1980 and 2003, AZA was associated with an increased risk of serious infections requiring hospitalizations (RR, 1.52; 95% CI, 1.18–1.97).[20] This risk was less than that of patients receiving CS (RR, 2.56; 95% CI, 2.29–2.85).

In patients with IBD, the risk of infection associated with thiopurines is less clear. A meta-analysis of patients with Crohn disease treated with AZA and 6-MP found that adverse events requiring withdrawal from a trial were increased as compared with placebo (OR, 3.01; 95% CI, 1.30–6.96).[18] The most common side effects were allergic reactions (2.3%); leukopenia (1.4%); and nausea (1.4%). In a recent review of 66 studies (8302 patients), the cumulative incidence rate of drug-induced myelotoxicity with AZA and 6-MP in 9103 years of patient follow-up was 7% (95% CI, 6%–8%).[21] Leukopenia was not associated with drug dosage and occurred most frequently within the first year of treatment. The cumulative incidence of infections in patients with AZA and 6-MP–induced myelotoxicity was 6.5% (95% CI, 3.2–9.8).

Whether leukopenia is directly associated with infectious complications is somewhat unclear. Many infectious complications in patients on AZA and 6-MP can occur in the absence of leukopenia, and as such it is difficult to assess the rate of infection based on risk of leukopenia alone.[22]

The rate of adverse events and infection may be higher in the "real-world" clinical setting when there is longer follow-up. In one study of 396 patients on 6-MP with 1800 patient-years of follow-up, the adverse event rate was reported to be as high as 15%.[23] In this same study, the reported incidence of infection was found to be 7.4% and the incidence of serious infection to be 1.8%. In another study, 410 patients with IBD treated with 6-MP were assessed from 1980 to 1999.[24] Fifty-eight (14.1%) patients experienced an infection while on 6-MP. Pneumonia was seen in 16 patients (3.9%), which is similar to the normal population (1.2%–5%).[25] Herpes zoster was seen in 12 patients (2.9%) and occurred at a mean of 32.5 months (range, 0.6–226 months) after initiation of treatment. Upper respiratory infections were seen in 29 patients (7.1% of patients).

In the two retrospective studies just mentioned, the risk of infection may be increased, but this is difficult to confirm because there was no specific control group. Data from the TREAT registry showed that in multivariate analysis, the use of immuno-modulator therapy did not play a role in the development of serious infections.[3] The limitation of this database analysis is that it does not take into account likely contributing risk factors, such as the duration of use or cumulative exposure to a particular agent.[6]

In the previously described study by Agrawal and colleagues,[14] which assessed the risk of abdominal abscess in patients with Crohn disease, there was no increased risk of infection in those treated with AZA. Another study assessed the risk of developing benign infections in 230 IBD patients receiving AZA.[26] The incidence of benign viral upper respiratory tract infections (compared with controls) was 2.1 ± 2.2 per observation year and there was no increased risk in patients on AZA ($P = 0.77$). There was an increased incidence of benign oral and genital herpes simplex virus flares in patients on AZA (1 ± 2.6 vs 0.2 ± 0.8 per year; $P = 0.04$), however, and an increased rate of worsening viral warts (human papillomavirus [HPV]) (17.2% vs 3.3%; $P = 0.004$).

Together, these studies suggest that the risk of infectious complications with AZA and 6-MP in patients with IBD may be limited to mild infections in most cases.

MTX

MTX is a folate antimetabolite that inhibits DNA synthesis and has been shown to be effective in the induction and maintenance of remission in two separate trials in patients with Crohn disease.[27,28] Although these trials were not powered to assess safety, of the 134 patients who received intramuscular and oral MTX, there was only one infectious complication reported (mycoplasma pneumonia). In one study of 54 patients with Crohn disease that compared 6 months of treatment with AZA with MTX (intramuscular followed by oral), no serious infectious complications were identified.[29] Another study involving 49 Crohn disease patients who received MTX (intramuscular) for a median duration of 18 months (range, 7–59 months) showed that although adverse reactions occurred in 24 patients (49%) and five patients (10%) withdrew from the study, no infections complications were identified.[30] A retrospective study of 39 Crohn disease patients receiving intramuscular followed by oral MTX, however, showed that 10 (26%) patients developed infections and 2 (5%) withdrew secondary to infectious compilations.[31] In this study population, however, more than 50% were taking concomitant CS, which could certainly confound the risk of infectious complications.

The safety experience with MTX in the RA literature is vast and lessons can be drawn from this literature. In the previously described nested case-control study of more than 23,000 RA patients, MTX treatment was associated with a modestly increased risk of pneumonia (RR, 1.6; 95% CI, 1.02–1.33), but not with serious infections requiring hospitalizations.[20] An extensive review of the infectious complications of MTX in RA concluded that MTX was associated with a minimal increased risk of infections, and that treatment was likely not associated with an increased risk of opportunistic or serious infections.[32] In RA registry data including almost 8000 patients, although there was a slightly increased risk of developing an infection compared with patients not on biologic or MTX therapy (RR, 1.3; 95% CI, 1.12–1.50), there was no increased risk of developing opportunistic infections.[33] This latter finding was in contrast to patients on CS (>10 mg/day) who did have an increased risk of opportunistic infections (RR, 1.30; 95% CI, 1.11–1.53).[33]

Overall, the data from the RA and Crohn disease literature demonstrate that treatment with MTX in patients with Crohn disease is likely safe from an infectious point of view, and does not increase the risk of serious or opportunistic infections. The use of MTX can be associated with liver and lung toxicity. Although MTX may be relatively safe to use in patients with CD, thiopurines have been used preferentially because they have been more extensively studied.

ANTI–TNF-α THERAPY

At present there are three different anti–TNF-α agents approved for the treatment of Crohn disease: (1) infliximab (Remicade, Centocor, Horsham, Pennsylvania); (2) adalimumab (Humira, Abbott Laboratories, North Chicago, Illinois); and (3) certolizumab pegol (Cimzia, UCB, Smyrna, Georgia).[34] Infliximab is the only anti–TNF-α agent approved for use in the treatment of UC.[35] There has been increasing use of these agents over the last decade, and multiple studies have examined the risk of infectious complications.

There is definite evidence that anti–TNF-α agents are associated with an increased rate of serious infections in patients with RA. A meta-analysis of nine placebo-controlled trials of infliximab and adalimumab in RA involving over 5000 patients yielded a pooled OR for serious infection of 2.01 (95% CI, 1.31–3.09).[36]

In terms of patients with IBD, the association between anti-TNF therapy and serious infection is not as clear and may relate to the fact that the patients with IBD are generally younger and have less comorbid disease, compared with patients with RA. Individual randomized trials in Crohn disease have not demonstrated an elevated risk of serious infection. In a recently published meta-analysis, 21 trials with a total of 5356 patients were reviewed to assess the safety of anti–TNF-α agents.[37] There were 3341 patients in the anti–TNF-α group and 2015 patients in the control group, with a median follow-up of 24 weeks (range, 4–60 weeks). There was no significant difference in the risk of serious infection in the anti-TNF group versus the control group (2.09% versus 2.13%, respectively; 95% CI, 0.45–0.65). In subgroup analysis, there were no differences in infectious risk between anti–TNF-α and control groups whether they were induction or maintenance trials.[37]

Data from the TREAT registry assessed the infectious complications of IBD therapeutic medications. The risk of serious infection 3 months after an infliximab infusion was compared with the risk of infection 3 months before an infusion. In univariate analysis, serious infections were more than twice as likely to occur in the 3 months after an infliximab infusion (OR, 2.15; 95 CI, 1.44–3.21).[3] After controlling for other factors, however, such as disease duration and severity, concurrent use of CS, immunomodulators, and narcotic analgesics, the association between infliximab and serious infection was no longer significant (OR, 0.99; 95% CI, 0.64–1.53).[3] An update of the TREAT registry, now with 24,575 patient years of follow-up, was recently presented in abstract form.[38] Infliximab-treated patients had an increased risk of serious infections (RR, 1.57; 95%

CI, 1.16–2.14); however, multivariate analysis again suggested that this increased risk was independently associated with prednisone and not infliximab.

Several retrospective referral center–based studies have assessed the risk of anti–TNF-α agents in patients with IBD. In one study, among the first 500 Crohn disease patients treated with infliximab at Mayo Clinic, serious infections occurred in 20 (4%), including four deaths caused by infection (0.8%).[5] In a study of 202 patients with UC and Crohn disease who had a median follow-up of 2.4 years (range, 1–4.9; 620 patient-years), 42 patients (20.8%) experienced an infectious event including 22 patients (10.9%) with a serious infection.[39] The safety of more than 3000 patients treated with adalimumab in clinical trials was recently assessed.[40] The incidence of opportunistic infections was 1.8%, with oral candidiasis being the most commonly reported infection (1.2%). Serious infections were seen 5.8% of patients (incidence rate of 6.6 cases per 100 person-years) but almost half of those were intra-abdominal (2.5%). It is important to note that these three studies had no control group and did not take into account concomitant medications and so direct causality cannot be established.

More recently, in a single-center experience from Leuven, Belgium, the long-term safety of anti–TNF-α agents was assessed in 1400 patients with Crohn disease (of whom 734 received infliximab).[41] Patients who received anti-TNF therapy were followed for a median of 58 months (interquartile ratio, 33–88 months). The percentage of patients who developed serious infections was 6% in the infliximab group and 9% in the control group. The incidence rate of serious infections in the two groups was not significantly different (1.6 per 100 patient-years in infliximab group versus 1.1 per 100 patient-years in control group).

Two population-based studies have reported on the safety of infliximab. The first, a population-based cohort from Stockholm County, examined 217 patients who received infliximab between 1999 and 2001.[42] Eighteen patients (8.3%) developed severe infectious complications (seven were postoperative) and there were two deaths related to infection (both on CS, none on AZA and 6MP). In this cohort, 51% of the patients were on concomitant immunomodulators, 54% were being treated with CS, and 25% were on both immunomodulators and CS. Given that both of these agents increase infectious risk, the exact role of infliximab with regards to infection can not be determined from this study. The second population-based cohort examined the association between infliximab and other immunosuppressive agents in a cohort of 10,662 IBD patients in British Columbia, Canada.[43] In patients receiving infliximab, the event rate of serious bacterial infection was 4.28 per 1000 patient-years (95% CI, 0.11–23.8) but this was not significantly increased compared with patients receiving CS or immunomodulators.

The risk of infectious complications with anti–TNF-α monotherapy in patients with Crohn disease does not seem to be increased in terms of overall infections. These studies may not be large enough, however, to detect rarer opportunistic infections (see later sections on TB and fungal infections). In a referral center–based case-control study of risk factors for opportunistic infections in patients with IBD, infliximab was associated with a fourfold increased risk of opportunistic infection (OR, 4.4; 95% CI, 1.2–17.1).[4]

COMBINATION THERAPY

A recent randomized controlled trial published in abstract form demonstrated that in patients with moderate to severe Crohn disease, combination therapy with AZA and infliximab was superior in achieving clinical and endoscopic remission compared with either drug alone.[44] Other studies have shown that the combination therapy reduces the immunogenicity of anti–TNF-α agents, especially when the latter are administered episodically.[45,46] Although combination therapy with biologic therapy and concomitant immunomodulators may be more effective, this increased efficacy may come at the cost of increased infectious complications.

A randomized trial of infliximab with concomitant MTX in more than 1000 RA patients was designed specifically to assess safety end points.[47] Patients in the study were randomized to placebo infusion to week 22, then 3 mg/kg every 8 weeks to week 54; 3 mg/kg infliximab infusions to week 22 with escalation by 1.5 mg/kg as needed to control symptoms; and lastly to 10 mg/kg infliximab infusions for the length of the study. There was greater than a threefold increased risk of serious infections in the 10 mg/kg group at week 22 compared with those patients who received MTX alone ($P = 0.013$), but not in those who received 3 mg/kg on infliximab.

In patients with IBD, the evidence of increased risk with concomitant therapy is unclear. In one study, data from four prospective randomized phase 3 trials in IBD patients were used to assess the efficacy of concomitant immunomodulators with infliximab.[46] In the pooled safety analysis of 1007 infliximab-treated patients, similar proportions of patients with and without combination therapy had infections (44.1% and 44.5) or serious infections (3.7% and 3.2%). In the earlier referenced population-based study out of British Columbia, an increased risk of serious infections was not found in patients receiving concomitant therapy with infliximab and an immunomodulator.[43] In the study by Fidder and colleagues,[41] only the concomitant use of steroids (and not immunomodulators) was associated with an increased risk of serious infection (OR, 2.7; 95% CI, 1.2–6.1). Throwing caution to these results, the case-control study by Toruner and colleagues[4] demonstrated the OR for opportunistic infections in patients on two or more immunosuppressive medications simultaneously was 14.5 (95% CI, 4.9–43) and was "infinite" in patients with three immunosuppressive medications (CS, immunomodulators, and anti–TNF-α agent). Further examination of this study suggests, however, that much of the increased risk was driven by the use of CS.

Although concomitant therapy may increase the risk of infection, it seems that it is the use of that CS plays the largest role in the development of serious or opportunistic infections.

CYCLOSPORINE

The use of cyclosporine in IBD is at present limited to rescue therapy for patients with fulminant UC. There are limited data on the safety of cyclosporine in this setting, and underlying disease severity complicates the assessment of safety.

In patients receiving cyclosporine for the prevention of liver allograft rejection, therapy was associated with a risk of infection of approximately 40%, sepsis in 20%, and cytomegalovirus in 15% to 25%.[48] A study assessing the long-term outcome of treatment with intravenous cyclosporine in patients with severe UC demonstrated that in 86 patients treated with cyclosporine between 1992 and 2000, five (5.8%) patients had opportunistic infections, and three patients (3.5%) died (one from *Pneumocystis jiroveci (carinii)* pneumonia [PCP] and two from *Aspergillus* pneumonia).[49] In addition, there were catheter-related infections in eight patients (9.3%). In a separate retrospective study, 19 patients with CS-refractory UC who received cyclosporine after infliximab or infliximab after cyclosporine were assessed.[50] In total, three patients (15.8%) developed severe complications and one patient died (gram-negative bacterial sepsis with death, herpetic esophagitis, and pancreatitis with *Enterococcus* and *Klebsiella* bacteremia). Overall, these limited data suggest that treatment with cyclosporine leads to an increased risk of serious infections.

NATALIZUMAB

Natalizumab (Tysabri, Biogen Idec, Cambridge, Massachusetts, and Elan Pharmaceuticals, South San Francisco, California), a humanized IgG4 monoclonal antibody against α_4 integrin–mediated leukocyte migration, was approved by the FDA in 2008 for use in patients with Crohn disease with evidence of active inflammation who have had an inadequate response to or cannot tolerate anti-TNF therapy.[51] In the ENACT-1 and ENACT-2 trials of natalizumab in Crohn disease, subjects in the treatment arm had a significantly increased risk of developing influenza or an influenza-like illness (12% vs 5%; $P<.05$).[52] One case of varicella pneumonia and cytomegalovirus hepatitis was also reported in the natalizumab group. In two earlier trials with natalizumab in Crohn disease and in one smaller trial in patients with UC, an increased risk of serious infections was not found.[53–55]

After publication of the ENACT trials, a fatal case of JC virus–induced progressive multifocal leukoencephalopathy was reported in one patient who had been enrolled in this trial.[56] Two further cases were identified in patients receiving natalizumab for multiple sclerosis, and the drug was withdrawn temporarily from commercial use.[57,58] Natalizumab was reintroduced under restrictive rules prohibiting concurrent therapy with an immunomodulator or long-term CS therapy. Since being reintroduced to the market, of the 52,000 patients who have taken the drug, there are, as of early June 2009, six additional cases of progressive multifocal leukoencephalopathy (four cases occurred in patients not on any concurrent therapy) resulting in an incidence of approximately 1.2 cases per 10,000 patients treated.[59]

POSTOPERATIVE COMPLICATIONS

Several studies have examined the risk of preoperative CS in patients undergoing abdominal surgery. A recent meta-analysis of five observational studies involving 1714 patients assessed the risk of postsurgical infectious complications.[60] Pooled analysis showed an increased risk of postoperative infectious complications in patients on CS (OR, 1.68; 95% CI, 1.24–2.28), with an increased risk in patients on higher perioperative oral CS (>40 mg) (OR, 2.04; 95% CI, 1.28–3.26).

A retrospective cohort study that was included in this meta-analysis assessed 159 postoperative IBD patients and assessed the risk of infectious complications with AZA and 6-MP.[61] Both univariate and multivariate analysis failed to demonstrate an increased risk of postsurgical complications in patients receiving AZA and 6-MP. In addition, studies assessing postoperative complications in 270 patients with Crohn disease and 151 patients with UC did not demonstrate an increased risk of postoperative complications in patients taking AZA, 6-MP, and MTX.[62,63]

In terms of anti–TNF-α medications, a retrospective cohort study of 141 UC patients compared preoperative infliximab exposure with those not previously exposed.[64] The use of infliximab did not play a role in the development of postoperative complications but a moderate to high dose of CS ($\geq$20 mg methylprednisone for $\geq$2 months) was associated with an increased risk of short-term postoperative complications (OR, 5.19; 95% CI, 2.12–19.64; $P = .001$). In addition, four other studies have failed to show an increase in postoperative infectious complications in patients treated with anti-TNF agents preoperatively.[62,65–67] One of these studies assessed a total of 413 patients with both UC and Crohn disease undergoing abdominal surgery. One hundred twenty-one (24.5%) received preoperative infliximab and no increased risk of infectious complication was identified compared with patients who had not received prior infliximab.[65]

Three separate studies, however, have demonstrated an increased risk of infection in patients with UC who were exposed to infliximab preoperatively. One small study, which assessed 47 postoperative UC patients, suggested that anti-TNF agents may increase infectious complications (adjusted OR, 2.7; 95% CI, 1.1–6.7).[68] Another retrospective case-control study assessed 523 patients who underwent restorative proctocolectomy and found that preoperative infliximab use was associated with an increased risk of early complications (adjusted OR, 3.5; 95% CI, 1.51–8.31) and sepsis (adjusted OR, 13.8; 95% CI, 1.82–105).[69] In a recently published abstract of a retrospective study of 436 patients who underwent ileal pouch–anal anastomosis (IPAA), infliximab use (within 12 weeks of surgery) was associated with a significant increase in early (<30 days) infectious complications (adjusted OR, 2.5; 95% CI, 1–6.1), but not overall early or late complications.[70] In addition, these studies demonstrated that in patients on infliximab, a two-stage IPAA (proctocolectomy with formation of IPAA and protecting loop ileostomy, followed by ileostomy closure) resulted in increased infectious complications compared with those who underwent a three-stage IPAA (subtotal colectomy with Hartmann pouch and end ileostomy, followed by completion proctectomy and formation of IPAA with protecting loop ileostomy, followed by ileostomy closure).[69,70]

Given the conflicting results of these studies, the postoperative infectious risk of prior anti–TNF-α treatment remains unclear and further studies are needed to clarify the risk of these agents.

Overall, it seems that CS increases the risk of postoperative infectious complications and should generally be tapered to the lowest possible dose before surgery. Immunomodulators do not seem to confer an increased risk in the postoperative setting and can be continued perioperatively. Preoperative infliximab use may independently increase the risk of early infectious complications in patients with UC (no evidence in Crohn disease), and these patients should be considered for a three-stage IPAA rather than a two-stage surgical procedure.

BACTERIAL INFECTIONS
Tuberculosis

CS seems to play a role in the development of active TB. A retrospective study using the General Practice Research Database from the United Kingdom assessed 16,213 IBD patients and 66,512 controls for the development of active TB.[71] The annual incidence of active TB was 20 cases per 100,000 person-years in IBD patients and 9 per 100,000 in control subjects, leading to an unadjusted relative risk for active TB of 2.36 (95% CI, 1.17–4.74). Exposure to CS was found to be a significant independent risk factor for active TB. In this study, no increased risk was found in patients on immunomodulatory medications.

The risk of reactivation of TB is significantly elevated in patients receiving anti–TNF-α medications. Mycobacteria (and other granulomatous infections) are sequestered within granulomas, and because TNF-α is required for the continued maintenance of granuloma structure, it is thought that anti–TNF-α agents may predispose to TB reactivation.[72]

A Spanish safety registry of over 1500 patients treated with anti–TNF-α drugs noted a TB incidence rate approximately 50 to 90 times higher than expected in the general Spanish population.[73] A Swedish study of RA patients showed that those on anti–TNF-α agents were four times more likely than those not on anti–TNF-α agents to develop TB.[74] A United States study including more than 10,000 RA patients demonstrated an eightfold elevation in TB risk among infliximab-treated patients.[75]

In 70 cases reported by the Food and Drug Administration (FDA) among 147,000 patients treated with infliximab (both IBD and RA), most cases of TB were extrapulmonary, and 24% presented with disseminated disease.[76] Most of these cases occurred within 2 to 4 months of starting therapy in regions with a low prevalence of TB, and in patients with a limited recent exposure to TB. These findings suggest that these patients had reactivation of latent infection rather than newly acquired infection. In patients who have developed active TB while on anti–TNF-α therapy, mortality has been reported to be as high as 13%.[77]

This increased risk of TB is now incorporated into the black-box warning section on the prescribing information for all commercially available anti–TNF-α agents. Recommendations indicate that latent TB should be assessed with a tuberculin skin test and chest radiograph before initiating anti–TNF-α treatment.[15] There are no prospective data on when anti-TNF therapy can be safely started (or restarted) once TB treatment is initiated. Patients with latent TB should ideally receive chemoprophylaxis with isoniazid for 9 months before anti-TNF therapy and should be supervised by a thoracic or infectious disease physician.[78] At the minimum, if anti-TNF therapy needs to be started, patients should be receiving at least 1 to 2 months of TB treatment.[15,72,79,80]

Other Granulomatous Infections

Listeria monocytogenes has been described in patients receiving anti–TNF-α therapy. The FDA reported 38 cases of *Listeria* infections in patients receiving anti-TNF therapy from 1998 to 2002 (15.5 cases [versus 1.8 expected] per 100,000 patients).[81] *Listeria* infections of the bloodstream and central nervous system usually occurred in patients who were on concomitant immunosuppression.[82–84] Other granulomatous infections, such as nocardiosis and nontuberculous mycobacteria, have also been reported in patients on anti-TNF agents.[81,85]

Clostridium Difficile

In the population-based study by Schneeweiss and colleagues[43] the incidence of *Clostridium difficile* was 14 cases per 1000 person-years (95% CI, 10.6–18.2) in patients on CS. This risk of infection was triple that of other immunosuppressive agents (RR, 3.4; 95% CI, 1.9–6.1). Anti–TNF-α therapy did not seem to increase the risk of *C difficile* infection. There are no prospective data on the use of immunomodulators or biologics in the setting of active *C difficile* infection. Given the association between immunomodulators and *C difficile* infection, the risk/benefit of continuing these medications should be carefully considered, especially in the setting of recurrent-resistant infections.[78]

FUNGAL INFECTIONS
PCP

Several case series and reports of IBD patients developing PCP after being treated with AZA and 6-MP have been published.[86–88] PCP has also been reported in patients receiving cyclosporine for severe UC[49,89,90] and in patients receiving anti–TNF-α agents for Crohn disease or RA.[42,86,91–93] A review of the FDA Adverse Event Reporting System found 84 cases of infliximab-associated PCP between 1998 and 2003 and 23 deaths (27%).[86] In a case-control study, older age, pulmonary disease, and high doses of CS were risk factors for the development of PCP in patients taking anti–TNF-α agents.[94]

Granulomatous Fungal Infections

Histoplasmosis and coccidioidomycosis infections have been reported in patients on anti–TNF-α therapy.[95,96] In 2008, the FDA issued a black-box warning with regards to the risk of pulmonary and disseminated fungal granulomatous infections (including blastomycosis) in patients who are being treated with anti–TNF-α agents.[97] This warning stems from the fact that as of September 2008, 240 cases of anti–TNF-α associated histoplasmosis were reported (17 cases per 100,000 patients in infliximab-treated groups), whereas the number of cases from the late 1990s through July 2001 was only 10.[95]

Among cases of anti–TNF-α associated histoplasmosis in the United States, most patients had resided in areas endemic for the infection (Ohio and Mississippi River valleys), and virtually all were receiving other immunosuppressive agents.[95,96]

Similarly, symptomatic coccidioidomycosis following anti–TNF-α therapy has been reported in the endemic areas of Arizona, California, and Nevada, and virtually all patients were on concomitant immunosuppression.[98]

Other Fungal Infections

The FDA Adverse Event Reporting System listed 11 *Cryptococcus neoformans* infections in patents receiving infliximab therapy from 1998 to 2002 (4.7 per 100,000 patients).[81] Most reports indicate that patients were on concomitant medications.

In the same database, aspergillosis was reported in 39 patients on infliximab therapy (12.4 per 100,000 patients).[81] There have been reports of invasive pulmonary aspergillosis, systemic candidiasis, and disseminated sporotrichosis in patients receiving anti–TNF-α therapy.[99–102]

VIRAL INFECTIONS
Hepatitis B and C

The impact of CS, immunomodulators, or anti–TNF-α therapy on the course of hepatitis B virus (HBV) infection or hepatitis C virus (HCV) infection has not been studied prospectively.[78]

Recently published guidelines suggest that all IBD patients should be tested for HBV infection and that vaccination should be recommended to all patients who are seronegative.[78] Immunomodulator and anti–TNF-α therapy may negatively affect the efficacy of vaccination and higher doses of HBV vaccine may be required to achieve immunity. In addition, serologic response should be measured after vaccination. There are case reports of patients with stable HBV infection who have had reactivation (both asymptomatic and severe) during treatment with infliximab.[103,104] Of note, reactivation of HBV is more commonly seen in patients on chemotherapeutic regimens containing CS who are being treated for lymphoma.[105] Data from patients being treated with immunosuppressive chemotherapy have shown that HBV replication and reactivation can occur in up to 20% to 50% of cases.[106] Patients with chronic HBV (HBsAg$^+$) should receive prophylaxis with antiviral agents (nucleoside-nucleotide analogues) to avoid a HBV flare of disease.[78] Immunomodulator and anti–TNF-α therapy should be delayed in patients with acute HBV infections.

There is no consensus with regards to HCV screening before starting immunomodulator or anti–TNF-α therapy in patients with IBD.[78] There are no data to suggest that treatment with any IBD therapeutic medication increases the risk of developing HCV or exacerbates existing HCV infection.[78]

HIV

There are no data to suggest a role for CS, immunomodulator, or anti–TNF-α therapy in the development or progression of HIV infection in patients with IBD.[78] Several case reports and small studies have shown no detrimental effects when using anti–TNF-α therapy in patients with established HIV.[107–109]

Human Papillomavirus

There is an increased incidence of HPV-associated warts or condylomata in patients receiving immunomodulator therapy.[26] Current or previous infection with HPV is not a contraindication to patients receiving immunomodulator or biologic therapy.[78] Routine prophylactic immunization has been recommended in all females greater that 11 years of age and vaccination is most effective before onset of sexual activity.[110,111] There are no specific guidelines for the use of HPV vaccine in patients with IBD, but it is a nonlive vaccine and can safely be used in female patients on immunomodulator or anti–TNF-α therapy.

Other Viral Infections

Viral infections, including herpes simplex virus, primary varicella infection, herpes zoster, Epstein-Barr virus, and cytomegalovirus, have been reported following CS, immunomodulatory, or anti–TNF-α therapy in both Crohn disease and RA.[98,112–118] In cases of disseminated cytomegalovirus or varicella, these infections have been life-threatening.[113,115–119] In a small prospective study of RA patients who were tested serially for viral loads for cytomegalovirus, Epstein-Barr virus, and human herpesvirus-6, infliximab did not result in reactivation.[120]

RECOMMENDED VACCINATIONS

In addition to the vaccinations recommended to the general population, recently published European guidelines suggest that patients with IBD should be considered for five additional vaccines.[78]

Vaccinations for HBV-seronegative patients and HPV in young women have been discussed previously. In addition, vaccinations should be considered for influenza, pneumococcus, and varicella (specifically in those who are seronegative). Given the potential for decreased seroconversion in immunosuppressed patients, vaccination should be considered before therapy is instituted (at diagnosis) and patients on immunomodulatory-biologic agents should only receive inactivated vaccines.

REFERENCES

1. D'Haens G, Baert F, van Assche G, et al. Early combined immunosuppression or conventional management in patients with newly diagnosed Crohn disease: an open randomised trial. Lancet 2008;371(9613):660–7.
2. Sandborn WJ. Initial combination therapy in early Crohn disease. Lancet 2008; 371(9613):635–6.
3. Lichtenstein GR, Feagan BG, Cohen RD, et al. Serious infections and mortality in association with therapies for Crohn disease: TREAT registry. Clin Gastroenterol Hepatol 2006;4(5):621–30.
4. Toruner M, Loftus EV Jr, Harmsen WS, et al. Risk factors for opportunistic infections in patients with inflammatory bowel disease. Gastroenterology 2008; 134(4):929–36.

5. Colombel JF, Loftus EV Jr, Tremaine WJ, et al. The safety profile of infliximab in patients with Crohn disease: the Mayo Clinic experience in 500 patients. Gastroenterology 2004;126(1):19–31.
6. Reddy JG, Loftus EV Jr. Safety of infliximab and other biologic agents in the inflammatory bowel diseases. Gastroenterol Clin North Am 2006;35(4):837–55.
7. Faubion WA Jr, Loftus EV Jr, Harmsen WS, et al. The natural history of corticosteroid therapy for inflammatory bowel disease: a population-based study. Gastroenterology 2001;121(2):255–60.
8. Munkholm P, Langholz E, Davidsen M, et al. Frequency of glucocorticoid resistance and dependency in Crohn disease. Gut 1994;35(3):360–2.
9. Silverstein MD, Loftus EV, Sandborn WJ, et al. Clinical course and costs of care for Crohn disease: Markov model analysis of a population-based cohort. Gastroenterology 1999;117(1):49–57.
10. Munkholm P, Langholz E, Davidsen M, et al. Disease activity courses in a regional cohort of Crohn disease patients. Scand J Gastroenterol 1995; 30(7):699–706.
11. Lewis JD, Bilker WB, Brensinger C, et al. Inflammatory bowel disease is not associated with an increased risk of lymphoma. Gastroenterology 2001; 121(5):1080–7.
12. Stuck AE, Minder CE, Frey FJ. Risk of infectious complications in patients taking glucocorticosteroids. Rev Infect Dis 1989;11(6):954–63.
13. Malchow H, Ewe K, Brandes JW, et al. European Cooperative Crohn Disease Study (ECCDS): results of drug treatment. Gastroenterology 1984;86(2): 249–66.
14. Agrawal A, Durrani S, Leiper K, et al. Effect of systemic corticosteroid therapy on risk for intra-abdominal or pelvic abscess in non-operated Crohn disease. Clin Gastroenterol Hepatol 2005;3(12):1215–20.
15. Lichtenstein GR, Abreu MT, Cohen R, et al. American Gastroenterological Association Institute medical position statement on corticosteroids, immunomodulators, and infliximab in inflammatory bowel disease. Gastroenterology 2006; 130(3):935–9, 940–87.
16. Papi C, Luchetti R, Gili L, et al. Budesonide in the treatment of Crohn disease: a meta-analysis. Aliment Pharmacol Ther 2000;14(11):1419–28.
17. Pearson DC, May GR, Fick G, et al. Azathioprine for maintaining remission of Crohn disease. Cochrane Database Syst Rev 2000;(2):CD000067.
18. Sandborn W, Sutherland L, Pearson D, et al. Azathioprine or 6-mercaptopurine for inducing remission of Crohn disease. Cochrane Database Syst Rev 2000;(2):CD000545.
19. Timmer A, McDonald JW, Macdonald JK. Azathioprine and 6-mercaptopurine for maintenance of remission in ulcerative colitis. Cochrane Database Syst Rev 2007;(1):CD000478.
20. Bernatsky S, Hudson M, Suissa S. Anti-rheumatic drug use and risk of serious infections in rheumatoid arthritis. Rheumatology (Oxford) 2007;46(7):1157–60.
21. Gisbert JP, Gomollon F. Thiopurine-induced myelotoxicity in patients with inflammatory bowel disease: a review. Am J Gastroenterol 2008;103(7):1783–800.
22. Lichtenstein GR, Abreu MT, Cohen R, et al. American Gastroenterological Associate Institute technical review on corticosteroids, immunomodulators, and infliximab in inflammatory bowel disease. Gastroenterology 2006;130(3):940–87.
23. Present DH, Meltzer SJ, Krumholz MP, et al. 6-Mercaptopurine in the management of inflammatory bowel disease: short- and long-term toxicity. Ann Intern Med 1989;111(8):641–9.

24. Warman JI, Korelitz BI, Fleisher MR, et al. Cumulative experience with short- and long-term toxicity to 6-mercaptopurine in the treatment of Crohn disease and ulcerative colitis. J Clin Gastroenterol 2003;37(3):220–5.
25. Marrie TJ. [Community acquired pneumonia]. Praxis (Bern 1994) 2001;90(21): 935–40 [in German].
26. Seksik P, Cosnes J, Sokol H, et al. Incidence of benign upper respiratory tract infections, HSV and HPV cutaneous infections in inflammatory bowel disease patients treated with azathioprine. Aliment Pharmacol Ther 2009;29(10): 1106–13.
27. Feagan BG, Fedorak RN, Irvine EJ, et al. A comparison of methotrexate with placebo for the maintenance of remission in Crohn disease. North American Crohn Study Group Investigators. N Engl J Med 2000;342(22):1627–32.
28. Feagan BG, Rochon J, Fedorak RN, et al. Methotrexate for the treatment of Crohn disease. The North American Crohn Study Group Investigators. N Engl J Med 1995;332(5):292–7.
29. Ardizzone S, Bollani S, Manzionna G, et al. Comparison between methotrexate and azathioprine in the treatment of chronic active Crohn disease: a randomised, investigator-blind study. Dig Liver Dis 2003;35(9):619–27.
30. Lemann M, Zenjari T, Bouhnik Y, et al. Methotrexate in Crohn disease: long-term efficacy and toxicity. Am J Gastroenterol 2000;95(7):1730–4.
31. Din S, Dahele A, Fennel J, et al. Use of methotrexate in refractory Crohn disease: the Edinburgh experience. Inflamm Bowel Dis 2008;14(6):756–62.
32. McLean-Tooke A, Aldridge C, Waugh S, et al. Methotrexate, rheumatoid arthritis and infection risk: what is the evidence? Rheumatology (Oxford) 2009;48(8): 867–71.
33. Greenberg JD, Reed G, Kremer JM, et al. Association of Methotrexate and TNF antagonists with risk of infection outcomes including opportunistic infections in the CORRONA registry. Ann Rheum Dis 2009; [Epub ahead of print].
34. Blonski W, Lichtenstein GR. Safety of biologic therapy. Inflamm Bowel Dis 2007; 13(6):769–96.
35. Rutgeerts P, Sandborn WJ, Feagan BG, et al. Infliximab for induction and maintenance therapy for ulcerative colitis. N Engl J Med 2005;353(23):2462–76.
36. Bongartz T, Sutton AJ, Sweeting MJ, et al. Anti-TNF antibody therapy in rheumatoid arthritis and the risk of serious infections and malignancies: systematic review and meta-analysis of rare harmful effects in randomized controlled trials. JAMA 2006;295(19):2275–85.
37. Peyrin-Biroulet L, Deltenre P, de Suray N, et al. Efficacy and safety of tumor necrosis factor antagonists in Crohn disease: meta-analysis of placebo-controlled trials. Clin Gastroenterol Hepatol 2008;6(6):644–53.
38. Lichtenstein GR, Cohen R, Feagan B, et al. Safety of infliximab and other Crohn disease therapies-TREAT registry data with nearly 24,575 patient years of follow-up [abstract]. Am J Gastroenterol 2008;104(S1):5436.
39. Lees CW, Ali AI, Thompson AI, et al. The safety profile of anti-tumour necrosis factor therapy in inflammatory bowel disease in clinical practice: analysis of 620 patient-years follow-up. Aliment Pharmacol Ther 2009;29(3):286–97.
40. Colombel JF, Sandborn WJ, Panaccione R, et al. Adalimumab safety in global clinical trials of patients with Crohn disease. Inflamm Bowel Dis 2009; [Epub ahead of print].
41. Fidder H, Schnitzler F, Ferrante M, et al. Long-term safety of infliximab for the treatment of inflammatory bowel disease: a single-centre cohort study. Gut 2009;58(4):501–8.

42. Ljung T, Karlen P, Schmidt D, et al. Infliximab in inflammatory bowel disease: clinical outcome in a population based cohort from Stockholm County. Gut 2004;53(6):849–53.

43. Schneeweiss S, Korzenik J, Solomon DH, et al. Infliximab and other immunomodulating drugs in patients with inflammatory bowel disease and the risk of serious bacterial infections. Aliment Pharmacol Ther 2009;30(3):253–64.

44. Sandborn W, Rutgeerts P, Reinisch W, et al. SONIC: a randomized, double-blind, controlled trial comparing infliximab and infliximab plus azathioprine to azathioprine in patients with Crohn disease naïve to immunomodulators and biologic therapy [abstract]. Am J Gastroenterol 2008;103(S1):5436.

45. Vermeire S, Noman M, Van Assche G, et al. Effectiveness of concomitant immunosuppressive therapy in suppressing the formation of antibodies to infliximab in Crohn disease. Gut 2007;56(9):1226–31.

46. Lichtenstein GR, Diamond RH, Wagner CL, et al. Benefits and risks of immunomodulators and maintenance infliximab for IBD: subgroup analyses across four randomized trials. Aliment Pharmacol Ther 2009;30(3):210–26.

47. Westhovens R, Yocum D, Han J, et al. The safety of infliximab, combined with background treatments, among patients with rheumatoid arthritis and various comorbidities: a large, randomized, placebo-controlled trial. Arthritis Rheum 2006;54(4):1075–86.

48. Randomised trial comparing tacrolimus (FK506) and cyclosporin in prevention of liver allograft rejection. European FK506 Multicentre Liver Study Group. Lancet 1994;344(8920):423–8.

49. Arts J, D'Haens G, Zeegers M, et al. Long-term outcome of treatment with intravenous cyclosporin in patients with severe ulcerative colitis. Inflamm Bowel Dis 2004;10(2):73–8.

50. Maser EA, Deconda D, Lichtiger S, et al. Cyclosporine and infliximab as rescue therapy for each other in patients with steroid-refractory ulcerative colitis. Clin Gastroenterol Hepatol 2008;6(10):1112–6.

51. Natalizumab: AN 100226, anti-4alpha integrin monoclonal antibody. Drugs R D 2004;5(2):102–7.

52. Sandborn WJ, Colombel JF, Enns R, et al. Natalizumab induction and maintenance therapy for Crohn disease. N Engl J Med 2005;353(18):1912–25.

53. Ghosh S, Goldin E, Gordon FH, et al. Natalizumab for active Crohn disease. N Engl J Med 2003;348(1):24–32.

54. Gordon FH, Hamilton MI, Donoghue S, et al. A pilot study of treatment of active ulcerative colitis with natalizumab, a humanized monoclonal antibody to alpha-4 integrin. Aliment Pharmacol Ther 2002;16(4):699–705.

55. Gordon FH, Lai CW, Hamilton MI, et al. A randomized placebo-controlled trial of a humanized monoclonal antibody to alpha4 integrin in active Crohn disease. Gastroenterology 2001;121(2):268–74.

56. Van Assche G, Van Ranst M, Sciot R, et al. Progressive multifocal leukoencephalopathy after natalizumab therapy for Crohn disease. N Engl J Med 2005;353(4):362–8.

57. Kleinschmidt-DeMasters BK, Tyler KL. Progressive multifocal leukoencephalopathy complicating treatment with natalizumab and interferon beta-1a for multiple sclerosis. N Engl J Med 2005;353(4):369–74.

58. Langer-Gould A, Atlas SW, Green AJ, et al. Progressive multifocal leukoencephalopathy in a patient treated with natalizumab. N Engl J Med 2005;353(4):375–81.

59. Tysabri update. Available at: http://www.biogenidec.com/site/tysabri-information-center.html. Accessed June 9, 2009.

60. Subramanian V, Saxena S, Kang JY, et al. Preoperative steroid use and risk of postoperative complications in patients with inflammatory bowel disease undergoing abdominal surgery. Am J Gastroenterol 2008;103(9):2373–81.

61. Aberra FN, Lewis JD, Hass D, et al. Corticosteroids and immunomodulators: postoperative infectious complication risk in inflammatory bowel disease patients. Gastroenterology 2003;125(2):320–7.

62. Colombel JF, Loftus EV Jr, Tremaine WJ, et al. Early postoperative complications are not increased in patients with Crohn disease treated perioperatively with infliximab or immunosuppressive therapy. Am J Gastroenterol 2004; 99(5):878–83.

63. Mahadevan U, Loftus EV Jr, Tremaine WJ, et al. Azathioprine or 6-mercaptopurine before colectomy for ulcerative colitis is not associated with increased postoperative complications. Inflamm Bowel Dis 2002;8(5):311–6.

64. Ferrante M, D'Hoore A, Vermeire S, et al. Corticosteroids but not infliximab increase short-term postoperative infectious complications in patients with ulcerative colitis. Inflamm Bowel Dis 2009;15(7):1062–70.

65. Kunitake H, Hodin R, Shellito PC, et al. Perioperative treatment with infliximab in patients with Crohn disease and ulcerative colitis is not associated with an increased rate of postoperative complications. J Gastrointest Surg 2008; 12(10):1730–6 [discussion: 1736–7].

66. Marchal L, D'Haens G, Van Assche G, et al. The risk of post-operative complications associated with infliximab therapy for Crohn disease: a controlled cohort study. Aliment Pharmacol Ther 2004;19(7):749–54.

67. Schluender SJ, Ippoliti A, Dubinsky M, et al. Does infliximab influence surgical morbidity of ileal pouch-anal anastomosis in patients with ulcerative colitis? Dis Colon Rectum 2007;50(11):1747–53.

68. Selvasekar CR, Cima RR, Larson DW, et al. Effect of infliximab on short-term complications in patients undergoing operation for chronic ulcerative colitis. J Am Coll Surg 2007;204(5):956–62 [discussion: 962–3].

69. Mor IJ, Vogel JD, da Luz Moreira A, et al. Infliximab in ulcerative colitis is associated with an increased risk of postoperative complications after restorative proctocolectomy. Dis Colon Rectum 2008;51(8):1202–7 [discussion: 1207–10].

70. Swoger JM, Loftus EV Jr, Pardi DS, et al. Pre-operative infliximab exposure and the occurrence of post-operative complications following proctocolectomy and ileal pouch-anal anastomosis (IPAA) for ulcerative colitis [abstract]. Gastroenterology 2009;136:A188.

71. Aberra FN, Stettler N, Brensinger C, et al. Risk for active tuberculosis in inflammatory bowel disease patients. Clin Gastroenterol Hepatol 2007;5(9):1070–5.

72. Gardam MA, Keystone EC, Menzies R, et al. Anti-tumour necrosis factor agents and tuberculosis risk: mechanisms of action and clinical management. Lancet Infect Dis 2003;3(3):148–55.

73. Gomez-Reino JJ, Carmona L, Valverde VR, et al. Treatment of rheumatoid arthritis with tumor necrosis factor inhibitors may predispose to significant increase in tuberculosis risk: a multicenter active-surveillance report. Arthritis Rheum 2003;48(8):2122–7.

74. Askling J, Fored CM, Brandt L, et al. Risk and case characteristics of tuberculosis in rheumatoid arthritis associated with tumor necrosis factor antagonists in Sweden. Arthritis Rheum 2005;52(7):1986–92.

75. Wolfe F, Michaud K, Anderson J, et al. Tuberculosis infection in patients with rheumatoid arthritis and the effect of infliximab therapy. Arthritis Rheum 2004; 50(2):372–9.

76. Keane J, Gershon S, Wise RP, et al. Tuberculosis associated with infliximab, a tumor necrosis factor alpha-neutralizing agent. N Engl J Med 2001;345(15): 1098–104.

77. Sichletidis L, Settas L, Spyratos D, et al. Tuberculosis in patients receiving anti-TNF agents despite chemoprophylaxis. Int J Tuberc Lung Dis 2006;10(10): 1127–32.

78. Rahier JF, Ben-Horin S, Chowers Y, et al. European evidence-based consensus on the prevention, diagnosis and management of opportunistic infections in inflammatory bowel disease. J Crohn Colitis 2009, doi:10.1016/j.crohns.2009.02.010.

79. British Thoracic Society Standards of Care Committee. BTS recommendations for assessing risk and for managing *Mycobacterium tuberculosis* infection and disease in patients due to start anti-TNF-alpha treatment. Thorax 2005; 60:800–5.

80. Theis VS, Rhodes JM. Review article: minimizing tuberculosis during anti-tumour necrosis factor-alpha treatment of inflammatory bowel disease. Aliment Pharmacol Ther 2008;27:19–30.

81. Wallis RS, Broder MS, Wong JY, et al. Granulomatous infectious diseases associated with tumor necrosis factor antagonists. Clin Infect Dis 2004; 38(9):1261–5.

82. Gluck T, Linde HJ, Scholmerich J, et al. Anti-tumor necrosis factor therapy and *Listeria monocytogenes* infection: report of two cases. Arthritis Rheum 2002; 46(8):2255–7 [author reply 2257].

83. Kamath BM, Mamula P, Baldassano RN, et al. Listeria meningitis after treatment with infliximab. J Pediatr Gastroenterol Nutr 2002;34(4):410–2.

84. Slifman NR, Gershon SK, Lee JH, et al. Listeria monocytogenes infection as a complication of treatment with tumor necrosis factor alpha-neutralizing agents. Arthritis Rheum 2003;48(2):319–24.

85. Singh SM, Rau NV, Cohen LB, et al. Cutaneous nocardiosis complicating management of Crohn disease with infliximab and prednisone. CMAJ 2004; 171(9):1063–4.

86. Kaur N, Mahl TC. *Pneumocystis jiroveci (carinii)* pneumonia after infliximab therapy: a review of 84 cases. Dig Dis Sci 2007;52(6):1481–4.

87. Khatchatourian M, Seaton TL. An unusual complication of immunosuppressive therapy in inflammatory bowel disease. Am J Gastroenterol 1997;92(9): 1558–60.

88. Takenaka R, Okada H, Mizuno M, et al. *Pneumocystis carinii* pneumonia in patients with ulcerative colitis. J Gastroenterol 2004;39(11):1114–5.

89. Smith MB, Hanauer SB. *Pneumocystis carinii* pneumonia during cyclosporine therapy for ulcerative colitis. N Engl J Med 1992;327(7):497–8.

90. Quan VA, Saunders BP, Hicks BH, et al. Cyclosporin treatment for ulcerative colitis complicated by fatal *Pneumocystis carinii* pneumonia. BMJ 1997; 314(7077):363–4.

91. Seddik M, Meliez H, Seguy D, et al. *Pneumocystis jiroveci (carinii)* pneumonia following initiation of infliximab and azathioprine therapy in a patient with Crohn disease. Inflamm Bowel Dis 2004;10(4):436–7.

92. Tai TL, O'Rourke KP, McWeeney M, et al. *Pneumocystis carinii* pneumonia following a second infusion of infliximab. Rheumatology (Oxford) 2002;41(8): 951–2.

93. Velayos FS, Sandborn WJ. *Pneumocystis carinii* pneumonia during maintenance anti-tumor necrosis factor-alpha therapy with infliximab for Crohn sdisease. Inflamm Bowel Dis 2004;10(5):657–60.

94. Harigai M, Koike R, Miyasaka N. Pneumocystis pneumonia associated with infliximab in Japan. N Engl J Med 2007;357(18):1874–6.

95. Lee JH, Slifman NR, Gershon SK, et al. Life-threatening histoplasmosis complicating immunotherapy with tumor necrosis factor alpha antagonists infliximab and etanercept. Arthritis Rheum 2002;46(10):2565–70.

96. Wood KL, Hage CA, Knox KS, et al. Histoplasmosis after treatment with antitumor necrosis factor-alpha therapy. Am J Respir Crit Care Med 2003;167(9):1279–82.

97. Food and drug administration Medwatch. Available at: http://www.fda.gov/cder/drug/InfoSheets/HCP/TNF_blockersHCP.htm. Accessed June 9, 2009.

98. Bergstrom L, Yocum DE, Ampel NM, et al. Increased risk of coccidioidomycosis in patients treated with tumor necrosis factor alpha antagonists. Arthritis Rheum 2004;50(6):1959–66.

99. Belda A, Hinojosa J, Serra B, et al. [Systemic candidiasis and infliximab therapy]. Gastroenterol Hepatol 2004;27(6):365–7 [in Spanish].

100. De Rosa FG, Shaz D, Campagna AC, et al. Invasive pulmonary aspergillosis soon after therapy with infliximab, a tumor necrosis factor-alpha-neutralizing antibody: a possible healthcare-associated case? Infect Control Hosp Epidemiol 2003;24(7):477–82.

101. Gottlieb GS, Lesser CF, Holmes KK, et al. Disseminated sporotrichosis associated with treatment with immunosuppressants and tumor necrosis factor-alpha antagonists. Clin Infect Dis 2003;37(6):838–40.

102. van der Klooster JM, Bosman RJ, Oudemans-van Straaten HM, et al. Disseminated tuberculosis, pulmonary aspergillosis and cutaneous herpes simplex infection in a patient with infliximab and methotrexate. Intensive Care Med 2003;29(12):2327–9.

103. del Valle Garcia-Sanchez M, Gomez-Camacho F, Poyato-Gonzalez A, et al. Infliximab therapy in a patient with Crohn disease and chronic hepatitis B virus infection. Inflamm Bowel Dis 2004;10(5):701–2.

104. Millonig G, Kern M, Ludwiczek O, et al. Subfulminant hepatitis B after infliximab in Crohn disease: need for HBV-screening? World J Gastroenterol 2006;12(6):974–6.

105. Cheng AL, Hsiung CA, Su IJ, et al. Steroid-free chemotherapy decreases risk of hepatitis B virus (HBV) reactivation in HBV-carriers with lymphoma. Hepatology 2003;37(6):1320–8.

106. Lok AS, McMahon BJ. Chronic hepatitis B. Hepatology 2007;45(2):507–39.

107. Cepeda EJ, Williams FM, Ishimori ML, et al. The use of anti-tumour necrosis factor therapy in HIV-positive individuals with rheumatic disease. Ann Rheum Dis 2008;67(5):710–2.

108. Kaur PP, Chan VC, Berney SN. Successful etanercept use in an HIV-positive patient with rheumatoid arthritis. J Clin Rheumatol 2007;13(2):79–80.

109. Wallis RS, Kyambadde P, Johnson JL, et al. A study of the safety, immunology, virology, and microbiology of adjunctive etanercept in HIV-1-associated tuberculosis. AIDS 2004;18(2):257–64.

110. Markowitz LE, Dunne EF, Saraiya M, et al. Quadrivalent human papillomavirus vaccine: recommendations of the Advisory Committee on Immunization Practices (ACIP). MMWR Recomm Rep 2007;56(RR-2):1–24.

111. Advisory Committee on Immunization Practices. Recommended adult immunization schedule: United States, 2009. Ann Intern Med 2009;150(1):40–4.

112. Saag KG, Koehnke R, Caldwell JR, et al. Low dose long-term corticosteroid therapy in rheumatoid arthritis: an analysis of serious adverse events. Am J Med 1994;96(2):115–23.
113. Bargallo A, Carrion S, Domenech E, et al. [Infectious mononucleosis in patients with inflammatory bowel disease under treatment with azathioprine]. Gastroenterol Hepatol 2008;31(5):289–92 [in Spanish].
114. Reijasse D, Le Pendeven C, Cosnes J, et al. Epstein-Barr virus viral load in Crohn disease: effect of immunosuppressive therapy. Inflamm Bowel Dis 2004;10(2):85–90.
115. Haerter G, Manfras BJ, de Jong-Hesse Y, et al. Cytomegalovirus retinitis in a patient treated with anti-tumor necrosis factor alpha antibody therapy for rheumatoid arthritis. Clin Infect Dis 2004;39(9):e88–94.
116. Helbling D, Breitbach TH, Krause M. Disseminated cytomegalovirus infection in Crohn disease following anti-tumour necrosis factor therapy. Eur J Gastroenterol Hepatol 2002;14(12):1393–5.
117. Kandiel A, Lashner B. Cytomegalovirus colitis complicating inflammatory bowel disease. Am J Gastroenterol 2006;101(12):2857–65.
118. Papadakis KA, Tung JK, Binder SW, et al. Outcome of cytomegalovirus infections in patients with inflammatory bowel disease. Am J Gastroenterol 2001; 96(7):2137–42.
119. Sands BE, Anderson FH, Bernstein CN, et al. Infliximab maintenance therapy for fistulizing Crohn disease. N Engl J Med 2004;350(9):876–85.
120. Torre-Cisneros J, Del Castillo M, Caston JJ, et al. Infliximab does not activate replication of lymphotropic herpesviruses in patients with refractory rheumatoid arthritis. Rheumatology (Oxford) 2005;44(9):1132–5.

Clostridium Difficile and Inflammatory Bowel Disease

Ashwin N. Ananthakrishnan, MD, MPH[a], Mazen Issa, MD[a],
David G. Binion, MD[b],*

KEYWORDS

- *Clostridium difficile* • Inflammatory bowel disease
- Crohn disease • Ulcerative colitis • Colectomy

The past decade has seen an alarming increase in the burden of disease associated with *Clostridium difficile*.[1–4] Studies from North America have demonstrated a doubling of incidence during this time period.[3,4] The estimated economic costs associated with *C difficile* infection (CDI) range from $436 million to $3 billion in the United States annually.[5,6] Initially considered to play a key role in the development of antibiotic-associated pseudomembranous colitis,[7] *C difficile* is now known to cause a wide range of disease presentations ranging from asymptomatic carriage to fulminant colitis, toxic megacolon, sepsis, multiorgan failure, and death. Recent antibiotic exposure or hospitalization were previously considered key in the acquisition of CDI but recent data suggest an increasing number of CDI not associated with antibiotic use and infections being acquired in the community.

Inflammatory bowel diseases (IBD; Crohn disease [CD], ulcerative colitis [UC]) are chronic, lifelong, immunologically mediated inflammatory disorders of the gut that present typically with symptoms of abdominal pain, diarrhea, or rectal bleeding.[8] Several studies have now demonstrated an increasing incidence of CDI in patients with IBD with a more severe course of disease compared with the non-IBD population.[9–14] The similarity in symptoms between the two conditions (CDI and an IBD flare) but markedly divergent treatment plans (specific-antibiotic therapy and potential reduction of immunosuppression for CDI in the setting of IBD compared with escalation of immunosuppressive therapy for an IBD flare) makes it essential for treating physicians to be aware of the impact of CDI on patients with IBD, have a high index

This article originally appeared in *Gastroenterology Clinics of North America*, Volume 38, issue 4.
[a] Division of Gastroenterology and Hepatology, Medical College of Wisconsin, Milwaukee, WI, USA
[b] Division of Gastroenterology, Hepatology and Nutrition, University of Pittsburgh School of Medicine, UPMC IBD Center, Mezzanine Level C Wing, 200 Lothrop Street, Pittsburgh, PA 15226, USA
* Corresponding author.
E-mail address: binion@pitt.edu (D.G. Binion).

Med Clin N Am 94 (2010) 135–153
doi:10.1016/j.mcna.2009.08.013

of suspicion, and institute early diagnostic testing and appropriate therapy to ensure optimal outcomes.

This article summarizes the available literature on the impact of CDI on IBD and discusses the various diagnostic testing and treatment options available. Also reviewed are clinical situations that may be specific to patients with IBD that are important for the treating physician to recognize.

PATHOGENESIS OF CDI

Clostridium difficile is a gram-positive spore-forming anaerobe that exerts its effect on tissue through active toxin production. There are two toxins associated with *C difficile* (toxin A and toxin B), which are coded by the *tcd A* and *tcd B* genes, respectively.[15,16] These loci are located on a 19.6-kg base locus, the pathogenicity locus. The toxins act by binding to receptors on the enterocyte with subsequent endocytosis. This leads to pore formation, which further facilitates intracellular entry of the toxins. This is followed by glycosylation of Rho and Ras proteins leading to disruption of the epithelial cytoskeleton. As a result, there is loosening of the intercellular tight junction, increasing secretory losses, and voluminous diarrhea.[15–22] In addition, toxin A also exerts a cytotoxic effect. Although most of the strains causing CDI produce both toxins A and B, a small fraction of CDI is caused by strains that either produce toxin A (11% of infections) or toxin B alone (7% of infections).[23,24] Up to six other toxins are produced by *C difficile*. Important among these is a recently identified toxin, the binary toxin,[25–27] which may be associated with more severe disease. The exact role of the binary toxin in the pathogenesis of CDI has not yet been defined.

NAP1/027 Epidemic Strain of Clostridium difficile

Between 2002 and 2005, outbreaks of CDI were identified in the province of Quebec, Canada.[4] The strain of *C difficile* associated with these outbreaks demonstrated greater virulence than previously described strains. Over 150 ribotypes of CDI have been described so far. This epidemic strain of hypervirulent *C difficile* was identified to be the BI/NAP1/027 strain (restriction-endonuclease analysis group BI; pulsed-field gel electrophoresis type NAP1 [North American pulsed-field gel electrophoresis type 1]; and polymerase chain reaction ribotype 027).[28,29] This strain carries the binary toxin in addition to producing 16 times the amount of toxin A and 23 times the amount of toxin B compared with typical strains.[30] This epidemic strain has also been identified subsequently from several countries, forming an increasingly important cause of regional outbreaks of *C difficile*. The specific impact of this epidemic strain on patients with IBD is still unknown. Bossuyt and colleagues[10] in examining the rising IBD-associated CDI in their institution did not find it to be disproportionately caused by the epidemic strain, but did not describe a prevalence of BI/NAP/027 ribotype among all their cases of CDI.

PREVALENCE OF CDI IN PATIENTS WITH IBD

Two decades ago *C difficile* was believed to be an infrequent infectious complication in patients with IBD. More recent reports have noted higher rates of infection, however, but more importantly, a rising temporal trend in CDI complicating the course of patients with IBD across several institutions and study populations.[9–11,13,14] Rodemann and colleagues[14] in a single center retrospective study identified a doubling of the incidence of CDI in patients with CD (from 9.5 to 22.3 per 1000 admissions) and a tripling in incidence among UC patients (from 18.4 to 57.6 per 1000 admissions) from 1998 to 2004. At the Medical College of Wisconsin, the authors identified a similar rise in the proportion of *C difficile* cases complicating IBD from 1.8% in 2004 to 4.6% in 2005.[11] The data from these single-center reports have been corroborated by larger studies using nationwide representative hospitalization population sampling in the United States.[9,13] In a study using the Agency for Healthcare Research and Quality's Nationwide Inpatient Sample from the United States, Ananthakrishnan and colleagues[9] identified similar increases in CDI complicating hospitalization for IBD occurring nationally (UC, from 24 per 1000 to 39 per 1000; CD, from 8 per 1000 to 12 per 1000) between 1998 and 2004. Extending this study to 2006 reveals a continuing increase in the proportion of IBD hospitalizations being complicated by CDI (**Fig. 1**). The similar frequency estimates in the previously mentioned single-center and national studies suggest that the issue of CDI complicating hospitalizations in patients with IBD is widespread and not restricted to specific hospitals, tertiary referral centers, or regions within the United States.

Although these studies used the entire United States inpatient IBD cohort as the denominator in calculating the rates of infection, the frequency of *C difficile* complicating disease course in IBD patients who present with typical symptoms of colitis or disease flare, such as diarrhea and rectal bleeding, is much higher. Early reports found CDI infrequently in this population. Rolny and colleagues[31] identified *C difficile* in only 5% of patients admitted for a flare. Subsequent reports placed the frequency of CDI between 5% and 18% among patients presenting with disease flare.[32–35] More recently, among 99 patients who were admitted to Mount Sinai hospital with symptoms of a UC flare and had stool testing for *C difficile* toxin, 47% were positive, emphasizing the importance of a having a high index of suspicion for CDI in IBD patients presenting with typical symptoms.[12] Adult IBD patients are not the only cohort impacted by *C difficile*. A recent study from Italy identified *C difficile* in 24.7% of patients with diarrhea or abdominal pain from within their pediatric IBD cohort.[36] Although most studies on *C difficile* in IBD have focused on the hospitalized population, the prevalence of *C difficile* identified through stool culture was as high as 8.2% in an asymptomatic outpatient IBD cohort.[37] Whether this represents asymptomatic

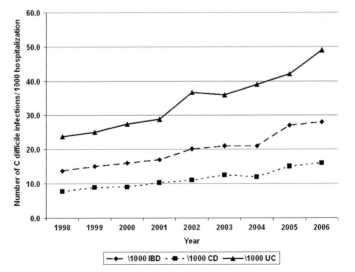

Fig. 1. Trends in *Clostridium difficile* infection complicating hospitalizations in patients with inflammatory bowel disease in the United States. *Data from* the Nationwide Inpatient Sample 1998–2006.

colonization or has true disease-modifying effect by affecting the future disease course of IBD is still unclear. The rising frequency of CDI complicating IBD has paralleled the alarming increases in *C difficile* seen in the non-IBD population. In some institutions, the rate of increase of *C difficile* in the younger, healthier patients with IBD has outpaced that in the older non-IBD population with a greater comorbid burden, a traditionally higher-risk cohort.

RISK FACTORS FOR CDI
Environmental Risk Factors

Environmental exposure is the most common route of acquisition of CDI, which is frequently the result of person-to-person transfer of infectious spores.[15,38,39] Exposure to a health care environment including recent hospitalizations increases the risk for nosocomial acquisition of CDI, the most common source of infection. Health care personnel are both at a greater risk for acquisition of infection and potentially transferring infection between patients if appropriate infection control measures are not followed.

Prior antibiotic exposure remains a key risk factor for the acquisition and development of CDI.[38,40–42] Emerging data suggest, however, it no longer remains the only or even a necessary risk factor.[43] Clindamycin was the antibiotic initially associated with CDI[7] but since then multiple other antibiotics have been identified to confer a higher risk for CDI. These more commonly include broad-spectrum antibiotics, particularly fluoroquinolones,[44,45] but the risk is not restricted to any specific antibiotic class. *C difficile* has even been described during the use of such antibiotics as vancomycin and metronidazole,[46] agents typically used to treat CDI. The mechanism through which antibiotic use seems to increase the risk for CDI may be through the disruption of the normal intestinal flora and a subsequent proliferation of *C difficile*, a more resistant organism.[39] Antibiotic use seems to be less essential for development of CDI in the IBD population. Antibiotic use within 3 months before CDI was seen in only 40% of IBD patients compared with 69% in the non-IBD population in one study,[10] whereas another study was not able to identify any recent antibiotic exposure in 39% of IBD patients developing *C difficile*.[11]

Immunosuppression is another well-recognized risk factor for acquisition of *C difficile* with greater frequency of CDI recognized in cancer patients undergoing chemotherapy or patients with organ transplantation on immunosuppression.[38,39] Being chronic immunologically mediated inflammatory diseases, both CD and UC require long-term immunosuppressive therapy in a significant proportion of patients. Issa and colleagues[11] identified maintenance immunosuppression to be associated with twofold risk of CDI (odds ratio [OR] 2.58; 95% confidence interval [CI], 1.28–5.12), a finding corroborated by a second study from Belgium.[10] One other study failed to demonstrate this association, but may have been limited by a small sample size.[36] Aminosalicylates (5-aminosalicylic acid compounds, such as mesalamine) have not been associated with CDI.

Other potential offending drugs that have been proposed include gastric acid suppressive therapy, such as with proton pump inhibitors.[43,47] Some initial studies demonstrated a higher risk of development of CDI with proton pump inhibitor therapy but this finding has not been universally demonstrated. Recent studies of CDI in IBD populations also did not confirm this association of proton pump inhibitors with CDI.[10,48]

Nosocomial or health care associated–infection is the most common modality of acquisition of CDI. Several recent studies in IBD population have shown, however, that a significant proportion of CDI in this cohort is community acquired.[14] Lack of recent health care environment should also not deter the treating physician from suspecting CDI.

Host Risk Factors

Increasing age and greater comorbid burden increase the risk of CDI in the IBD and non-IBD populations.[15,38–40,49] IBD patients who develop CDI tend to be younger, however, than the corresponding non-IBD population who develop CDI. Nguyen and colleagues[13] from an analysis of the Nationwide Inpatient Sample demonstrated a 13% greater risk of CDI with each 1 point increase in the Charlson's comorbidity burden index. In addition to immunosuppressive medication, host immunity may play a role in determining susceptibility to CDI with patients who are able to mount a greater antibody response against the toxin being less likely to develop overt disease.[50,51]

IBD-specific Risk Factors for CDI

Recent studies have shown that underlying IBD itself seems to be a risk factor for the development of CDI. Among IBD patients, involvement of the colon (compared with small bowel disease) seems to be a risk factor for CDI.[11,13,52] Several studies have documented a greater rate of *C difficile* complicating UC compared with CD.[9] Issa and colleagues[11] identified colonic involvement in nearly 93% of IBD patients with CDI; on multivariate analysis, colonic disease conferred threefold greater risk (OR 3.12; 95% CI, 1.28–5.12) for CDI. Among CD, patients within colonic involvement seem to be at a greater risk for CDI than those with isolated small bowel disease.[13] Also, among the subgroup of patients with colonic disease, left-sided or pancolonic involvement is more frequently complicated with CDI than those with limited colonic involvement.[52] This suggests that extent of colonic disease may also be an additional risk factor. Patients with a greater disease activity may also be at a higher risk for CDI.[36] Whether this elevated risk in colonic IBD is attributable to the extent of disruption of the mucosal barrier, alteration in gut flora, or other mechanisms has not yet been well defined. Because most studies on this topic have been retrospective, it has been difficult to tease out whether these associations represent true causation and are risk factors, or actually represent a consequence of the CDI complicating IBD. Further prospective studies are essential to identify if there are any IBD-specific risk factors that may increase the risk for CDI.

CLINICAL FEATURES
Symptoms and Signs

CDI typically presents with symptoms of diarrhea, lower abdominal pain, and tenderness. Although CDI itself presents with voluminous, watery diarrhea without gross blood or mucous, in the setting of underlying active IBD colitis overt rectal bleeding may not be infrequent.[15,38] Patients may also have systemic symptoms, such as fever, malaise, and anorexia, and in the right setting these symptoms should raise suspicion for *C difficile* in the absence of an alternative explanation, even if diarrhea is not a prominent symptom. Laboratory evaluation may reveal leukocystosis with left shift; anemia (caused by bleeding or chronic inflammation); or hypoalbuminemia. Stool microscopy can reveal the presence of polymorphonuclear leukocytes and is also essential to rule out other bacterial or parasitic causes of diarrhea.

The frequency and impact of asymptomatic carriage of *C difficile* in patients with IBD remains under investigation. Between 1% and 4% of healthy adults may carry *C difficile*.[15] In a study of 122 outpatients with quiescent, mild IBD not on immunosuppression, Clayton and colleagues[37] identified asymptomatic carriage of C difficile (by stool culture) in 8.2% of the cohort; this was statistically higher than the rate in their control population of healthy volunteers. They identified no clinically evident CDI during a follow-up of 6 months, but whether the same lack of clinical CDI holds true in patients with greater severity of underlying IBD including those on maintenance immunomodulatory or biologic therapy has not yet been defined and merits future investigation.

Radiologic Evaluation

Radiologic evaluation is not required in most patients with CDI but it can be an important tool to aid in the assessment of complications of severe CDI.[38,39] Plain abdominal radiography or abdominal CT scans may demonstrate colonic dilatation, wall thickening, or overt perforation and free air in those with complications or severe CDI, with CT scans being the more sensitive of the two modalities. Abdominal imaging can also help in the diagnosis of toxic megacolon or reveal alternative etiology to the patients' symptoms, such as partial small bowel obstruction or internal penetrating disease.

Endoscopy

Lower gastrointestinal endoscopic evaluation is a key modality for assessment of CDI. The classic endoscopic appearance of CDI, described in about 50% of patients,[53,54] is the pseudomembrane formation caused by sloughing and necrosis of the mucosa with ulceration. Histologic examination of this pseudomembrane may reveal a "volcano" lesion, focal ulceration with an eruption of necrotic debris and inflammatory cell infiltrate through the area of ulceration. The use of endoscopy in differentiating active colitis related to IBD from CDI has remained disappointing, however, because of the lack of typical features of pseudomembranous colitis in many patients with CDI associated with IBD. Both Issa and colleagues[11] and Bossuyt and colleagues[10] identified no pseudomembranes in any of the IBD patients with CDI who underwent endoscopic evaluation. In the right clinical scenario, the absence of pseudomembranes on lower gastrointestinal endoscopy should not deter the treating clinician from entertaining the diagnosis of CDI in IBD patients. Given the low discriminatory power of endoscopy in distinguishing active IBD colitis from CDI, the authors do not tend to evaluate patients endoscopically solely for the purpose of diagnosis CDI. In patients with fulminant disease, endoscopic evaluation may help objectively assess disease activity and look for other complicating infections, such as cytomegalovirus colitis. In this situation, the authors also obtain stool samples for C difficile toxin testing using suction and a collection trap.

DIAGNOSIS OF CDI

The diagnosis of CDI relies on the demonstration of the organism by stool culture or the identification of the toxins in the stool.[38,39,54] The most commonly performed and widely available test for C difficile is the stool ELISA for toxins A and B. Although the first-generation ELISA tests detected only toxin A, more recent ELISA tests detect both toxins. This has improved sensitivity because in a small group of patients, CDI is caused by strains producing only toxin B. A minimum of 100 to 1000 pg of either toxin is required for detection by ELISA. The false-negative rate is between 10% and 20% with some studies demonstrating sensitivity as low as 66%.[15,18,38]

Stool culture is the most sensitive method for the identification of C difficile and is the gold standard but fails to differentiate toxin-producing from nontoxigenic strains.[38]

It requires additional testing for toxins A and B with either cell cytotoxicity assays or ELISA. In addition, it has a prolonged turnaround time of 48 hours and is not widely available. Stool cultures have the advantage of allowing for antibiotic susceptibility testing and molecular typing (especially in outbreak investigations). Cell cytotoxicity assays have sensitivity and specificity approaching 98% and detect much lower levels of toxin than the ELISA.[38] Similar to stool culture, however, they too require significant laboratory support and have a turnaround time of 24 to 48 hours precluding their wide-spread adoption in routine clinical practice.

It is also important for the treating clinician to recognize the need for testing of multiple consecutive samples because a single sample, particularly with ELISA, may fail to have adequate sensitivity to diagnose CDI.[15] In the authors' experience, the initial stool ELISA for toxins A and B identified only 54% of cases with the second, third, and fourth specimens identifying 75%, 78%, and 92% of cases, respectively.[11]

COMPLICATIONS AND OUTCOMES
Short-term Outcomes

Important and life-threatening complications of CDI include toxic megacolon, colonic perforation, and peritonitis with sepsis. Complicating the clinical picture, many patients who acquire CDI may do so during prolonged hospital stays and have significant underlying comorbid illness, contributing to the higher risk of death associated with CDI.

There are now several single-center and nationwide studies defining the short-term impact of CDI on patients with IBD. Although some studies found shorter hospital stays related to CDI in IBD compared with non-IBD patients,[10] in contrast other studies found similar[12] or longer duration of hospitalization[9,11] among IBD patients with CDI compared with those with isolated CDI or IBD-related hospitalizations. In one study, CDI-IBD was associated with a 3-day longer hospital stay compared with IBD hospitalizations not complicated by *C difficile* (3 days; 95% CI, 2.3–3.7 days) and $11,406 higher adjusted hospitalization charges.[9]

Studies have reported varying rates of colectomy for CDI in the setting of IBD. One study reported low rates for urgent or semiurgent colectomy after CDI (1 of 15 patients).[10] Jodorkovsky and colleagues,[12] however, found a 23% rate of emergent colectomy in their CDI-UC population with the indications being toxic complications (4 of 11) or medically refractory disease (7 of 11). This rate was higher than in the *C difficile*–negative IBD population. In the authors' center, the rate of colectomy in hospitalized IBD patients with CDI was similarly high at 45% in 2004, but decreased to 25% in 2005 despite similar rates of requirements for hospitalization.[11] Analysis of the nationwide inpatient sample corroborated these single-center studies demonstrating that underlying IBD was associated with sixfold (OR 6.6; 95% CI, 4.7–9.3) greater risk of bowel surgery compared with patients with CDI without underlying IBD.[9]

Long-term Outcomes

Despite this information on the short-term outcomes of IBD patients with CDI, there are far more limited data on the long-term outcomes following CDI in IBD patients. A report from Mount Sinai hospital demonstrated worse outcomes in IBD patients with associated CDI for as long as 1 year after the initial infection, although this study was limited by its inability to tease out recurrent CDI versus a true change in the behavior of underlying IBD.[12] In the previously mentioned study, UC patients with CDI had a significantly higher number of hospitalizations for UC-related causes (58 vs 27; P = .001) or emergency room visits at 1 year following the initial hospitalization for *C difficile*. They also had a twofold (OR 2.38; 95% CI, 1.01–5.6) higher risk for colectomy at 1 year. At the authors' institution, they performed a case-control study comparing the disease course for 1 year before and 1 year after the initial infection in 81 patients with IBD who developed *C difficile*.[55] They found that the mean difference in hospitalizations between the year prior and the year following CDI was 0.89 (95% CI, 0.51–1.27). Forty patients (46%) had at least one more hospitalization in the year following *C difficile* infection (range 1–9) compared with the year prior. Over half the patients with IBD and CDI required an escalation in the medical therapy for IBD after treatment of *C difficile* (46 patients, 52.9%). This included new initiation of biologic therapy (23 patients); escalation of current biologic (seven patients); escalation or initiation of azathioprine and 6-MP (10 patients); or methotrexate (six patients). There were 10 documented cases of recurrent *C difficile* documented by positive toxin assay in this cohort.

The limitations of these retrospective studies remain, however, specifically in teasing out if underlying disease severity is a confounding factor, predisposing to these worse outcomes. It remains undefined whether more severe IBD is associated with acquisition of *C difficile* and subsequent CDI, although the study by Issa and colleagues[11] indirectly suggested that the use of maintenance immunosuppression and potentially more severe illness was associated with the development of CDI. Likewise, it is unknown if CDI itself truly exerts a disease-modifying effect in patients with IBD.

TREATMENT
General Measures

Entertaining a high suspicion for *C difficile* and initiating early and appropriate testing is essential in the management of CDI. Infection control measures, such as hand washing and contact isolation for hospitalized patients, help in preventing patient-to-patient transfer of infection and prevent transfer through health care providers.[15,39] Among patients who develop CDI in the setting of antibiotic use, a small proportion (10%–20%) may respond completely simply with the cessation of the offending antibiotic.[15,56] Bossuyt and colleagues[10] found that in 18% of IBD patients with CDI, this approach resulted in resolution of symptoms. Most patients, however, require specific directed antimicrobial therapy in addition to the previously mentioned steps.

MEDICAL THERAPY
Metronidazole

Metronidazole has historically been the first choice for the treatment of CDI, including infection in the setting of IBD. Despite the lack of Food and Drug Administration approval for this indication, several small randomized controlled trials have demonstrated success rates with metronidazole in the range of 75% to 90% and it remains a widely used antibiotic for treatment of CDI.[15,39,42,57,58] Guidelines from the Infectious Disease Society of America recommend a dose of 500 mg orally three times daily for 10 days. In patients unable to take oral agents, metronidazole is also the only agent that can be administered intravenously (in doses of 500 mg four times daily) and attain sufficient concentration in the colon following biliary excretion for the treatment of CDI. Metronidazole also offers several advantages over vancomycin, namely a lower cost and less likelihood for the development and spread of vancomycin-resistant enterococci. Peripheral neuropathy, pancreatitis, and gastrointestinal side effects, however, including a metallic taste are not uncommon with metronidazole and limit its tolerability.

More recently, other important concerns have arisen regarding the use of metronidazole and its use in CDI.[59] Failure rates before the emergence of the epidemic *C difficile* BI/NAP1/027 strain were 16%, but more recent failure rates are alarmingly high at 35%.[57,60] Although it has efficacy comparable with vancomycin in the treatment of mild *C difficile*–associated diarrhea, it is inferior for severe *C difficile*–associated diarrhea[61] and should not be used as first-line therapy in such circumstances. This is an important consideration for hospitalized IBD patients, who face a double challenge of infection and concomitant exacerbation of their idiopathic inflammatory colitis. Its efficacy specifically in the IBD population with CDI is unknown, but one study reported that just less than one quarter of the IBD patients with CDI required to be initiated on oral vancomycin because of lack of sufficient response with metronidazole.[10]

Vancomycin

The only Food and Drug Administration approved agent for the treatment of CDI, vancomycin is typically dosed at 125 mg orally four times daily for a 10-day course.[15,39,57,62] Alternate dosing schedules include doses of 250 or 500 mg orally every 6 hours, with a trial by Fekety and colleagues[63] demonstrating equivalent efficacy with both the 125- and 500-mg doses. It is important for clinicians to remember that intravenous vancomycin has no role in the treatment of CDI because it fails to achieve a sufficient concentration in the colon. Numerous clinical trials have documented efficacy of vancomycin in treating CDI with the relative risk of initial symptomatic resolution compared with placebo of 6.75 (95% CI, 1.16–48.43).[64] Vancomycin is the agent of choice in patients unable to tolerate oral metronidazole, pregnant or lactating patients, and those with recurrent episodes or CDI refractory to metronidazole therapy. Overall, vancomycin is as effective as metronidazole in terms of achieving initial symptomatic resolution or bacteriologic cure, and slightly inferior to teicoplanin.[64] A recent randomized trial has demonstrated superiority of vancomycin over metronidazole, however, in the treatment of severe CDI.[61] In that study, severity of CDI was assessed by giving a score of 1 point each for age greater than 60 years, a temperature of greater than 38.3°C, albumin level greater than 2.5 mg/dL, and WBC count of greater than 15,000 cells/mm^3, and 2 points each for pseudomembranous colitis or hospitalization in the intensive care unit. Patients with a severity score of 2 or more were considered as having severe CDI. In patients with mild disease (N = 81), vancomycin (125 mg four times a day) and metronidazole (250 mg four times a day) had similar clinical cure rates of 98% and 90%, respectively (P = .36), but in those with severe *C difficile*–associated diarrhea (N = 69), vancomycin had a superior cure rate of 97% compared with only 76% with metronidazole (P = .02). Given the demonstrated higher rate of adverse outcomes with CDI in the IBD compared with a non-IBD population, it has not yet been defined how underlying IBD affects this severity stratification. Physicians involved in treating IBD patients must recognize the potential compounding effect of these conditions and promptly consider switching therapy to vancomycin if there is no response to metronidazole in 2 to 3 days, particularly in patients requiring hospitalization.

Vancomycin is available in pill formulation, but this formulation is often more expensive and poses challenges for patients with inadequate health care coverage. An alternative solution is to use parenteral formulations of vancomycin that are routinely available for hospitalized patients as an orally ingested solution. For outpatients, this strategy can also be arranged, typically through the assistance of hospital-based pharmacies to provide the medication, at significant cost savings. The unpalatability of oral vancomycin solution can be lessened with the oral dosing being followed by apple juice or alternatively having the patient rinse their mouth with mouthwash to diminish drug aftertaste.

Although it is appropriate to wait for the confirmation of CDI with a positive *C difficile* toxin assay in most patients before starting therapy, there are a few situations where the authors consider starting empiric therapy on suspicion of underlying CDI while waiting for the stool toxin assay and testing of multiple samples after an initial negative result. These include patients with fulminant colitis, especially those who remain unresponsive to steroids, or in those with unexplained clinical deterioration despite previously stable, mild disease in the right setting. In ambulatory patients with mild CDI, therapy is started with oral metronidazole. In most IBD patients with CDI severe enough to require hospitalization, the authors start treatment with oral vancomycin, typically 125 to 500 mg four times a day. In hospitalized patients with ileus or inability to consistently take oral antibiotics, they add intravenous metronidazole for severe CDI.

A more difficult issue has been the management of ongoing immunosuppressive therapy in the setting of IBD complicated by CDI with limited data on this topic. In most patients with CDI, the authors tend to not escalate immunosuppressive therapy during the acute CDI episode while the patient is being treated with metronidazole-vancomycin, and sometimes even decrease the dose of corticosteroids. Patients who have persistent disease activity after an episode of CDI who have documented negative toxin assays after completion of antibiotic course, however, may merit escalation of their immunosuppression. For hospitalized, fulminant IBD colitis patients this may involve initiation of anti–tumor necrosis factor-a therapy with infliximab. The rationale for the use of infliximab stems from concern regarding the broad immunosuppressive effect of high-dose intravenous corticosteroids, which may exert an inhibitory effect on humoral immunity, which is required to effectively clear the *C difficile* infection. In addition, *C difficile* infection elicits a tumor necrosis factor-a response in the gut, and this inflammatory mechanism may be targeted with the use of an anti–tumor necrosis factor-a antibody rescue strategy for hospitalized, severely ill IBD patients.

Probiotics

One proposed theory for the development of CDI has been disruption of the normal gut flora by the inciting antibiotics with subsequent proliferation of *C difficile*. Probiotics are nonpathogenic microorganisms that theoretically may help restoration of gut flora, and decrease the incidence of CDI and potentially may be used in the treatment of CDI. There are several studies that have examined the role of probiotics in this setting.[65] Interpretation of these studies is limited by small sample sizes, however, or variation in either the types of microbes studied or study population. The most promising results have been for *Saccharomyces boulardii*, with two studies demonstrating efficacy in the treatment of initial infection or recurrent disease.[66] A recent Cochrane review concluded, however, that there was insufficient data to recommend use of probiotics either as the sole agent or in conjunction with antibiotics for the treatment of CDI.[65]

Other Agents

Rifaximin is a nonabsorbed rifamycin-derived antibiotic that is used in the treatment of travelers' diarrhea and has good in vitro activity against *C difficile*.[67] There are no randomized double-blind controlled trials yet examining its efficacy in the treatment of CDI. A single open-label trial comparing rifaximin with vancomycin demonstrated an efficacy of 90% in the treatment of CDI. Several studies have also demonstrated in vitro resistance of C difficile to rifaximin, however, particularly among the epidemic BI/NAP1/027 strain.[18,57,58,68,69]

Teicoplanin is a glycopeptide antibiotic that has shown comparable or slightly superior efficacy than oral vancomycin in the treatment of CDI.[57,64] It is not commercially available, however, in the United States. Other antibiotics that have demonstrated efficacy in treatment of CDI include nitazoxonide, fusidic acid, and bacitracin with none of the agents being used widely.

Anion-binding resins, such as cholestyramine and colestipol, may bind to the C difficile toxin and be used in conjunction with antibiotic therapy.[39] It is important to give these agents at least 2 to 3 hours apart from other oral agents to prevent binding to the antibiotics.

SURGICAL TREATMENT

In patients with CDI refractory to medical therapy or fulminant disease, surgery may be required for management.[70,71] Surgery for CDI may have increased temporally over the past decade with a greater proportion of severe disease. Studies have also demonstrated a greater need for colectomy in patients with IBD and CDI compared with those without underlying IBD.[9] Early involvement of surgeons with experience in the management of fulminant colitis is essential to ensure optimal outcomes. Total colectomy is the procedure of choice for patients requiring surgical treatment with inferior outcomes after hemicolectomy or limited resection. The optimal timing of surgery in IBD patients has not yet been well-defined. Patients with toxic megacolon or perforated bowel require emergent surgery. Patients who do not improve with medical therapy within 3 to 5 days with worsening symptoms may also require more urgent surgery.

SEVERE OR REFRACTORY CDI

Metronidazole or vancomycin achieve clinical and bacteriologic cure in most patients with CDI, but a small cohort of patients may not respond and have refractory disease. Vancomycin has superior efficacy compared with metronidazole in the treatment of severe CDI.[61] A combination of oral vancomycin and intravenous metronidazole can also be tried in patients who do not respond to either antibiotic or have adynamic ileus as a means of ensuring adequate colonic antibiotic concentration.[15,57,58] There are no randomized trials, however, of intravenous metronidazole in the treatment of CDI. In patients with severe CDI, intraluminal administration of vancomycin by intracolonic delivery or rectal administration using a retention enema administered through a Foley catheter has shown success in a small number of patients.[15,57]

Intravenous immunoglobulin (IVIG) has been used successfully for the treatment of CDI in a series of 14 patients,[72] all of whom had failed a median of three courses of treatment with either vancomycin or metronidazole. They were administered a single dose of IVIG in doses ranging from 150 to 400 mg/kg. Six patients responded with a median time to response of 10 days. This success has been replicated in another small series and is a therapeutic option in this cohort of patients. IVIG may have a more important role in a subset of patients who develop IBD as a complication of an underlying congenital immunodeficiency state, such as hypogammaglobulinemia or common variable immunodeficiency. In patients with a history suspicious for common variable immunodeficiency, the authors check quantitative immunoglobulins and in patients with low levels, consultation with an allergy or immunology specialist and an initiation of an immunoglobulin replacement regimen may help treat the underlying colitis. They also check quantitative immunoglobulin levels in hospitalized patients who are unresponsive to standard CDI therapy and use IVIG to treat refractory disease in patients with low immunoglobulin levels.

Rectal infusion of feces obtained from healthy hosts (fecal biotherapy) has shown benefit in some patients.[39] Early surgical consultation is essential for patients with severe or refractory CDI.

RECURRENT CDI

After a single episode of CDI, patients may either develop a relapse (if symptoms recur within 7–14 days of cessation of therapy) or a true recurrence if symptoms reappear at a more distant time interval. Recurrence may be seen in 15% to 35% of patients after an initial episode, with this rate rising to 35% to 65% after the first recurrence.[15,57,73] Some recurrences may last for several months. A recent meta-analysis of 12 studies including 1382 patients identified continued use of non–C difficile antibiotics after diagnosis of CDI (OR 4.23; 95% CI, 2.10–8.55; $P<.001$), concomitant receipt of antacid medications (OR 2.15; 95% CI, 1.13–4.08; $P = .019$), and older age (OR 1.62; 95% CI, 1.11–2.36; $P = .0012$) to be risk factors for recurrent disease.[74] There are limited data on CDI recurrence rates in an IBD population. At the authors' center, among 81 IBD patients who had a positive stool C difficile toxin assay in 2005 to 2006, 10 patients had documented toxin positive recurrence within the subsequent year.[75]

There are several treatment options available for the treatment of recurrent disease.[15,39,57] Patients with the first recurrence after treatment with metronidazole can be treated with a course of vancomycin, whereas those who fail vancomycin may be tried on a second course.[57] For multiply recurrent disease, there are several nonrandomized series documenting efficacy of various treatment regimens. A longer course of vancomycin administered with gradual taper over 6 weeks was effective in a small cohort of patients.[57,76,77] Higher doses of vancomycin (500 mg four times a day) may be effective but may also be associated with a high rate of relapse. IVIG may be useful in patients with accompanying hypogammaglobulinemia.[72,78] One study reported on use of rifaximin in eight patients with more than three recurrences each. Oral vancomycin was used until symptomatic cure followed by a 2-week course of rifaximin. This regimen achieved success in seven of eight patients.[79] There are limited data on treatment of recurrent disease in IBD patients. In a study from the authors' center of 14 IBD patients, rifaximin was administered at a dose of 200 mg three times a day for 2 weeks, followed by 200 mg once daily for 2 weeks and 200 mg every other day for the final 2 weeks of the taper.[75] They were able to prevent recurrent CDI in all patients with this regimen. Probiotics have also shown a benefit in preventing recurrent CDI with two randomized studies showing a benefit with the addition of S boulardii to standard treatment.[66]

In patients with recurrent CDI, in addition to the previously mentioned therapeutic options, it is important to remove potential external sources of reinfection. Cessation of the offending antimicrobial agent, if possible, is important. Use of more targeted antimicrobial therapy may decrease disruption of gut flora. The treating physician should also inquire about all potential environmental sources of recurrent disease including exposure to a health care setting or patients who may be caregivers to people who are carriers of C difficile. All patients should be instructed on the importance of strict hand hygiene measures.

INFECTION CONTROL AND PREVENTION

Clostridium difficile is transmitted through spores that are relatively resistant to environmental degradation.[80] The spores can persist for as long as 5 months on hard surfaces. One study found C difficile in 49% of sites in rooms occupied by those with CDI.[81] Commonly used quaternary-ammonium–based or surfactant-based detergents may not adequately eradicate C difficile spores and may actually increase sporulation.[80,82] In addition, the epidemic BI/NAP1/O27 epidemic strain may hypersporulate, producing more spores than other C difficile strains. A 10% sodium hypochlorite solution has been shown to have good efficacy in decreasing environmental spore burden and reducing the number of cases of CDI.[80]

In addition to environmental precautions, hand washing and hygiene are keys in preventing transmission of C difficile. Soap-and-water hand washing effectively mechanically dislodges spores. Alcohol-based hand gels do not eradicate spores or reduce transmission with a mean of 30% of spores being transferred by a handshake even after use of these gels.[80] Although institution-wide use of alcohol-based gels has not been shown to increase the rate of CDI, experts suggest use of soap-and-water hand washing techniques after the care of patients with CDI. Contact isolation may help prevention of patient-to-patient transfer of infection within hospitals and health care institutions. The use of gloves and gowns in the care of patients with CDI may also help prevent transmission and reduce cases of CDI. Standard endoscope decontamination procedures may be followed after lower gastrointestinal endoscopy in patients with CDI.[80]

CDI IN SPECIAL SITUATIONS IN IBD
Clostridium difficile Enteritis

Infection with C difficile has been reported in the small bowel in patients with colectomy. Such infection may carry high morbidity and mortality in the range of 60% to 93%.[83–86] The authors reported a series of six patients with C difficile enteritis from 2004 to 2006.[83] All patients had undergone colectomy for severe UC and had developed high-volume ileostomy output (six of six), fever and leukocytosis (four of six), and ileus (five of six) in the postoperative period. Ileostomy output tested positive for C difficile toxin and there were no other likely explanations for the patient's symptoms. All patients responded to treatment with oral and intravenous metronidazole or oral vancomycin.

Clostridium difficile Pouchitis

Total proctocolectomy with ileo-anal pouch anastomosis is the procedure of choice in patients with severe UC who require surgery for dysplasia or refractory medical disease. The ileal pouch is also susceptible to infection with C difficile and may be associated with either C difficile enteritis above the reconstruction or C difficile–associated inflammation of the pouch. Because as many as half the patients develop acute or chronic pouchitis after ileo-anal pouch anastomosis and require treatment with antibiotics, this may predispose them to developing CDI. There are now several reports of infection with C difficile causing pouchitis that is refractory to broad-spectrum antibiotic therapy.[87–89] Administration of oral vancomycin in such patients with a positive C difficile toxin assay has shown benefit in some. A recent study of 115 patients with ileo-anal pouch anastomosis from the Cleveland Clinic identified 21 patients (18.3%) to be positive for C difficile toxin by ELISA.[89] Male gender (OR 5.12; 95% CI, 1.38–20.46) and preoperative left-sided colitis (OR 8.4; 95% CI, 1.25–56.4) were independent risk factors for C difficile infection. Interestingly, there was no difference in antibiotic or immunomodulator use between the two groups, again serving to emphasize that prior antibiotic use should not be considered essential to entertain a suspicion for C difficile infection in IBD patients.[89]

Clostridium difficile infection has also been reported in segments of diverted bowel[90] and responds to topical therapy with metronidazole or vancomycin.

DIRECTIONS FOR FUTURE RESEARCH

Although there are growing data on the incidence and impact of CDI on patients with IBD, there are several areas that have yet remained undefined. Most studies have been retrospective in design, which has precluded moving identifying associated factors to defining true causative risk factors. The studies have also focused on hospitalized cohorts of IBD patients, an important subgroup given the higher rate of adverse outcomes in this cohort. Further research is essential, however, to examine the impact of CDI in those with milder IBD or ambulatory cohorts to truly define the impact of CDI on IBD. There is need for research on the role of asymptomatic carriage of *C difficile* and examination of longer-term outcomes of CDI in IBD. There are preliminary data suggesting that an episode of CDI can affect disease activity for even as long as 1 year after the initial infection. This needs to be examined prospectively, however, with better identification of recurrences, standard protocols of measuring disease activity at periodic intervals after the initial infection, and using an appropriate control population. There is also a significant dearth of data on the therapeutic efficacy of various treatment regimens for CDI including recurrent and refractory disease in the setting of underlying IBD. Multicenter cohorts and randomized trials in the IBD population are essential to satisfy this need.

SUMMARY

Infection with *C difficile* is an increasingly common complication in patients with IBD and can have severe consequences in some patients. There has been a temporal escalation of burden of CDI over the past decade with higher rates of surgery and mortality in the IBD population compared with the non-IBD cohort. A high index of suspicion should be maintained even in the absence of traditional risk factors, such as antibiotic use or health care exposure, and should be followed by testing including testing of multiple stool samples in appropriate clinical situations. Directed antibiotic therapy should be initiated early after a positive test; in select patients with severe presentation, empiric antibiotic therapy should be considered. Comanagement with surgeons is a key in those with severe disease.

REFERENCES

1. Jarvis WR, Schlosser J, Jarvis AA, et al. National point prevalence of *Clostridium difficile* in US health care facility inpatients, 2008. Am J Infect Control 2009;37: 263–70.
2. Kuijper EJ, Coignard B, Tull P. Emergence of *Clostridium difficile*-associated disease in North America and Europe. Clin Microbiol Infect 2006;12(Suppl 6): 2–18.
3. McDonald LC, Owings M, Jernigan DB. *Clostridium difficile* infection in patients discharged from US short-stay hospitals, 1996–2003. Emerg Infect Dis 2006; 12:409–15.
4. Pepin J, Valiquette L, Alary ME, et al. *Clostridium difficile*-associated diarrhea in a region of Quebec from 1991 to 2003: a changing pattern of disease severity. CMAJ 2004;171:466–72.

5. Dubberke ER, Wertheimer AI. Review of current literature on the economic burden of *Clostridium difficile* infection. Infect Control Hosp Epidemiol 2009;30: 57–66.
6. Kyne L, Hamel MB, Polavaram R, et al. Health care costs and mortality associated with nosocomial diarrhea due to *Clostridium difficile*. Clin Infect Dis 2002; 34:346–53.
7. Bartlett JG, Chang TW, Gurwith M, et al. Antibiotic-associated pseudomembranous colitis due to toxin-producing clostridia. N Engl J Med 1978;298:531–4.
8. Podolsky DK. Inflammatory bowel disease. N Engl J Med 2002;347:417–29.
9. Ananthakrishnan AN, McGinley EL, Binion DG. Excess hospitalisation burden associated with *Clostridium difficile* in patients with inflammatory bowel disease. Gut 2008;57:205–10.
10. Bossuyt P, Verhaegen J, Van Assche G, et al. Increasing incidence of *Clostridium difficile*-associated diarrhea in inflammatory bowel disease. J Crohns Colitis 2009;3:4–7.
11. Issa M, Vijayapal A, Graham MB, et al. Impact of *Clostridium difficile* on inflammatory bowel disease. Clin Gastroenterol Hepatol 2007;5:345–51.
12. Jodorkovsky D, Young Y, Abreu MT. Clinical outcomes of patients with ulcerative colitis and co-existing *Clostridium difficile* infection. Dig Dis Sci 2009. [Epub ahead of print].
13. Nguyen GC, Kaplan GG, Harris ML, et al. A national survey of the prevalence and impact of *Clostridium difficile* infection among hospitalized inflammatory bowel disease patients. Am J Gastroenterol 2008;103:1443–50.
14. Rodemann JF, Dubberke ER, Reske KA, et al. Incidence of *Clostridium difficile* infection in inflammatory bowel disease. Clin Gastroenterol Hepatol 2007;5: 339–44.
15. Kelly CP. A 76-year-old man with recurrent *Clostridium difficile*-associated diarrhea: review of *C. difficile* infection. JAMA 2009;301:954–62.
16. Voth DE, Ballard JD. *Clostridium difficile* toxins: mechanism of action and role in disease. Clin Microbiol Rev 2005;18:247–63.
17. Giesemann T, Egerer M, Jank T, et al. Processing of *Clostridium difficile* toxins. J Med Microbiol 2008;57:690–6.
18. Issa M, Ananthakrishnan AN, Binion DG. *Clostridium difficile* and inflammatory bowel disease. Inflamm Bowel Dis 2008;14:1432–42.
19. Jank T, Giesemann T, Aktories K. *Clostridium difficile* glucosyltransferase toxin B-essential amino acids for substrate binding. J Biol Chem 2007;282: 35222–31.
20. Taylor NS, Thorne GM, Bartlett JG. Comparison of two toxins produced by *Clostridium difficile*. Infect Immun 1981;34:1036–43.
21. Borriello SP. Pathogenesis of *Clostridium difficile* infection. J Antimicrob Chemother 1998;41(Suppl C):13–9.
22. Bongaerts GP, Lyerly DM. Role of toxins A and B in the pathogenesis of *Clostridium difficile* disease. Microb Pathog 1994;17:1–12.
23. Drudy D, Harnedy N, Fanning S, et al. Isolation and characterisation of toxin A-negative, toxin B-positive *Clostridium difficile* in Dublin, Ireland. Clin Microbiol Infect 2007;13:298–304.
24. Johnson S, Kent SA, O'Leary KJ, et al. Fatal pseudomembranous colitis associated with a variant *Clostridium difficile* strain not detected by toxin A immunoassay. Ann Intern Med 2001;135:434–8.
25. Rupnik M, Grabnar M, Geric B. Binary toxin producing *Clostridium difficile* strains. Anaerobe 2003;9:289–94.

26. Barbut F, Decre D, Lalande V, et al. Clinical features of *Clostridium difficile*-associated diarrhoea due to binary toxin (actin-specific ADP-ribosyltransferase)-producing strains. J Med Microbiol 2005;54:181–5.

27. McEllistrem MC, Carman RJ, Gerding DN, et al. A hospital outbreak of *Clostridium difficile* disease associated with isolates carrying binary toxin genes. Clin Infect Dis 2005;40:265–72.

28. Loo VG, Poirier L, Miller MA, et al. A predominantly clonal multi-institutional outbreak of *Clostridium difficile*-associated diarrhea with high morbidity and mortality. N Engl J Med 2005;353:2442–9.

29. McDonald LC, Killgore GE, Thompson A, et al. An epidemic, toxin gene-variant strain of *Clostridium difficile*. N Engl J Med 2005;353:2433–41.

30. Warny M, Pepin J, Fang A, et al. Toxin production by an emerging strain of *Clostridium difficile* associated with outbreaks of severe disease in North America and Europe. Lancet 2005;366:1079–84.

31. Rolny P, Jarnerot G, Mollby R. Occurrence of *Clostridium difficile* toxin in inflammatory bowel disease. Scand J Gastroenterol 1983;18:61–4.

32. Bolton RP, Sherriff RJ, Read AE. *Clostridium difficile* associated diarrhoea: a role in inflammatory bowel disease? Lancet 1980;1:383–4.

33. Gryboski JD. *Clostridium difficile* in inflammatory bowel disease relapse. J Pediatr Gastroenterol Nutr 1991;13:39–41.

34. Meyer AM, Ramzan NN, Loftus EV Jr, et al. The diagnostic yield of stool pathogen studies during relapses of inflammatory bowel disease. J Clin Gastroenterol 2004;38:772–5.

35. Mylonaki M, Langmead L, Pantes A, et al. Enteric infection in relapse of inflammatory bowel disease: importance of microbiological examination of stool. Eur J Gastroenterol Hepatol 2004;16:775–8.

36. Pascarella F, Martinelli M, Miele E, et al. Impact of *Clostridium difficile* infection on pediatric inflammatory bowel disease. J Pediatr 2009;154:854–8.

37. Clayton EM, Rea MC, Shanahan F, et al. The vexed relationship between *Clostridium difficile* and inflammatory bowel disease: an assessment of carriage in an outpatient setting among patients in remission. Am J Gastroenterol 2009; 104:1162–9.

38. Bartlett JG, Gerding DN. Clinical recognition and diagnosis of *Clostridium difficile* infection. Clin Infect Dis 2008;46(Suppl 1):S12–8.

39. McFarland LV. Renewed interest in a difficult disease: *Clostridium difficile* infections–epidemiology and current treatment strategies. Curr Opin Gastroenterol 2009;25:24–35.

40. Bartlett JG. Clinical practice: antibiotic-associated diarrhea. N Engl J Med 2002; 346:334–9.

41. Bignardi GE. Risk factors for *Clostridium difficile* infection. J Hosp Infect 1998;40: 1–15.

42. Gerding DN, Johnson S, Peterson LR, et al. *Clostridium difficile*-associated diarrhea and colitis. Infect Control Hosp Epidemiol 1995;16:459–77.

43. Dial S, Alrasadi K, Manoukian C, et al. Risk of *Clostridium difficile* diarrhea among hospital inpatients prescribed proton pump inhibitors: cohort and case-control studies. CMAJ 2004;171:33–8.

44. Gaynes R, Rimland D, Killum E, et al. Outbreak of *Clostridium difficile* infection in a long-term care facility: association with gatifloxacin use. Clin Infect Dis 2004;38: 640–5.

45. Pepin J, Saheb N, Coulombe MA, et al. Emergence of fluoroquinolones as the predominant risk factor for *Clostridium difficile*-associated diarrhea: a cohort study during an epidemic in Quebec. Clin Infect Dis 2005;41:1254–60.
46. Bingley PJ, Harding GM. *Clostridium difficile* colitis following treatment with metronidazole and vancomycin. Postgrad Med J 1987;63:993–4.
47. Dial S, Delaney JA, Barkun AN, et al. Use of gastric acid-suppressive agents and the risk of community-acquired *Clostridium difficile*-associated disease. JAMA 2005;294:2989–95.
48. Arif M, Weber LR, Knox JF, et al. Patterns of proton pump inhibitor use in inflammatory bowel disease and concomitant risk of *Clostridium difficile* infection. Gastroenterology 2007;132:A513.
49. Kyne L, Sougioultzis S, McFarland LV, et al. Underlying disease severity as a major risk factor for nosocomial *Clostridium difficile* diarrhea. Infect Control Hosp Epidemiol 2002;23:653–9.
50. Kyne L, Warny M, Qamar A, et al. Asymptomatic carriage of *Clostridium difficile* and serum levels of IgG antibody against toxin A. N Engl J Med 2000;342:390–7.
51. Kyne L, Warny M, Qamar A, et al. Association between antibody response to toxin A and protection against recurrent *Clostridium difficile* diarrhoea. Lancet 2001;357:189–93.
52. Powell N, Jung SE, Krishnan B. *Clostridium difficile* infection and inflammatory bowel disease: a marker for disease extent? Gut 2008;57:1183–4 author reply 1184.
53. Fekety R, Shah AB. Diagnosis and treatment of *Clostridium difficile* colitis. JAMA 1993;269:71–5.
54. Kelly CP, LaMont JT. *Clostridium difficile* infection. Annu Rev Med 1998;49:375–90.
55. Chiplunker A, Ananthakrishnan AN, Beaulieu DB, et al. Long-term impact of *Clostridium difficile* on inflammatory bowel disease. Gastroenterology 2009;136(Suppl 1):S1145.
56. Teasley DG, Gerding DN, Olson MM, et al. Prospective randomised trial of metronidazole versus vancomycin for *Clostridium-difficile*-associated diarrhoea and colitis. Lancet 1983;2:1043–6.
57. Gerding DN, Muto CA, Owens RC Jr. Treatment of *Clostridium difficile* infection. Clin Infect Dis 2008;46(Suppl 1):S32–42.
58. Leffler DA, Lamont JT. Treatment of *Clostridium difficile*-associated disease. Gastroenterology 2009;136:1899–912.
59. Musher DM, Aslam S, Logan N, et al. Relatively poor outcome after treatment of *Clostridium difficile* colitis with metronidazole. Clin Infect Dis 2005;40:1586–90.
60. Pepin J, Alary ME, Valiquette L, et al. Increasing risk of relapse after treatment of *Clostridium difficile* colitis in Quebec, Canada. Clin Infect Dis 2005;40:1591–7.
61. Zar FA, Bakkanagari SR, Moorthi KM, et al. A comparison of vancomycin and metronidazole for the treatment of *Clostridium difficile*-associated diarrhea, stratified by disease severity. Clin Infect Dis 2007;45:302–7.
62. Fekety R. Guidelines for the diagnosis and management of *Clostridium difficile*-associated diarrhea and colitis. American college of gastroenterology, Practice Parameters Committee. Am J Gastroenterol 1997;92:739–50.
63. Fekety R, Silva J, Kauffman C, et al. Treatment of antibiotic-associated *Clostridium difficile* colitis with oral vancomycin: comparison of two dosage regimens. Am J Med 1989;86:15–9.
64. Nelson R. Antibiotic treatment for *Clostridium difficile*-associated diarrhea in adults. Cochrane Database Syst Rev 2007;3:CD004610.

65. Pillai A, Nelson R. Probiotics for treatment of *Clostridium difficile*-associated colitis in adults. Cochrane Database Syst Rev 2008;1:CD004611.
66. McFarland LV. Meta-analysis of probiotics for the prevention of antibiotic associated diarrhea and the treatment of *Clostridium difficile* disease. Am J Gastroenterol 2006;101:812–22.
67. Jiang ZD, Dupont HL, La Rocco M, et al. In vitro activity of rifaximin and rifampin against clinical isolates of *Clostridium difficile* in Houston, Texas. Anaerobe 2009. [Epub ahead of print].
68. Garey KW, Jiang ZD, Bellard A, et al. Rifaximin in treatment of recurrent *Clostridium difficile*-associated diarrhea: an uncontrolled pilot study. J Clin Gastroenterol 2008. [Epub ahead of print].
69. Oldfield EC III. Use of a rifaximin chaser in the treatment of recurrent *Clostridium difficile*-associated diarrhea. Rev Gastroenterol Disord 2008;8:157–8.
70. Hall JF, Berger D. Outcome of colectomy for *Clostridium difficile* colitis: a plea for early surgical management. Am J Surg 2008;196:384–8.
71. Koss K, Clark MA, Sanders DS, et al. The outcome of surgery in fulminant *Clostridium difficile* colitis. Colorectal Dis 2006;8:149–54.
72. McPherson S, Rees CJ, Ellis R, et al. Intravenous immunoglobulin for the treatment of severe, refractory, and recurrent *Clostridium difficile* diarrhea. Dis Colon Rectum 2006;49:640–5.
73. Aslam S, Hamill RJ, Musher DM. Treatment of *Clostridium difficile*-associated disease: old therapies and new strategies. Lancet Infect Dis 2005;5:549–57.
74. Garey KW, Sethi S, Yadav Y, et al. Meta-analysis to assess risk factors for recurrent *Clostridium difficile* infection. J Hosp Infect 2008;70:298–304.
75. Issa M, Weber LR, Brandenburg H, et al. Rifaximin and treatment of recurrent *Clostridium difficile* infection in patients with inflammatory bowel disease. Am J Gastroenterol 2006;101:S469.
76. McFarland LV, Elmer GW, Surawicz CM. Breaking the cycle: treatment strategies for 163 cases of recurrent *Clostridium difficile* disease. Am J Gastroenterol 2002; 97:1769–75.
77. Tedesco FJ, Gordon D, Fortson WC. Approach to patients with multiple relapses of antibiotic-associated pseudomembranous colitis. Am J Gastroenterol 1985;80: 867–8.
78. Hassett J, Meyers S, McFarland L, et al. Recurrent *Clostridium difficile* infection in a patient with selective IgG1 deficiency treated with intravenous immune globulin and *Saccharomyces boulardii*. Clin Infect Dis 1995;20(Suppl 2):S266–8.
79. Johnson S, Schriever C, Galang M, et al. Interruption of recurrent *Clostridium difficile*-associated diarrhea episodes by serial therapy with vancomycin and rifaximin. Clin Infect Dis 2007;44:846–8.
80. Gerding DN, Muto CA, Owens RC Jr. Measures to control and prevent *Clostridium difficile* infection. Clin Infect Dis 2008;46(Suppl 1):S43–9.
81. McFarland LV, Mulligan ME, Kwok RY, et al. Nosocomial acquisition of *Clostridium difficile* infection. N Engl J Med 1989;320:204–10.
82. Wilcox MH, Fawley WN. Hospital disinfectants and spore formation by *Clostridium difficile*. Lancet 2000;356:1324.
83. Lundeen SJ, Otterson MF, Binion DG, et al. *Clostridium difficile* enteritis: an early postoperative complication in inflammatory bowel disease patients after colectomy. J Gastrointest Surg 2007;11:138–42.
84. Vesoulis Z, Williams G, Matthews B. Pseudomembranous enteritis after proctocolectomy: report of a case. Dis Colon Rectum 2000;43:551–4.

85. Yee HF Jr, Brown RS Jr, Ostroff JW. Fatal *Clostridium difficile* enteritis after total abdominal colectomy. J Clin Gastroenterol 1996;22:45–7.
86. Miller DL, Sedlack JD, Holt RW. Perforation complicating rifampin-associated pseudomembranous enteritis. Arch Surg 1989;124:1082.
87. Mann SD, Pitt J, Springall RG, et al. *Clostridium difficile* infection–an unusual cause of refractory pouchitis: report of a case. Dis Colon Rectum 2003;46:267–70.
88. Shen B, Goldblum JR, Hull TL, et al. *Clostridium difficile*-associated pouchitis. Dig Dis Sci 2006;51:2361–4.
89. Shen BO, Jiang ZD, Fazio VW, et al. *Clostridium difficile* infection in patients with ileal pouch-anal anastomosis. Clin Gastroenterol Hepatol 2008;6:782–8.
90. Tsironi E, Irving PM, Feakins RM, et al. Diversion colitis caused by *Clostridium difficile* infection: report of a case. Dis Colon Rectum 2006;49:1074–7.

Novel Diagnostic and Prognostic Modalities in Inflammatory Bowel Disease

Timothy L. Zisman, MD, MPH[a], David T. Rubin, MD[b],*

KEYWORDS

- Inflammatory bowel disease • Diagnosis • Prognosis
- Serologies • Imaging • Fecal biomarkers

Inflammatory bowel disease (IBD) is a heterogenous group of diseases that can be broadly classified into Crohn disease and ulcerative colitis (UC). The term IBD-unclassified (IBDU) applies to the subset of 10% to 15% of patients with IBD in whom this subcategorization is not possible. There is no gold standard single test that provides the diagnosis of IBD, so assigning a diagnosis of IBD is often not straightforward and involves integration of historical factors, physical examination findings, and evidence of inflammation on endoscopic, histologic, and radiologic evaluations. Consequently, there is significant uncertainty both in establishing the initial diagnosis and, importantly, in assessing for disease relapse after a period of remission. These challenges are compounded by the increased appreciation of the importance of an accurate and timely diagnosis. Delay in diagnosis can result in complications of stricturing or penetrating disease, whereas an incorrect diagnosis has emotional and insurance implications and can expose patients to the modest but nonetheless real risks of medical therapy. The uncertainty in diagnosing IBD and the need to get the diagnosis right has fueled improvements in techniques to assess bowel inflammation, including serologic and fecal markers and novel endoscopic and radiologic tools for imaging the entire bowel. These new techniques for evaluating patients with IBD are developed with the goals of improving early and accurate diagnosis, clarifying disease type and distribution in order to select optimal therapy, identifying patients at high risk

This article originally appeared in the 38:4 issue of *Gastroenterology Clinics of North America*. Financial disclosures: Timothy L. Zisman: none; David T. Rubin: consultant and receives grant support from Prometheus Laboratories, consultant for Given Imaging.

[a] Division of Gastroenterology, University of Washington Medical Center, 1959 NE Pacific Street, Box 356424, Seattle, WA 98195, USA

[b] Inflammatory Bowel Disease Center, University of Chicago Medical Center, 5841 South Maryland Avenue, MC 4076, Chicago, IL 60637, USA

* Corresponding author.

E-mail address: drubin@medicine.bsd.uchicago.edu (D.T. Rubin).

Med Clin N Am 94 (2010) 155–178

doi:10.1016/j.mcna.2009.10.003

medical.theclinics.com

for aggressive disease, and detecting complications such as abscess or malignancy. The past decade has seen a dramatic advancement in diagnostic and prognostic modalities in IBD, and these novel instruments are reviewed in this article.

SEROLOGIC BIOMARKERS

Serologic biomarkers in IBD include an enlarging panel of antibodies directed against microbial and self-antigens and acute phase reactants. It is unclear whether these antimicrobial antibodies are mechanistically related to the pathogenesis of IBD. They may represent a loss of immune tolerance to commensal organisms, or they may simply be an indicator of increased bowel permeability with consequent exposure to luminal antigens. A variety of uses for these markers have been explored in IBD patients, including as potential diagnostic tools, follow-up parameters, prognostic indicators for phenotypic stratification, or subclinical disease markers in IBD patients or their family members. Serologic tests have several advantages in that they are easy to obtain, noninvasive, and objectively quantified.

Antineutrophil Cytoplasmic Antibodies

Antineutrophil cytoplasmic antibodies (ANCA) are detected on peripheral blood neutrophils by indirect immunofluorescence (IIF) techniques. Two major staining patterns have been described. A cytoplasmic (c-ANCA) staining pattern characterized by diffuse granularity of the cytoplasm is classically seen in patients with Wegener granulomatosis. These c-ANCA antibodies typically recognize proteinase-3 on enzyme-linked immunosorbent assay (ELISA) testing. By contrast, a thin homogeneous rim-like staining of the perinuclear cytoplasm (p-ANCA) is associated with microscopic polyangiitis and antibodies directed against myeloperoxidase. A third pattern exists, often referred to as atypical p-ANCA, that appears as a broad heterogeneous staining of the nuclear periphery, often with intranuclear inclusions to suggest that the antigen may be in the periphery of the nucleus rather than in the perinuclear cytoplasm. This atypical p-ANCA is associated with IBD[1] and primary sclerosing cholangitis[2] and autoimmune hepatitis type I.[3] Atypical p-ANCA is present in 40% to 80% of patients with UC [4,5] and 5% to 25% of patients with Crohn disease.[1] The target antigens of atypical p-ANCA have not been identified, but several have been explored, including cathepsin G, elastase, β-glucuronidase, lactoferrin, and the natural antibiotic bactericidal permeability increasing protein. Myeloperoxidase and proteinase-3, the antigens recognized by typical p-ANCA and c-ANCA, respectively, are not autoantigens in IBD. Because the target antigens of atypical p-ANCA have not been identified, there is no ELISA test to distinguish these antibodies from typical p-ANCA. Rather one must rely on IIF, which has drawbacks, including differences in methodology and subjective interpretation of staining pattern that result in substantial variability of results among laboratories.[6,7] Consequently, the numerous studies describing the performance characteristics of atypical p-ANCA in the detection of IBD have yielded heterogeneous and discrepant results.[1] Given this variability, an alternative methodology was developed by Targan and colleagues[8] to distinguish atypical p-ANCA from the typical vasculitis-associated p-ANCA by a 3-step process that involves IIF staining before and after treatment of neutrophils with deoxyribonuclease (DNase). Addition of DNase abolishes the fluorescent staining of atypical, UC-associated p-ANCA, allowing distinction from the typical p-ANCA pattern. In a large meta-analysis, the overall sensitivity of atypical p-ANCA for detecting UC was 55%, with a specificity of 89%, a positive likelihood ratio of 4.5, and a negative likelihood ratio of −0.5.[9]

Anti-Saccharomyces Cerevisiae Antibodies

Anti-*Saccharomyces cerevisiae* antibodies (ASCAs) are antibodies directed against a cell wall component of the baker's and brewer's yeast *S cerevisiae*.[10] This antigen is not unique to the cell wall of *S cerevisiae*, however. Recently it has been discovered that *Candida albicans* is an immunogen for ASCAs.[11] ASCAs are present in 50% to 60% of patients with Crohn disease, 10% to 15% of those with UC,[12–14] 20% of healthy first-degree relatives of patients with Crohn disease,[15,16] and 0% to 5% of healthy controls.[17] IgG and IgA antibodies are produced, and the specificity for Crohn disease increases if both antibodies are positive. As with atypical p-ANCA, there is substantial heterogeneity of ASCA results among laboratories, attributable to a lack of standardization of the assay methodology and defined cutoff values.[16]

Newer Serologic Biomarkers

Anti-OmpC antibody is an IgA antibody directed against the outer membrane porin C protein of *Escherichia coli* and is present in 55% of patients with Crohn disease but only in 5% to 11% of patients with UC and in 5% of healthy controls.[18] In the pediatric population with Crohn disease, however, the prevalence of anti-OmpC antibodies is markedly reduced.[19] Anti-OmpC antibodies are present in 5% to 15% of patients with Crohn disease who are ASCA negative, and they can help to identify a subset of patients that would otherwise be missed by conventional serologic testing.

Antibodies to I2, a bacterial sequence derived from *Pseudomonas fluorescens*, are associated with Crohn disease.[20] Anti-I2 IgA antibodies are present in 30% to 50% of patients with Crohn disease, 10% of patients with UC, 19% of patients with other inflammatory conditions of the intestine, and 5% of healthy controls.[21,22] The sensitivity and specificity of I2 antibodies for detecting Crohn disease are 42% and 76%, respectively. The low sensitivity and modest specificity limit the clinical utility of this antimicrobial marker.

Antipancreatic antibodies (PAB) are more common in Crohn disease (30%) than in UC (2%–6%) or healthy subjects (0%–2%).[23] PAB antibodies are directed against an unidentified antigen on exocrine pancreatic tissue. Their utility in IBD diagnosis and management remains to be demonstrated.

CBir1 flagellin is a dominant antigen of the enteric microbial flora that induces an immune response in colitic mice. Approximately half of Crohn patients have anti-CBir1 antibodies compared with only 6% of patients with UC and 8% of control subjects.[24,25] The presence of anti-CBir1 antibodies is independent of the presence of other antimicrobial or autoantigens in IBD patients. Among the subset of Crohn patients who are positive only for p-ANCA, 40% to 44% express anti-CBir1 antibodies compared with only 4% of p-ANCA–positive UC patients.[25]

There has been increasing interest in exploring antibodies to carbohydrate (glycan)-based antigens because mucosal immune responses involve interaction with the glycosylated cell wall components of luminal fungi, yeast, and bacteria. Three novel antiglycan antibodies have been described in IBD patients. Antilaminaribioside carbohydrate IgG antibodies (ALCA), antichitobioside carbohydrate IgA antibodies (ACCA), and antimannobioside carbohydrate IgA antibodies (AMCA) are all associated with Crohn disease and are present in 44% to 50% of ASCA-negative patients. Although highly specific for Crohn disease, these carbohydrate antibodies demonstrate lackluster sensitivity (18%–28%) for distinguishing Crohn disease from UC.[26,27] In a Hungarian cohort of patients, these antiglycan antibodies were shown to be associated with the *NOD2/CARD15* genotype in Crohn disease.[28] Seow and colleagues[29] demonstrated that antichitin IgA (anti-C) and antilaminarin IgA (anti-L) antibodies improve differentiation of Crohn disease from UC and are independently associated with complicated Crohn disease. These latter anticarbohydrate antibodies are related to, but distinct from, ALCA and ACCA.

Applications of Serologic Biomarkers

Diagnosis of IBD

The diagnostic precision of ASCA and p-ANCA profiles was evaluated in a meta-analysis of 60 studies, including a total of 4019 patients with Crohn disease, 3841 patients with UC, and 3748 controls.[9] This analysis demonstrated that the serologic profile of positive ASCA and negative p-ANCA was associated with a 93% specificity and 55% sensitivity for detection of Crohn disease. A positive p-ANCA test, independent of ASCA result, was associated with a sensitivity of 55% and specificity of 89% for UC. In a subgroup of pediatric patients with a negative ASCA, the results improved to a sensitivity of 73% and specificity of 93% for atypical p-ANCA in detecting UC. Given the substantial heterogeneity in the results of individual studies, this pooled analysis may represent the most accurate estimate of the performance characteristics of these serologic biomarkers.

The suboptimal sensitivity of atypical p-ANCA and ASCA limits their clinical utility for excluding IBD with a negative test. Although the specificity of atypical p-ANCA and ASCA is high, a positive test must still be interpreted with caution and is reliable only in patients with a moderate-to-high pretest probability of having IBD. This point is underscored in an article by Austin and colleagues,[30] in which the authors assumed a 94% specificity for serologic markers and applied the test to hypothetical populations with varying prevalence of disease. When applied to patients with a pretest probability of 5%, the positive predictive value was only 35%, indicating that most results are falsely positive. Consequently, the optimal use of serologic tests in the diagnostic workup of IBD remains unclear, but these tests should not supplant clinical judgment in assigning a diagnosis.

In the setting of established IBD, serologic profiles can assist in distinguishing Crohn disease from UC. The combination of positive ASCA in the absence of atypical p-ANCA is highly specific for Crohn disease, whereas the reverse serologic profile (ASCA-negative, atypical p-ANCA–positive) is strongly associated with UC.[1] However, this does not hold true among Crohn patients with isolated colonic disease, many of whom have a serologic profile similar to that of UC with presence of atypical p-ANCA.

IBD-unclassified

Although most patients with IBD can be categorized as having either Crohn disease or UC using standard clinical, endoscopic, and radiologic techniques, this distinction is not possible in approximately 10% to 15% of patients, and a diagnosis of IBD-U is assigned. Serologic markers have been explored as a potential tool to aid in this distinction. A prospective study of patients with IBD-U analyzed the value of ASCA and atypical p-ANCA in clarifying disease subtype.[31] After 1 year of follow-up, only 31 of the 97 patients could be categorized clinically as having definite UC or Crohn disease. The profile of positive ASCA with negative atypical p-ANCA predicted Crohn disease in 80% of these patients, whereas negative ASCA with positive atypical p-ANCA detected UC in 64% of patients. An important finding in this study was that nearly half of patients with IBD-U did not have either ASCA or atypical p-ANCA antibodies and they remained "seronegative" for a mean duration of 10 years. This highlights an important limitation to the utility of serologic tests in this context.

In the meta-analysis by Reese and colleagues[9] the authors reported that ASCA is less reliable for diagnosing Crohn disease in patients with exclusively colonic involvement, suggesting that ASCA and p-ANCA may be less useful in clarifying disease subtype in patients with IBD-U. Many of these patients have a "UC-like Crohn disease" with left-sided colonic inflammation and often have positive p-ANCA. However, anti-CBir1 antibody may assist in discriminating the "UC-like Crohn disease" from UC. Up to 44% of patients with Crohn disease who are ASCA negative and atypical p-ANCA positive will have anti-CBir1 antibodies as opposed to just 4% of patients with UC who have the identical ASCA/p-ANCA profile.[25] The application of anti-CBir1 in the setting of IBD-U has not been specifically evaluated, however.

Tool for disease monitoring

There does not appear to be a relationship between disease activity and atypical p-ANCA titer in UC, and p-ANCA remains positive after colectomy.[32] Likewise, ASCA levels do not correlate with disease activity in Crohn disease and do not decrease in the setting of clinical response to treatment.[16] These data indicate that serial measurement of atypical p-ANCA and ASCA titers cannot be used to monitor disease activity or to predict impending disease exacerbations.

Predicting disease behavior

The capacity of serologic markers to identify IBD phenotypes and predict disease behavior is becoming increasingly well established. Among UC patients, atypical p-ANCA is associated with left-sided colitis, poor response to medical therapy, and higher rates of colectomy.[33] In addition, several investigators have described an association between high titers of atypical p-ANCA and chronic pouchitis after ileal pouch-anal anastomosis surgery.[34,35] Among patients with Crohn disease, a positive atypical p-ANCA characterizes a distinct phenotype of left-sided colonic inflammation and a generally favorable response to medical therapy.[36]

Several studies have shown that ASCA correlates with distinct clinical phenotypes in Crohn disease. Presence of ASCA is associated with ileal disease, young age at onset, fibrostenotic and penetrating behavior, and multiple bowel surgeries.[12,37–39] In a cohort of children, ASCA was demonstrated to be associated with disease of the ileum and right colon and to correlate with increased likelihood of ileocecal resection.[19] Among patients with UC undergoing ileal pouch-anal anastomosis, ASCA positivity predicts a greater likelihood of developing fistula complications or a change in disease diagnosis to Crohn disease.[22,40,41]

The presence of anti-OmpC antibodies in Crohn disease is associated with internal perforating disease and requirement for surgery in adults[38] and with fibrostenotic and penetrating disease in children.[42] Patients with Crohn disease with anti-I2 are more likely to have stenosing ileal disease and to require surgical resection.[38,42] An increasing number of positive serologic markers portends a more aggressive disease behavior with a higher frequency of complications and surgery, such that a patient with 4 positive antimicrobial antibodies has an elevenfold increased risk of internal penetrating or stenosing disease when compared with seronegative patients with Crohn disease.[38,42] Similar to the other antimicrobial antibodies, anti-CBir1 expression is associated independently with small bowel, internal penetrating, and fibrostenosing disease features.[25] Presence of anti-CBir1 antibodies is associated with ileal disease, fibrostenotic and fistulizing complications.[25] The combination of NOD2 and anti-CBir1 antibodies increases the strength of association with complicated Crohn disease.[43,44] Among the newer antiglycan antibodies, ALCA is more common in perforating disease, whereas ACCA is associated with fibrostenotic complications.[28] However, the magnitude of association with these antibodies is modest, and the additive value to disease prognosis over the older antimicrobial antibodies is correspondingly small.

Subclinical markers

Some authors have reported that 16% to 30% of healthy first-degree relatives of patients with UC are positive for atypical p-ANCA.[45,46] However, other authors were not able to confirm this finding.[47,48] Among patients with Crohn disease, it has been consistently shown that 20% to 25% of healthy first-degree family members are ASCA positive.[14–16] It remains to be determined whether this finding foreshadows an increased risk of future disease for these family members.

Among Israeli military recruits who eventually developed IBD, many were found to have positive serologic findings on blood specimens that were drawn as part of a biorepository, well before the onset of clinical disease.[49] ASCAs were present in 31% of patients with Crohn disease (vs 0% in controls), and atypical p-ANCA was present in 25% of patients with UC (vs 0% of controls) at an average interval of 38 months before clinical diagnosis. These intriguing data highlight a potential role of these tests in the early identification of patients at risk for IBD and stress the need for further investigation on this topic.

C-Reactive Protein

C-reactive protein (CRP) is an acute phase protein, produced by hepatocytes under the stimulation of interleukin-6, interleukin-1β, and tumor necrosis factor-α[50] and is well known as a marker of systemic inflammation. The rapid production of CRP in response to an acute-phase stimulus within hours and its short half-life make it well suited as a marker for monitoring of disease activity in IBD.[50] However, CRP upregulation is not specific to IBD, and occurs in response to other inflammatory diseases, infectious stimuli, tissue necrosis, malignancy, and other conditions. Some patients have polymorphisms in the CRP gene that result in lower CRP levels,[51] rendering CRP an unreliable measure of inflammatory activity in those patients.

CRP is elevated in 70% to 100% of patients with Crohn disease and 50% to 60% of patients with UC,[52] and the level correlates with disease severity such that mean CRP concentration is higher in patients with severe Crohn disease than those with moderate disease and is even lower in patients with mild disease.[53] The same trend is evident for UC, but the absolute levels of CRP are much lower than in Crohn disease.[53] A study from the Mayo Clinic demonstrated a correlation between CRP levels and evidence of inflammation as assessed by endoscopy and histology in patients with Crohn disease.[54] Among the patients with UC, elevated CRP was associated with clinical disease activity and endoscopic severity, but not histologic degree of inflammation.

CRP may also be useful in prognosticating disease course. A prospective study followed 71 patients with Crohn disease in remission with serial measurements of CRP and other biomarkers every 6 weeks.[55] Elevated CRP (>20 mg/L) forecasted clinical disease exacerbation within 6 weeks. In the setting of severe UC requiring parenteral steroids, a high CRP level has been demonstrated in several predictive models to portend a poor prognosis and higher rate of colectomy.[56,57] A population-based study from Norway showed that elevated CRP at diagnosis predicted nearly a fivefold increase in the odds of subsequent surgery among patients with UC.[58] A similar association between CRP level at diagnosis and surgery was demonstrated for patients with Crohn ileitis.

Although CRP has been used for decades, it has received increased attention lately due to the finding in randomized controlled studies that elevated CRP levels are associated with lower placebo response and consequently increased treatment effect.[59,60] This may be explained by the observation that CRP can aid in the distinction between inflammatory and irritable bowel symptoms,[61] the latter being more likely to exhibit improvement with placebo. Other authors have confirmed the ability of CRP to predict treatment response. Louis and colleagues[62] demonstrated that an elevated CRP level (>5 mg/mL) is associated with a favorable response to infliximab. However, in using CRP as an inclusion criterion or stratification in clinical trials, one must remember that some patients with active IBD may not produce CRP and therefore will be excluded in those studies.

Summary and Recommendations

Serologic biomarkers represent a novel and exciting tool for evaluation of IBD, but currently they have limited clinical application. Insufficient sensitivity and specificity of these antibodies renders them unreliable for establishing the diagnosis of IBD, particularly in patients with a low pretest probability of disease. Likewise, their use in clarifying disease diagnosis among patients with IBDU is hampered by the observation that patients with Crohn disease with isolated colonic involvement have a serologic profile similar to UC. Consequently, serologic panels cannot be routinely recommended for diagnosing IBD or distinguishing between Crohn disease and UC. The potential for serologic biomarkers to predict disease onset or behavior is intriguing, and prospective studies are underway to assess whether these markers also predict response to therapies and warrant a different treatment approach that results in changed short- and long-term outcomes. However, there is insufficient evidence that serologic profiles should override careful clinical evaluation in determining therapeutic management decisions.

CRP is a helpful adjunct tool in evaluating patients with IBD. Although the lack of specificity of CRP limits its utility for initial diagnosis, CRP can be valuable for assessing disease relapse in patients with established IBD and who have demonstrated an elevated CRP at the time of clearly active disease. Thereafter, use of CRP to confirm or predict relapse is helpful. Whether it warrants an immediate change in therapy has not been prospectively studied, but it certainly can assist in the assessment of adherence with current therapy and discussions with the patient.

RADIOLOGIC IMAGING

Most patients with Crohn disease have involvement of the distal ileum, a region of the bowel that is challenging to evaluate. Moreover, IBD patients have chronic disease, which may be progressive over time or alternate between periods of activity and quiescence, necessitating repeat evaluations throughout their life to assess disease distribution and activity. Objective assessment of bowel inflammation is essential to assign a diagnosis of IBD and is critical to inform management decisions in patients with established disease. Although direct endoscopic visualization of the intestinal mucosa along with histologic confirmation remains the gold standard for identifying active inflammation, this approach is invasive and ileoscopy is not always technically feasible. Noninvasive imaging tests are a valuable alternative to endoscopic evaluation of the small intestine for the purposes of diagnosis, determination of disease activity, and identification of complications of disease, such as obstruction or infection.

Fluoroscopic barium studies, including small bowel follow through (SBFT) and small bowel enteroclysis (SBE), have traditionally been the mainstay of small bowel imaging. These studies can provide details about mucosal ulceration or irregularities, luminal narrowing or distention, and presence of fistulous communications. Sensitivity of 85% to 95% and specificity of 89% to 94% have been reported for SBFT in patients with ileal Crohn disease, although this is dependent on the experience of the radiologist.[63,64] SBFT and SBE have comparable sensitivities, but SBFT is preferred by patients because it avoids the need for nasojejunal intubation.[65] These conventional barium examinations serve as the benchmark for comparison in evaluating the performance of novel imaging studies. Advances in computed tomography (CT), magnetic resonance imaging (MRI), and ultrasound have overcome barriers that previously limited their application to image the small bowel. With these advancements, there is now an expanded array of diagnostic imaging techniques for evaluation of IBD.

CT

Cross-sectional imaging with CT offers several distinct advantages over conventional small bowel radiography. Multiplanar imaging allows clear delineation of superimposed bowel loops, and visualization of extraintestinal structures permits identification of disease complications, such as abscesses, fistulae, or phlegmonous changes. Traditional CT evaluation of the abdomen uses a positive contrast agent such as iodine or barium that highlights intraluminal filling defects such as polyps or masses. By comparison, CT enterography (CTE) uses the combination of neutral (low-density) oral contrast and intravenous (IV) contrast to provide optimal distinction between the enhancing small intestinal wall and the adjacent low-attenuation intestinal lumen. This technique facilitates evaluation of the bowel wall and mucosa. Bowel distention is typically achieved with a low-concentration barium solution mixed with sorbitol and water. The amount and timing of oral contrast ingestion has not been standardized, but volumes of 900 to 1800 mL have been described.[66]

CT enteroclysis involves placement of a nasojejunal tube and rapid infusion of enteric contrast directly into the proximal small bowel. This technique improves bowel distention, but it is time consuming and uncomfortable for patients, and the incremental yield of this approach over CTE is modest at best. Findings on CTE or CT enteroclysis that indicate active inflammation include segmental mural enhancement, wall thickening, and mural stratification. Likewise, fibrofatty proliferation, engorgement of the vasa recta (sometimes called a "comb sign"), and reactive mesenteric adenopathy are extraluminal findings that support a diagnosis of active inflammation. Luminal narrowing, if present, can be because of inflammation with edema or chronic fibrostenotic disease, and the distinction between these 2 conditions is not always possible with CT.

In a prospective study of 96 patients undergoing both ileoscopy and CTE, the findings of mural enhancement and wall thickness were able to detect active Crohn disease, with a sensitivity of 80% to 90%.[67] CTE and ileoscopy were equally accurate at predicting histologic inflammation,[67] and radiologic findings correlated with clinical disease activity. In comparison with conventional fluoroscopic imaging, at least 2 studies have found that CTE is more sensitive than SBFT for detecting active disease.[68,69] Studies that compared CTE with capsule endoscopy report varying results, attributable in part to differences in study design. A prospective study comparing multiple small bowel imaging modalities described a sensitivity of 53% for CTE compared with capsule endoscopy (71%), ileoscopy (65%), and SBFT (24%).[69] This study defined any positive small bowel finding consistent with Crohn disease as a true positive and calculated the diagnostic yield of each modality. This methodology does not allow calculation of specificity because each finding is by definition a true positive. A similar analysis by Solem and colleagues[70] prospectively compared CTE with capsule endoscopy, ileoscopy, and SBFT, using a consensus clinical diagnosis of Crohn disease as the reference standard. This study demonstrated equivalent sensitivities for CTE and capsule endoscopy (83%), but CTE was far more specific (89% vs 53%). The authors suggested an algorithm involving these modalities, in which ileocolonoscopy and biopsy is the first test, followed by CTE and, if necessary and if there are no obstructive symptoms or findings, capsule endoscopy.

CTE and CT enteroclysis offer several distinct advantages over conventional fluoroscopic barium studies. SBFT is prone to obscuration of findings because of superimposed bowel loops, but this can be overcome using multiplanar images on CT. In addition, CT can better detect extraintestinal processes that may be missed with SBFT or with endoscopic imaging. When compared with capsule endoscopy, CTE is similarly or slightly less sensitive but far more specific.

The benefits of CTE, however, must be weighed against the deleterious effects of cumulative ionizing radiation, particularly in patients who are young or pregnant.[71] A recent study drew attention to the alarming dose of radiation exposure that many patients with Crohn disease receive.[72] This radiation exposure was primarily attributable to the increased use of CT imaging. Factors associated with exposure to high levels of ionizing radiation included penetrating disease, upper gastrointestinal tract involvement, diagnosis at an early age, requirement for steroids or infliximab, and multiple surgeries.[72]

MRI

Concerns about diagnostic radiation exposure with CT have fueled interest in developing alternative imaging modalities that avoid this risk. Historically, MRI of the bowel was hampered by long image acquisition times resulting in respiratory and peristaltic motion artifact that compromised image quality. However, technologic advances in image acquisition combined with administration of bowel relaxant medication during the procedure have led to substantial improvements in the quality of MR images of the intestine. Administration of large-volume oral contrast results in luminal distention, facilitating evaluation of bowel wall thickness and regularity. MR enteroclysis can also be performed by distending the small intestine with enteric contrast administered through a nasojejunal tube. Analogous to CT or conventional enteroclysis, MR enteroclysis results in superior distention of the bowel but at the sacrifice of patient comfort, and the increased distention may not be necessary in many cases. A prospective study of patients randomized to MR enterography or MR enteroclysis showed identical sensitivity (88%) in both groups.[73]

Superior image quality requires adequate bowel distention with oral contrast, minimization of motion artifact with ultrafast sequences and bowel relaxants, and enhanced bowel wall visualization with IV contrast.[74] Several enteric contrast agents have been investigated for MR enterography. Most studies in Crohn disease use biphasic contrast agents that demonstrate low signal intensity on T1-weighted images, allowing clear delineation of the dark lumen from the hyperenhancing inflammatory segments of the bowel wall after IV contrast. Large volumes of water or even milk have been used effectively, but these liquids can be rapidly absorbed, resulting in suboptimal distention of the distal bowel.[75] Other centers have reported better success with osmotic and/or bulking agents that retain water in the lumen, including mannitol, sorbitol, and locust bean gum.[76,77] Reduction of peristalsis with IV administration of hyoscine butylbromide (Buscopan) or glucagon is integral to preventing motion artifact and preserving image quality. Multiple pulse sequences and multiphasic acquisitions are obtained, and each provides complementary information. Typical MRI findings that indicate active inflammatory disease include mural thickening; ulcerations; hyperenhancement; increased mesenteric vascularity (the "comb sign");

mesenteric inflammation; reactive adenopathy; and complications such as obstruction, perforation, or abscess.[74]

Several investigators have reported that MRI is more sensitive than conventional fluoroscopic barium studies for detecting transmural bowel inflammation and has a sensitivity of as high as 96%.[78–80] However, mild mucosal changes are better visualized with traditional small bowel series radiographs.[78] The multiphasic sequences obtained with MRI can be useful to distinguish inflammatory from fibrostenotic strictures by detecting the differential water content of edematous tissue.[81] Diffusion-weighted imaging has also been shown to be a feasible technique for the detection of inflammation in Crohn disease.[82] When compared with endoscopy, MR enterography demonstrates a sensitivity of 84% to 96% and a specificity of 92% to 100% for detection of IBD.[80,83] In a prospective comparison of MR enterography and CTE, the sensitivities were similar for detecting active Crohn disease (91% vs 95%, respectively).[84]

MRI can also provide detailed and anatomically important information about perianal fistulae, which guides operative management, and it has therefore become a dominant imaging modality for assessment and staging of perianal complications in Crohn disease.[85–87] Although MR colonography has been investigated, its role in IBD diagnosis and management remains undetermined, but it may potentially be of use in patients with Crohn colitis or UC in whom optical colonoscopy is incomplete, contraindicated, or declined by the patient.

MR enterography is a safe and accurate method of evaluating the small bowel and extraluminal structures in patients with Crohn disease. The advantages of this technique over CT include a lack of ionizing radiation, greater safety in renal insufficiency and in pregnancy, and superior evaluation of the pelvic soft tissues and perianal fistulae. The downside of MRI includes a lack of appropriately trained radiologists outside of specialized centers and a considerable cost to perform the examination. Some authors have proposed in a cost-utility analysis that MR imaging may be superior to SBFT because of improved diagnostic accuracy that outweighs the increased cost.[88] This assertion remains to be substantiated with prospective data (**Figs. 1** and **2**).

Ultrasound

Abdominal ultrasound is an evolving imaging modality with a variety of potential applications in patients with established or suspected IBD. There has been renewed interest in exploring ultrasound as a tool in IBD because of its lower cost, excellent safety profile, and ability to be used in pregnant patients. Improvements in ultrasound equipment allow high-resolution images with improved depth of penetration, permitting detailed visualization of the bowel wall and adjacent mesenteric structures.

Inflammation is identified by increased bowel wall diameter, alteration of the normal sonographic pattern of mural stratification, and increased blood flow as assessed by Doppler evaluation. In a meta-analysis, the sensitivity of ultrasound for the initial diagnosis of Crohn disease ranges from 75% to 94%, with a specificity of 67% to 100%, depending on the cutoff value for defining mural thickening.[89] Ultrasound is most sensitive for detecting disease of the ileum (95%), with decreased sensitivity for detecting disease in the left colon (88%), transverse colon (82%), or jejunum (72%).[90] Ultrasound can accurately identify bowel wall thickening and can distinguish fibrosis from acute edema.[91] In a thickened bowel segment, loss of mural stratification is associated with inflammation, whereas retained stratification suggests fibrosis.[92] Introduction of a new microbubble contrast agent that persists in the bloodstream for several minutes has facilitated development of contrast-enhanced ultrasound (CE-US) for imaging parenchymal organs. By evaluating the presence and distribution of blood

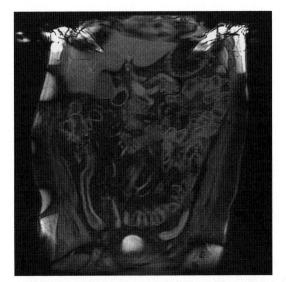

Fig. 1. Ileal stricture seen on magnetic resonance enterography, coronal view.

flow within the bowel wall, CE-US can assess disease activity with high sensitivity (93%) and specificity (93%) and has a strong correlation with clinical disease activity indices.[91]

Some challenges remain, however, that limit widespread application of abdominal ultrasound. Although ultrasound findings are sensitive for the bowel loop being examined, intraluminal gas can obscure visualization of some bowel loops altogether, and obese patients can be challenging to evaluate because of poor depth of penetration. Furthermore, an experienced operator and equipment with enhanced resolution are essential to obtaining high-quality images, and expertise in abdominal ultrasound is

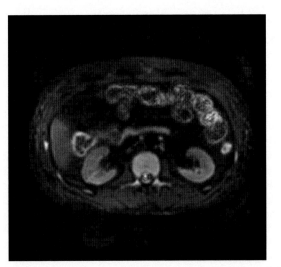

Fig. 2. Ileal inflammation seen on magnetic resonance enterography, axial view.

not pervasive. Nonetheless, these intriguing data suggest a developing role for ultrasound imaging in patients with IBD that warrants continued investigation.

Positron Emission Tomography

Positron emission tomography (PET) scanning is a nuclear medicine technique that uses [18F] fluoro-2-deoxy-D-glucose to identify areas of increased metabolic activity, and it has been used to evaluate multiple infectious, inflammatory, and malignant diseases. Several authors have demonstrated in prospective studies that PET, alone or in combination with CT, can successfully identify active inflammation in both children and adults with established or suspected IBD.[93] A study by Meisner and colleagues[94] reported that PET alone was sufficient to detect inflammation in UC, whereas PET/CT was more useful in Crohn disease. Although data are quite limited, PET appears to have excellent sensitivity and may even be able to detect subclinical inflammation in patients with UC.[95] However, questions remain about its specificity, and the practical application of PET in IBD management has not been established.

Summary and Recommendations

Novel imaging techniques represent a valuable noninvasive alternative to endoscopy for evaluation of the small bowel. CTE is preferable to SBFT as the initial radiologic imaging study in patients with ileal Crohn disease because of the capacity for multiplanar imaging and the ability to detect mural thickening and extraluminal findings. In addition, the utility of SBFT is declining, as the latest generation of radiologists has less experience with conventional barium techniques and interpretation. As the technology and experience with MR enterography imaging improves, MRE is favored over CTE not only due to the ability to distinguish active inflammation from fibrosis but also due to the avoidance of ionizing radiation. This is especially true for the evaluation of perianal Crohn disease, where MRI is clearly superior to other radiologic techniques. Abdominal ultrasound is an attractive and cost-effective option, but it remains substantially limiting by the absence of experience. PET scanning, although intriguing, remains investigational for the evaluation of patients with IBD.

ENDOSCOPIC EXAMINATION
Small Bowel Capsule Endoscopy

Small bowel capsule endoscopy (SBCE) was first introduced in 2001 and has emerged as a highly sensitive modality for the detection of small intestinal pathology, including Crohn disease. The principal advantage of SBCE over conventional endoscopy is the ability to visualize the entire small bowel. SBCE also has an easier preparation and is less invasive and better tolerated. In comparison to small bowel radiologic procedures, SBCE is very sensitive for detection of subtle mucosal lesions, but it provides no information about extraluminal processes.

Despite its many favorable attributes, SBCE also has some drawbacks. Biopsy or intervention is not possible, and there is no way to control the capsule; so significant pathology may be missed as a result of orientation of the camera away from a lesion, obscured visualization due to luminal bubbles or debris, or delayed intestinal transit resulting in an incomplete study. SBCE is contraindicated in patients with strictures because of the risk of capsule retention. However, even patients without symptoms or radiographic evidence of bowel obstruction are susceptible to capsule retention and the consequent need for surgical or advanced endoscopic intervention to retrieve the device.[96]

The performance of capsule endoscopy has been evaluated in multiple studies. Triester and colleagues[97] performed a meta-analysis of the yield of capsule compared to other diagnostic modalities in patients with nonstricturing small bowel Crohn disease. Pooled results of the 9 prospective studies comparing SBCE with barium radiography demonstrated a superior diagnostic yield of 69% for capsule endoscopy versus 30% for SBFT. Capsule endoscopy also outperformed ileocolonoscopy, push enteroscopy, CTE, and MR enterography. The diagnostic yield of SBCE was particularly high among patients with established disease who were being evaluated for disease recurrence or activity. These results may be exaggerated as a result of the "incremental yield" study design, which is biased to favor the most sensitive modality and does not account for false positives that may erode both the sensitivity and specificity of capsule endoscopy.[98] Underscoring this assertion is that false positives are known to be common with SBCE, as 14% of placebo patients and up to 75% of patients on nonsteroidal antiinflammatory drugs (NSAIDs) have mucosal lesions on SBCE.[99,100] Furthermore, there are no established diagnostic criteria for Crohn disease using SBCE, resulting in increased subjectivity and decreased diagnostic precision. Although most studies have defined the presence of more than 3 ulcerations in the absence of NSAID ingestion as a diagnostic criterion, as proposed by Mow and colleagues,[38] this has not been prospectively validated. Given the concerns about the specificity of SBCE, but recognizing that it has excellent sensitivity, some experts have proposed that it be used primarily for monitoring of patients with established IBD rather than for initial diagnosis.[98] Two studies have examined the potential of SBCE to aid in classification of disease among patients with IBD-U and suggest some modest utility in this context (**Fig. 3**).[101,102]

Balloon Enteroscopy

Double-balloon enteroscopy (DBE) was first described in 2001 as a technique that allows deep intubation of the small intestine with an endoscope.[103] A single-balloon device has also been developed with a similar intention. In contrast to push

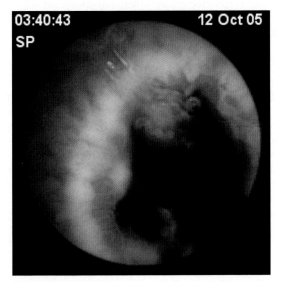

Fig. 3. Stricture in ileum seen with SBCE.

enteroscopy, in which the scope is advanced through a redundant and floppy small bowel, the balloon technique allows the endoscopist to pull and pleat the bowel over the scope using an overtube. The enteroscope can be inserted via the oral or anal route and, using the combination of these approaches, complete examination of the entire small bowel can be achieved in many patients.[104] Diagnostic sampling and therapeutic interventions are both possible with the double-balloon enteroscope.

A study by Mensink and colleagues[105] explored the utility of DBE in established Crohn disease. Of the 40 patients in the study, 24 patients (60%) had findings indicative of active inflammation, leading to a change in therapy in 18 patients (75%). Additional studies also support the utility of DBE in established Crohn disease as a complementary diagnostic modality.[106,107] Oshitani and colleagues[106] reported their outcomes in 40 patients with established Crohn who underwent DBE for evaluation of active disease. DBE was superior to radiologic evaluation for the detection of aphthae, erosions, and small ulcers in the ileum. The authors concluded that DBE is a useful complementary diagnostic modality in patients with Crohn disease. An international consensus statement on the role of small bowel endoscopy in the management of IBD concluded that there are not enough data to recommend DBE unless conventional diagnostic modalities have been inconclusive and histologic diagnosis would alter disease management.[108] This was primarily due to a paucity of data available about the application of this novel endoscopic modality in IBD patients. Nonetheless, the committee endorsed DBE and other device-assisted enteroscopy techniques as valid modalities for diagnosis of Crohn disease because histologic corroboration is available.[108] Balloon enteroscopy has the potential to affect management in select settings, but its exact role in the diagnosis and management of IBD remains to be established.

Summary and Recommendations

Capsule endoscopy is a highly sensitive modality for detecting small bowel erosions and ulcerations and is therefore useful to exclude active small bowel involvement in patients with known IBD. SBCE is currently reserved for patients with established IBD, in whom suspicion for small bowel inflammation remains despite negative findings on ileocolonoscopy and radiologic imaging. Balloon enteroscopy is most useful for obtaining mucosal biopsies of lesions detected with SBCE.

FECAL MARKERS OF INFLAMMATION

Endoscopy with biopsy and histologic evaluation remain the gold standard for identifying and quantifying bowel inflammation. However, endoscopy is expensive and invasive and comes with a small but real risk of complications. In IBD patients, especially, who require repeated evaluation throughout their lives, it would be helpful to have a noninvasive indicator of inflammation. This has driven investigation into surrogate markers of intestinal inflammation. The ideal marker would be simple to perform, noninvasive, inexpensive, rapid, and acceptable to patients and providers. It should also be accurate at identifying inflammation and should correlate well with disease state and prognosis. Fecal markers have a theoretical advantage over serologic markers in that they are more specific for intestinal processes and may reflect the entire intestinal tract. A variety of inflammatory diseases of the gastrointestinal tract, including IBD, are characterized by shedding of leukocytes in the feces. This observation led to the exploration of molecular methods to detect neutrophil-derived proteins in the stool as markers of bowel inflammation.

Calprotectin

Fecal calprotectin represents a promising noninvasive surrogate marker of intestinal inflammation in IBD. Calprotectin is a calcium-binding protein derived predominantly from neutrophils and to a lesser extent from monocytes and reactive macrophages.[109] It is excreted in the feces and can be readily measured using a commercially available ELISA immunoassay. The protein remains stable in stool specimens for up to a week at room temperature, and only 1 to 2 g of stool are needed to reliably perform the analysis.[110,111] These attributes add to the convenience of the test, allowing patients to collect a specimen at home and send it to a reference laboratory for analysis.[111]

Calprotectin is not specific for the cause of intestinal inflammation and may be elevated after the use of NSAIDs[112] or in the setting of enteric infection or intestinal malignancy.[113] Intestinal bleeding can also elevate calprotectin levels, although a significant amount of bleeding is necessary to cause a false-positive result.[114] The level of calprotectin fluctuates from one stool specimen to another in a single patient, and this fluctuation may be related to changes in diet or physical activity.[115]

Results of a meta-analysis showed that calprotectin has a sensitivity of 95% and specificity of 91% for diagnosis in adults and children with suspected IBD.[116] The 9 studies included in this meta-analysis were all prospective and used histologic diagnosis of IBD as the criterion standard. Calprotectin outperformed both CRP and erythrocyte sedimentation rate among the 4 studies in this meta-analysis that included these serum markers, and it is also more sensitive and specific than ASCA or atypical p-ANCA in this context.[9] One of the most promising attributes of calprotectin is its capacity to predict disease exacerbation. At least 2 studies have assessed the diagnostic accuracy of calprotectin in predicting relapse among IBD patients in remission.[117,118] Despite using different cutoff values, the results were remarkably similar, with a sensitivity of 89% to 90% and specificity of 82% to –83% for predicting relapse during a 12-month period. These findings were more robust for patients with UC as opposed to those with Crohn disease. Fecal excretion of calprotectin correlates closely with radiolabeled leukocyte excretion, a validated technique used to detect active inflammation in Crohn disease.[119] Calprotectin levels fluctuate correspondingly with disease activity and correlate with validated clinical, endoscopic, and histologic assessments of disease activity, more so in UC than Crohn disease.[114,120] Normalization of calprotectin has been shown to correspond to clinical improvement and mucosal healing in patients with UC.[121] This observation suggests that calprotectin could potentially play a role as a surrogate marker of response to therapy. Recent data suggest that dramatically elevated calprotectin levels in patients with severe UC predict medically refractory disease and colectomy.[122]

Lactoferrin

Lactoferrin is an iron-binding glycoprotein that is present in many body tissues, including human milk, tears, synovial fluid, and serum. It composes a major component of secondary granules in neutrophils. Leukocyte infiltration into the intestinal mucosa results in detectable increases in fecal lactoferrin concentration,[123] establishing its utility as a biomarker of intestinal inflammation. Much like calprotectin, lactoferrin remains stable in fecal specimens over days and can be detected using a simple and inexpensive ELISA assay.[124]

Lactoferrin has a sensitivity of 80% and a specificity of 82% for the diagnosis of IBD. Although these numbers suggest a slightly lower diagnostic accuracy of lactoferrin compared to calprotectin, direct comparison has not shown one to be consistently superior to the other.[125] In addition to its utility in initial diagnosis of IBD, lactoferrin also has a role in monitoring and management of established IBD patients. A correlation has been confirmed between fecal lactoferrin levels and disease activity, as assessed by standard clinical endoscopic and histologic instruments.[126–128] In a prospective multicenter study of 89 patients with Crohn disease and 74 patients with UC in remission, elevated lactoferrin was able to predict disease relapse (25% vs 10%; $P<.05$) within 12 months.[129] Among postoperative patients with Crohn disease, those with symptomatic recurrence have higher lactoferrin levels than patients without recurrence.[130] Even patients without symptomatic recurrence have persistently elevated lactoferrin levels at long-term follow-up. Two studies have shown a rapid and dramatic decline in fecal lactoferrin levels that paralleled clinical improvement after initiation of infliximab therapy in patients with Crohn disease.[131,132] These data highlight a potential role for lactoferrin as a tool for monitoring response to therapy.

Summary and Recommendations

The neutrophil-derived fecal markers hold enormous promise as noninvasive tools for detection and monitoring of bowel inflammation in IBD. However, despite this potential, their exact role in the diagnostic and management algorithm has not been clarified and they are not routinely used in clinical practice, with the exception of the patient with persistent symptoms and an otherwise negative work-up, in which case they may suggest occult inflammation.

SUMMARY

Advances in technology have ushered in a variety of novel diagnostic and prognostic modalities for evaluating IBD. Clinicians now have an expanded arsenal of strategies to assist with timely and accurate diagnosis, to assess disease distribution and activity, and to identify disease complications. Although serologic biomarkers are not reliable for disease diagnosis, they have a promising role in predicting disease behavior and the possibility of stratifying treatments. Improvements in imaging techniques offer complementary strategies for noninvasive evaluation of the bowel and extraluminal structures while avoiding ionizing radiation. Endoscopic advancements with capsule and balloon enteroscopy now permit detailed visualization, diagnostic sampling, and therapeutic intervention throughout the entire intestinal tract. Neutrophil-derived fecal markers hold promise as convenient and rapid tests to diagnose and monitor disease, but their exact place in the IBD management algorithm is not yet established. The future will undoubtedly deliver more exciting and innovative approaches to determining diagnosis and prognosis in patients with IBD.

REFERENCES

1. Bossuyt X. Serologic markers in inflammatory bowel disease. Clin Chem 2006; 52(2):171–81.
2. Terjung B, Worman HJ. Anti-neutrophil antibodies in primary sclerosing cholangitis. Best Pract Res Clin Gastroenterol 2001;15(4):629–42.
3. Terjung B, Bogsch F, Klein R, et al. Diagnostic accuracy of atypical p-ANCA in autoimmune hepatitis using ROC- and multivariate regression analysis. Eur J Med Res 2004;9(9):439–48.
4. Saxon A, Shanahan F, Landers C, et al. A distinct subset of antineutrophil cytoplasmic antibodies is associated with inflammatory bowel disease. J Allergy Clin Immunol 1990;86(2):202–10.

5. Rump JA, Scholmerich J, Gross V, et al. A new type of perinuclear anti-neutrophil cytoplasmic antibody (p-ANCA) in active ulcerative colitis but not in Crohn's disease. Immunobiology 1990;181(4–5):406–13.

6. Joossens S, Daperno M, Shums Z, et al. Interassay and interobserver variability in the detection of anti-neutrophil cytoplasmic antibodies in patients with ulcerative colitis. Clin Chem 2004;50(8):1422–5.

7. Sandborn WJ, Loftus EV Jr, Colombel JF, et al. Evaluation of serologic disease markers in a population-based cohort of patients with ulcerative colitis and Crohn's disease. Inflamm Bowel Dis 2001;7(3):192–201.

8. Vidrich A, Lee J, James E, et al. Segregation of pANCA antigenic recognition by DNase treatment of neutrophils: ulcerative colitis, type 1 autoimmune hepatitis, and primary sclerosing cholangitis. J Clin Immunol 1995;15(6):293–9.

9. Reese GE, Constantinides VA, Simillis C, et al. Diagnostic precision of anti-Saccharomyces cerevisiae antibodies and perinuclear antineutrophil cytoplasmic antibodies in inflammatory bowel disease. Am J Gastroenterol 2006; 101(10):2410–22.

10. Main J, McKenzie H, Yeaman GR, et al. Antibody to Saccharomyces cerevisiae (bakers' yeast) in Crohn's disease. BMJ 1988;297(6656):1105–6.

11. Standaert-Vitse A, Jouault T, Vandewalle P, et al. Candida albicans is an immunogen for anti-Saccharomyces cerevisiae antibody markers of Crohn's disease. Gastroenterology 2006;130(6):1764–75.

12. Quinton JF, Sendid B, Reumaux D, et al. Anti-Saccharomyces cerevisiae mannan antibodies combined with antineutrophil cytoplasmic autoantibodies in inflammatory bowel disease: prevalence and diagnostic role. Gut 1998;42(6):788–91.

13. Peeters M, Joossens S, Vermeire S, et al. Diagnostic value of anti-Saccharomyces cerevisiae and antineutrophil cytoplasmic autoantibodies in inflammatory bowel disease. Am J Gastroenterol 2001;96(3):730–4.

14. Seibold F, Stich O, Hufnagl R, et al. Anti-Saccharomyces cerevisiae antibodies in inflammatory bowel disease: a family study. Scand J Gastroenterol 2001; 36(2):196–201.

15. Sendid B, Quinton JF, Charrier G, et al. Anti-Saccharomyces cerevisiae mannan antibodies in familial Crohn's disease. Am J Gastroenterol 1998;93(8):1306–10.

16. Vermeire S, Peeters M, Vlietinck R, et al. Anti-Saccharomyces cerevisiae antibodies (ASCA), phenotypes of IBD, and intestinal permeability: a study in IBD families. Inflamm Bowel Dis 2001;7(1):8–15.

17. Poulain D, Sendid B, Fajardy I, et al. Mother to child transmission of anti-S cerevisiae mannan antibodies (ASCA) in non-IBD families. Gut 2000;47(6):870–1.

18. Landers CJ, Cohavy O, Misra R, et al. Selected loss of tolerance evidenced by Crohn's disease-associated immune responses to auto- and microbial antigens. Gastroenterology 2002;123(3):689–99.

19. Zholudev A, Zurakowski D, Young W, et al. Serologic testing with ANCA, ASCA, and anti-OmpC in children and young adults with Crohn's disease and ulcerative colitis: diagnostic value and correlation with disease phenotype. Am J Gastroenterol 2004;99(11):2235–41.

20. Sutton CL, Kim J, Yamane A, et al. Identification of a novel bacterial sequence associated with Crohn's disease. Gastroenterology 2000;119(1):23–31.

21. Joossens S, Colombel JF, Landers C, et al. Anti-outer membrane of porin C and anti-I2 antibodies in indeterminate colitis. Gut 2006;55(11):1667–9.

22. Hui T, Landers C, Vasiliauskas E, et al. Serologic responses in indeterminate colitis patients before ileal pouch-anal anastomosis may determine those at risk for continuous pouch inflammation. Dis Colon Rectum 2005;48(6):1254–62.

23. Lawrance IC, Hall A, Leong R, et al. A comparative study of goblet cell and pancreatic exocine autoantibodies combined with ASCA and pANCA in Chinese and Caucasian patients with IBD. Inflamm Bowel Dis 2005;11(10): 890–7.

24. Lodes MJ, Cong Y, Elson CO, et al. Bacterial flagellin is a dominant antigen in Crohn disease. J Clin Invest 2004;113(9):1296–306.

25. Targan SR, Landers CJ, Yang H, et al. Antibodies to CBir1 flagellin define a unique response that is associated independently with complicated Crohn's disease. Gastroenterology 2005;128(7):2020–8.

26. Ferrante M, Henckaerts L, Joossens M, et al. New serological markers in inflammatory bowel disease are associated with complicated disease behaviour. Gut 2007;56(10):1394–403.

27. Dotan I, Fishman S, Dgani Y, et al. Antibodies against laminaribioside and chitobioside are novel serologic markers in Crohn's disease. Gastroenterology 2006;131(2):366–78.

28. Papp M, Altorjay I, Dotan N, et al. New serological markers for inflammatory bowel disease are associated with earlier age at onset, complicated disease behavior, risk for surgery, and NOD2/CARD15 genotype in a Hungarian IBD cohort. Am J Gastroenterol 2008;103(3):665–81.

29. Seow CH, Stempak JM, Xu W, et al. Novel anti-glycan antibodies related to inflammatory bowel disease diagnosis and phenotype. Am J Gastroenterol 2009;104(6):1426–34.

30. Austin GL, Shaheen NJ, Sandler RS. Positive and negative predictive values: use of inflammatory bowel disease serologic markers. Am J Gastroenterol 2006;101(3):413–6.

31. Joossens S, Reinisch W, Vermeire S, et al. The value of serologic markers in indeterminate colitis: a prospective follow-up study. Gastroenterology 2002; 122(5):1242–7.

32. Reumaux D, Colombel JF, Masy E, et al. Anti-neutrophil cytoplasmic auto-antibodies (ANCA) in ulcerative colitis (UC): no relationship with disease activity. Inflamm Bowel Dis 2000;6(4):270–4.

33. Sandborn WJ, Landers CJ, Tremaine WJ, et al. Association of antineutrophil cytoplasmic antibodies with resistance to treatment of left-sided ulcerative colitis: results of a pilot study. Mayo Clin Proc 1996;71(5):431–6.

34. Sandborn WJ, Landers CJ, Tremaine WJ, et al. Antineutrophil cytoplasmic antibody correlates with chronic pouchitis after ileal pouch-anal anastomosis. Am J Gastroenterol 1995;90(5):740–7.

35. Fleshner PR, Vasiliauskas EA, Kam LY, et al. High level perinuclear antineutrophil cytoplasmic antibody (pANCA) in ulcerative colitis patients before colectomy predicts the development of chronic pouchitis after ileal pouch-anal anastomosis. Gut 2001;49(5):671–7.

36. Vasiliauskas EA, Plevy SE, Landers CJ, et al. Perinuclear antineutrophil cytoplasmic antibodies in patients with Crohn's disease define a clinical subgroup. Gastroenterology 1996;110(6):1810–9.

37. Vasiliauskas EA, Kam LY, Karp LC, et al. Marker antibody expression stratifies Crohn's disease into immunologically homogeneous subgroups with distinct clinical characteristics. Gut 2000;47(4):487–96.

38. Mow WS, Vasiliauskas EA, Lin YC, et al. Association of antibody responses to microbial antigens and complications of small bowel Crohn's disease. Gastroenterology 2004;126(2):414–24.

39. Walker LJ, Aldhous MC, Drummond HE, et al. Anti-Saccharomyces cerevisiae antibodies (ASCA) in Crohn's disease are associated with disease severity but not NOD2/CARD15 mutations. Clin Exp Immunol 2004;135(3):490–6.

40. Dendrinos KG, Becker JM, Stucchi AF, et al. Anti-Saccharomyces cerevisiae antibodies are associated with the development of postoperative fistulas following ileal pouch-anal anastomosis. J Gastrointest Surg 2006;10(7):1060–4.

41. Melmed GY, Fleshner PR, Bardakcioglu O, et al. Family history and serology predict Crohn's disease after ileal pouch-anal anastomosis for ulcerative colitis. Dis Colon Rectum 2008;51(1):100–8.

42. Dubinsky MC, Lin YC, Dutridge D, et al. Serum immune responses predict rapid disease progression among children with Crohn's disease: immune responses predict disease progression. Am J Gastroenterol 2006;101(2):360–7.

43. Papadakis KA, Yang H, Ippoliti A, et al. Anti-flagellin (CBir1) phenotypic and genetic Crohn's disease associations. Inflamm Bowel Dis 2007;13(5):524–30.

44. Devlin SM, Yang H, Ippoliti A, et al. NOD2 variants and antibody response to microbial antigens in Crohn's disease patients and their unaffected relatives. Gastroenterology 2007;132(2):576–86.

45. Seibold F, Slametschka D, Gregor M, et al. Neutrophil autoantibodies: a genetic marker in primary sclerosing cholangitis and ulcerative colitis. Gastroenterology 1994;107(2):532–6.

46. Shanahan F, Duerr RH, Rotter JI, et al. Neutrophil autoantibodies in ulcerative colitis: familial aggregation and genetic heterogeneity. Gastroenterology 1992; 103(2):456–61.

47. Lee JC, Lennard-Jones JE, Cambridge G. Antineutrophil antibodies in familial inflammatory bowel disease. Gastroenterology 1995;108(2):428–33.

48. Folwaczny C, Noehl N, Endres SP, et al. Antineutrophil and pancreatic autoantibodies in first-degree relatives of patients with inflammatory bowel disease. Scand J Gastroenterol 1998;33(5):523–8.

49. Israeli E, Grotto I, Gilburd B, et al. Anti-Saccharomyces cerevisiae and antineutrophil cytoplasmic antibodies as predictors of inflammatory bowel disease. Gut 2005;54(9):1232–6.

50. Vermeire S, Van Assche G, Rutgeerts P. C-reactive protein as a marker for inflammatory bowel disease. Inflamm Bowel Dis 2004;10(5):661–5.

51. Thalmaier D, Dambacher J, Seiderer J, et al. The +1059G/C polymorphism in the C-reactive protein (CRP) gene is associated with involvement of the terminal ileum and decreased serum CRP levels in patients with Crohn's disease. Aliment Pharmacol Ther 2006;24(7):1105–15.

52. Vermeire S, Van Assche G, Rutgeerts P. Laboratory markers in IBD: useful, magic, or unnecessary toys? Gut 2006;55(3):426–31.

53. Fagan EA, Dyck RF, Maton PN, et al. Serum levels of C-reactive protein in Crohn's disease and ulcerative colitis. Eur J Clin Invest 1982;12(4):351–9.

54. Solem CA, Loftus EV Jr, Tremaine WJ, et al. Correlation of C-reactive protein with clinical, endoscopic, histologic, and radiographic activity in inflammatory bowel disease. Inflamm Bowel Dis 2005;11(8):707–12.

55. Consigny Y, Modigliani R, Colombel JF, et al. A simple biological score for predicting low risk of short-term relapse in Crohn's disease. Inflamm Bowel Dis 2006;12(7):551–7.

56. Lindgren SC, Flood LM, Kilander AF, et al. Early predictors of glucocorticosteroid treatment failure in severe and moderately severe attacks of ulcerative colitis. Eur J Gastroenterol Hepatol 1998;10(10):831–5.

57. Travis SP, Farrant JM, Ricketts.C, et al. Predicting outcome in severe ulcerative colitis. Gut 1996;38(6):905–10.
58. Henriksen M, Jahnsen J, Lygren I, et al. C-reactive protein: a predictive factor and marker of inflammation in inflammatory bowel disease. Results from a prospective population-based study. Gut 2008;57(11):1518–23.
59. Schreiber S, Rutgeerts P, Fedorak RN, et al. A randomized, placebo-controlled trial of certolizumab pegol (CDP870) for treatment of Crohn's disease. Gastroenterology 2005;129(3):807–18.
60. Sandborn WJ, Colombel JF, Enns R, et al. Natalizumab induction and maintenance therapy for Crohn's disease. N Engl J Med 2005;353(18):1912–25.
61. Poullis AP, Zar S, Sundaram KK, et al. A new, highly sensitive assay for C-reactive protein can aid the differentiation of inflammatory bowel disorders from constipation- and diarrhoea-predominant functional bowel disorders. Eur J Gastroenterol Hepatol 2002;14(4):409–12.
62. Louis E, Vermeire S, Rutgeerts P, et al. A positive response to infliximab in Crohn disease: association with a higher systemic inflammation before treatment but not with -308 TNF gene polymorphism. Scand J Gastroenterol 2002;37(7):818–24.
63. Schreyer AG, Golder S, Seitz J, et al. New diagnostic avenues in inflammatory bowel diseases. Capsule endoscopy, magnetic resonance imaging and virtual enteroscopy. Dig Dis 2003;21(2):129–37.
64. Ott DJ, Chen YM, Gelfand DW, et al. Detailed per-oral small bowel examination vs. enteroclysis (Part II): Radiographic accuracy. Radiology 1985;155(1):31–4.
65. Bernstein CN, Boult IF, Greenberg HM, et al. A prospective randomized comparison between small bowel enteroclysis and small bowel follow-through in Crohn's disease. Gastroenterology 1997;113(2):390–8.
66. Paulsen SR, Huprich JE, Hara AK. CT enterography: noninvasive evaluation of Crohn's disease and obscure gastrointestinal bleed. Radiol Clin North Am 2007;45(2):303–15.
67. Bodily KD, Fletcher JG, Solem CA, et al. Crohn disease: mural attenuation and thickness at contrast-enhanced CT Enterography–correlation with endoscopic and histologic findings of inflammation. Radiology 2006;238(2):505–16.
68. Wold PB, Fletcher JG, Johnson CD, et al. Assessment of small bowel Crohn disease: noninvasive peroral CT enterography compared with other imaging methods and endoscopy–feasibility study. Radiology 2003;229(1):275–81.
69. Hara AK, Leighton JA, Heigh RI, et al. Crohn disease of the small bowel: preliminary comparison among CT enterography, capsule endoscopy, small-bowel follow-through, and ileoscopy. Radiology 2006;238(1):128–34.
70. Solem CA, Loftus EV Jr, Fletcher JG, et al. Small-bowel imaging in Crohn's disease: a prospective, blinded, 4-way comparison trial. Gastrointest Endosc 2008;68(2):255–66.
71. Brenner DJ, Hall EJ. Computed tomography–an increasing source of radiation exposure. N Engl J Med 2007;357(22):2277–84.
72. Desmond AN, O'Regan K, Curran C, et al. Crohn's disease: factors associated with exposure to high levels of diagnostic radiation. Gut 2008;57(11):1524–9.
73. Negaard A, Paulsen V, Sandvik L, et al. A prospective randomized comparison between two MRI studies of the small bowel in Crohn's disease, the oral contrast method and MR enteroclysis. Eur Radiol 2007;17(9):2294–301.
74. Siddiki H, Fidler J. MR imaging of the small bowel in Crohn's disease. Eur J Radiol 2009;69(3):409–17.

75. Lomas DJ, Graves MJ. Small bowel MRI using water as a contrast medium. Br J Radiol 1999;72(862):994–7.
76. Ajaj W, Goehde SC, Schneemann H, et al. Oral contrast agents for small bowel MRI: comparison of different additives to optimize bowel distension. Eur Radiol 2004;14(3):458–64.
77. Kuehle CA, Ajaj W, Ladd SC, et al. Hydro-MRI of the small bowel: effect of contrast volume, timing of contrast administration, and data acquisition on bowel distention. AJR Am J Roentgenol 2006;187(4):W375–85.
78. Gourtsoyiannis NC, Grammatikakis J, Papamastorakis G, et al. Imaging of small intestinal Crohn's disease: comparison between MR enteroclysis and conventional enteroclysis. Eur Radiol 2006;16(9):1915–25.
79. Rieber A, Wruk D, Potthast S, et al. Diagnostic imaging in Crohn's disease: comparison of magnetic resonance imaging and conventional imaging methods. Int J Colorectal Dis 2000;15(3):176–81.
80. Darbari A, Sena L, Argani P, et al. Gadolinium-enhanced magnetic resonance imaging: a useful radiological tool in diagnosing pediatric IBD. Inflamm Bowel Dis 2004;10(2):67–72.
81. Masselli G, Brizi GM, Parrella A, et al. Crohn disease: magnetic resonance enteroclysis. Abdom Imaging 2004;29(3):326–34.
82. Oto A, Zhu F, Kulkarni K, et al. Evaluation of diffusion-weighted MR imaging for detection of bowel inflammation in patients with Crohn's disease. Acad Radiol 2009;16(5):597–603.
83. Laghi A, Borrelli O, Paolantonio P, et al. Contrast enhanced magnetic resonance imaging of the terminal ileum in children with Crohn's disease. Gut 2003;52(3):393–7.
84. Siddiki HA, Fidler JL, Fletcher JG, et al. Prospective comparison of state-of-the-art MR enterography and CT enterography in small-bowel Crohn's disease. AJR Am J Roentgenol 2009;193(1):113–21.
85. Beets-Tan RG, Beets GL, van der Hoop AG, et al. Preoperative MR imaging of anal fistulas: does it really help the surgeon? Radiology 2001;218(1):75–84.
86. Koelbel G, Schmiedl U, Majer MC, et al. Diagnosis of fistulae and sinus tracts in patients with Crohn disease: value of MR imaging. AJR Am J Roentgenol 1989;152(5):999–1003.
87. Schwartz DA, Wiersema MJ, Dudiak KM, et al. A comparison of endoscopic ultrasound, magnetic resonance imaging, and exam under anesthesia for evaluation of Crohn's perianal fistulas. Gastroenterology 2001;121(5):1064–72.
88. Ebinger M, Rieber A, Leidl R. Cost-effectiveness of magnetic resonance imaging and enteroclysis in the diagnostic imaging of Crohn's disease. Int J Technol Assess Health Care 2002;18(3):711–7.
89. Fraquelli M, Colli A, Casazza G, et al. Role of US in detection of Crohn disease: meta-analysis. Radiology 2005;236(1):95–101.
90. Parente F, Maconi G, Bollani S, et al. Bowel ultrasound in assessment of Crohn's disease and detection of related small bowel strictures: a prospective comparative study versus x ray and intraoperative findings. Gut 2002;50(4):490–5.
91. Migaleddu V, Scanu AM, Quaia E, et al. Contrast-enhanced ultrasonographic evaluation of inflammatory activity in Crohn's disease. Gastroenterology 2009;137(1):43–52.
92. Maconi G, Carsana L, Fociani P, et al. Small bowel stenosis in Crohn's disease: clinical, biochemical and ultrasonographic evaluation of histological features. Aliment Pharmacol Ther 2003;18(7):749–56.

93. Spier BJ, Perlman SB, Reichelderfer M. FDG-PET in inflammatory bowel disease. Q J Nucl Med Mol Imaging 2009;53(1):64–71.
94. Meisner RS, Spier BJ, Einarsson S, et al. Pilot study using PET/CT as a novel, noninvasive assessment of disease activity in inflammatory bowel disease. Inflamm Bowel Dis 2007;13(8):993–1000.
95. Rubin DT, Surma BL, Gavzy SJ, et al. Positron emission tomography (PET) used to image subclinical inflammation associated with ulcerative colitis (UC) in remission. Inflamm Bowel Dis 2009;15(5):750–5.
96. Cheifetz AS, Kornbluth AA, Legnani P, et al. The risk of retention of the capsule endoscope in patients with known or suspected Crohn's disease. Am J Gastroenterol 2006;101(10):2218–22.
97. Triester SL, Leighton JA, Leontiadis GI, et al. A meta-analysis of the yield of capsule endoscopy compared to other diagnostic modalities in patients with non-stricturing small bowel Crohn's disease. Am J Gastroenterol 2006;101(5):954–64.
98. Lashner BA. Sensitivity-specificity trade-off for capsule endoscopy in IBD: is it worth it? Am J Gastroenterol 2006;101(5):965–6.
99. Goldstein JL, Eisen GM, Lewis B, et al. Video capsule endoscopy to prospectively assess small bowel injury with celecoxib, naproxen plus omeprazole, and placebo. Clin Gastroenterol Hepatol 2005;3(2):133–41.
100. Graham DY, Opekun AR, Willingham FF, et al. Visible small-intestinal mucosal injury in chronic NSAID users. Clin Gastroenterol Hepatol 2005;3(1):55–9.
101. Maunoury V, Savoye G, Bourreille A, et al. Value of wireless capsule endoscopy in patients with indeterminate colitis (inflammatory bowel disease type unclassified). Inflamm Bowel Dis 2007;13(2):152–5.
102. Mehdizadeh S, Chen G, Enayati PJ, et al. Diagnostic yield of capsule endoscopy in ulcerative colitis and inflammatory bowel disease of unclassified type (IBDU). Endoscopy 2008;40(1):30–5.
103. Yamamoto H, Kita H. Double-balloon endoscopy. Curr Opin Gastroenterol 2005;21(5):573–7.
104. Yamamoto H, Kita H, Sunada K, et al. Clinical outcomes of double-balloon endoscopy for the diagnosis and treatment of small-intestinal diseases. Clin Gastroenterol Hepatol 2004;2(11):1010–6.
105. Mensink PB, Groenen MJ, van Buuren HR, et al. Double-balloon enteroscopy in Crohn's disease patients suspected of small bowel activity: findings and clinical impact. J Gastroenterol 2009;44(4):271–6.
106. Oshitani N, Yukawa T, Yamagami H, et al. Evaluation of deep small bowel involvement by double-balloon enteroscopy in Crohn's disease. Am J Gastroenterol 2006;101(7):1484–9.
107. Manes G, Imbesi V, Ardizzone S, et al. Use of double-balloon enteroscopy in the management of patients with Crohn's disease: feasibility and diagnostic yield in a high-volume centre for inflammatory bowel disease. Surg Endosc 2009 May 23 [Epub ahead of print].
108. Bourreille A, Ignjatovic A, Aabakken L, et al. Role of small-bowel endoscopy in the management of patients with inflammatory bowel disease: an international OMED-ECCO consensus. Endoscopy 2009;41(7):618–37.
109. Bjerke K, Halstensen TS, Jahnsen F, et al. Distribution of macrophages and granulocytes expressing L1 protein (calprotectin) in human Peyer's patches compared with normal ileal lamina propria and mesenteric lymph nodes. Gut 1993;34(10):1357–63.

110. Roseth AG, Fagerhol MK, Aadland E, et al. Assessment of the neutrophil dominating protein calprotectin in feces. A methodologic study. Scand J Gastroenterol 1992;27(9):793–8.

111. Lundberg JO, Hellstrom PM, Fagerhol MK, et al. Technology insight: calprotectin, lactoferrin and nitric oxide as novel markers of inflammatory bowel disease. Nat Clin Pract Gastroenterol Hepatol 2005;2(2):96–102.

112. Meling TR, Aabakken L, Roseth A, et al. Faecal calprotectin shedding after short-term treatment with non-steroidal anti-inflammatory drugs. Scand J Gastroenterol 1996;31(4):339–44.

113. Costa F, Mumolo MG, Bellini M, et al. Role of faecal calprotectin as non-invasive marker of intestinal inflammation. Dig Liver Dis 2003;35(9):642–7.

114. Gisbert JP, McNicholl AG. Questions and answers on the role of faecal calprotectin as a biological marker in inflammatory bowel disease. Dig Liver Dis 2009; 41(1):56–66.

115. Poullis A, Foster R, Shetty A, et al. Bowel inflammation as measured by fecal calprotectin: a link between lifestyle factors and colorectal cancer risk. Cancer Epidemiol Biomarkers Prev 2004;13(2):279–84.

116. von Roon AC, Karamountzos L, Purkayastha S, et al. Diagnostic precision of fecal calprotectin for inflammatory bowel disease and colorectal malignancy. Am J Gastroenterol 2007;102(4):803–13.

117. Costa F, Mumolo MG, Ceccarelli L, et al. Calprotectin is a stronger predictive marker of relapse in ulcerative colitis than in Crohn's disease. Gut 2005;54(3): 364–8.

118. Tibble JA, Sigthorsson G, Bridger S, et al. Surrogate markers of intestinal inflammation are predictive of relapse in patients with inflammatory bowel disease. Gastroenterology 2000;119(1):15–22.

119. Roseth AG, Schmidt PN, Fagerhol MK. Correlation between faecal excretion of indium-111-labelled granulocytes and calprotectin, a granulocyte marker protein, in patients with inflammatory bowel disease. Scand J Gastroenterol 1999;34(1):50–4.

120. Roseth AG, Aadland E, Jahnsen J, et al. Assessment of disease activity in ulcerative colitis by faecal calprotectin, a novel granulocyte marker protein. Digestion 1997;58(2):176–80.

121. Roseth AG, Aadland E, Grzyb K. Normalization of faecal calprotectin: a predictor of mucosal healing in patients with inflammatory bowel disease. Scand J Gastroenterol 2004;39(10):1017–20.

122. Ho GT, Lee HM, Brydon G, et al. Fecal calprotectin predicts the clinical course of acute severe ulcerative colitis. Am J Gastroenterol 2009;104(3):673–8.

123. Guerrant RL, Araujo V, Soares E, et al. Measurement of fecal lactoferrin as a marker of fecal leukocytes. J Clin Microbiol 1992;30(5):1238–42.

124. Angriman I, Scarpa M, D'Inca R, et al. Enzymes in feces: useful markers of chronic inflammatory bowel disease. Clin Chim Acta 2007;381(1):63–8.

125. Langhorst J, Elsenbruch S, Koelzer J, et al. Noninvasive markers in the assessment of intestinal inflammation in inflammatory bowel diseases: performance of fecal lactoferrin, calprotectin, and PMN-elastase, CRP, and clinical indices. Am J Gastroenterol 2008;103(1):162–9.

126. Langhorst J, Elsenbruch S, Mueller T, et al. Comparison of 4 neutrophil-derived proteins in feces as indicators of disease activity in ulcerative colitis. Inflamm Bowel Dis 2005;11(12):1085–91.

127. Sipponen T, Savilahti E, Kolho KL, et al. Crohn's disease activity assessed by fecal calprotectin and lactoferrin: correlation with Crohn's disease activity index and endoscopic findings. Inflamm Bowel Dis 2008;14(1):40–6.

128. D'Inca R, Dal Pont E, Di Leo V, et al. Calprotectin and lactoferrin in the assessment of intestinal inflammation and organic disease. Int J Colorectal Dis 2007; 22(4):429–37.

129. Gisbert JP, Bermejo F, Perez-Calle JL, et al. Fecal calprotectin and lactoferrin for the prediction of inflammatory bowel disease relapse. Inflamm Bowel Dis 2009; 15(8):1190–8.

130. Scarpa M, D'Inca R, Basso D, et al. Fecal lactoferrin and calprotectin after ileocolonic resection for Crohn's disease. Dis Colon Rectum 2007;50(6):861–9.

131. Sipponen T, Savilahti E, Karkkainen P, et al. Fecal calprotectin, lactoferrin, and endoscopic disease activity in monitoring anti-TNF-alpha therapy for Crohn's disease. Inflamm Bowel Dis 2008;14(10):1392–8.

132. Buderus S, Boone J, Lyerly D, et al. Fecal lactoferrin: a new parameter to monitor infliximab therapy. Dig Dis Sci 2004;49(6):1036–9.

Postoperative Management of Crohn Disease

Su Min Cho, MBBS[a], Sung W. Cho, MBBS, MSc[b],
Miguel Regueiro, MD[c,d,e],*

KEYWORDS

• Crohn disease • Postoperative • Prevention • 5-ASA
• Immunomodulators • Infliximab

Crohn disease is a chronic relapsing inflammatory disease of the gastrointestinal tract with a myriad of systemic manifestations. The cause is unknown, but immunologic, genetic, and environmental factors are thought to be involved. Pathologically, it is characterized by noncaseating granuloma and transmural inflammation, which can affect the gut from the mouth to the anus. The most commonly affected sites of Crohn disease involvement in the gastrointestinal tract are the ileum and ascending colon. Thus, the most common surgery for Crohn disease is resection of the distal ileum and cecum.

It is estimated that 75% of patients with Crohn disease will eventually undergo surgery.[1] Indications for surgery include failure of medical management or complications of Crohn disease, such as perforation, obstruction, fistula formation, toxic megacolon, or malignancy. In recent years, "bowel-conserving" surgery has been advocated for Crohn disease, in which only the grossly involved bowel is removed.[2] This surgical strategy is based on radical surgery not being curative and on major advances in more effective medical therapies.

Approximately 30% of patients who have undergone bowel resection for Crohn disease will require another operation for recurrence within 5 years.[3] Moreover,

This article originally appeared in *Gastroenterology Clinics of North America*, Volume 38, Issue 4.

[a] Department of Gastroenterology, Hepatology, and Nutrition, University of Pittsburgh Medical Center, Pittsburgh, PA, USA

[b] Department of General Surgery, University of Pittsburgh Medical Center, Pittsburgh, PA, USA

[c] Department of Medicine, University of Pittsburgh School of Medicine, 200 Lothrop Street, PUH- C Wing Mezzanine Level, Pittsburgh, PA 15213, USA

[d] Inflammatory Bowel Disease Center, 200 Lothrop Street, PUH- C Wing Mezzanine Level, Pittsburgh, PA 15213, USA

[e] Gastroenterology, Hepatology, and Nutrition Fellowship Training Program, Division of Gastroenterology, Hepatology and Nutrition, University of Pittsburgh Medical Center, 200 Lothrop Street, PUH- C Wing Mezzanine Level, Pittsburgh, PA 15213, USA

* Corresponding Author. University of Pittsburgh Medical Center, 200 Lothrop Street, PUH- C Wing Mezzanine Level, Pittsburgh, PA 15213.

E-mail address: mdr7@pitt.edu (M. Regueiro).

Med Clin N Am 94 (2010) 179–188
doi:10.1016/j.mcna.2009.08.019
0025-7125/09/$ – see front matter © 2010 Elsevier Inc. All rights reserved.

medical.theclinics.com

optimal medical management of patients with Crohn disease after surgery is still controversial. In this article, the authors evaluate the literature on postoperative medications for Crohn disease and provide management recommendations.

NATURAL HISTORY

It is estimated that approximately 30% of patients who require surgery for Crohn disease will experience symptomatic recurrence within 3 years, and as high as 60%, within 10 years.[3] Relapse rates in the placebo group of randomized double-blind trials provide a reasonable guide of natural history of Crohn disease after surgery. In a meta-analysis, Renna and colleagues[4] found that the pooled estimate of 1-year relapse rates in the placebo groups was 10% to 38%. A logistic regression analysis of the factors associated with postoperative recurrence revealed that study duration was the only significant factor.

Endoscopic recurrence is more common than symptomatic relapse, approaching 90% one year after surgery.[5,6] Endoscopic findings that indicate recurrence include small aphthous ulcers, deep linear ulcers, mucosal inflammation, fistulae, and strictures. These varying degrees of endoscopic disease activity may be seen within 3 months of surgery in more than 70% of patients.[5] The most common site of recurrence is the surgical anastomosis, especially the proximal side of the anastomosis.[5] The cause for recurrence at this location is thought to be related to luminal contents, specifically intestinal flora.[7] Endoscopic recurrence precedes clinical recurrence, and the severity of endoscopic findings predicts the risk of clinical recurrence.[6]

RISK FACTORS FOR CLINICAL RECURRENCE

Various clinical variables, disease patterns, and surgical techniques have been studied to determine factors associated with recurrence and disease severity.

Active cigarette smoking has consistently been shown to be an independent risk factor for recurrence with relative risk ranges from 1.4 to 4.3.[8] The need for immunosuppressive drugs is associated with smoking in a dose-dependent fashion, and the adverse effect of smoking is more strongly associated with early recurrence in women than in men.[9] Several studies have found that the disease pattern that is seen at the initial surgery influences postoperative course.[10] Crohn disease can be divided into 2 subtypes, perforating and nonperforating. Patients with the perforating type require surgery for fistula, abscess, or free perforation, whereas for the nonperforating type, the indications include obstruction, failure of medical treatment, hemorrhage, or toxic megacolon.[11] In the multivariate analysis, surgery for the perforating indication was an independent predictor of early recurrence. In addition, recurrences requiring additional surgery occurred twice as fast in the perforating type as in the nonperforating type.[11,12] Patients tend to recur with a similar disease pattern and require repeat surgery for similar indications.[11]

The anatomic site that is affected by Crohn disease is another disease-specific variable that determines recurrence rates. Involvement of the small bowel was associated with an increased risk of recurrence requiring another surgery.[13]

Surgical techniques of anastomosis have also been studied. In several studies, side-to-side stapled ileocolic anastomosis was associated with a lower risk of recurrence than hand-sewn anastomosis. In one large case-control study, ileocolic anastomosis that was made in a side-to-side stapled fashion was associated with 24% recurrence rate, which was significantly lower than the 57% recurrence rate in the group with conventional end-to-end hand-sewn anastomosis.[14] Additional studies have confirmed these results, and they have found that side-to-side anastomosis after ileocolic resection was associated with lower recurrence rates than end-to-end anastomosis.[15,16]

Endoscopic recurrence has been established as one of the greatest objective predictors of clinical recurrence. An endoscopic recurrence score developed by Rutgeerts and colleagues[6] is the most widely accepted scoring system for measuring postoperative recurrence (**Table 1**, **Fig. 1**). It stratifies the endoscopic finding into 5 categories, reflecting a spectrum of disease severity. At 1 year, those with endoscopic findings of the i0 or i1 subtype had a 10% risk of clinical recurrence at 10 years; those with the i2 subtype had a 20% risk, at 10 years; and those with the i3 or i4 subtype had a 50% risk, as early as within 5 years, with many of them requiring surgery.[6]

SURVEILLANCE STRATEGY

Scheduled postoperative assessment for recurrence, to allow for early detection and intervention, is important. There are a range of clinical, laboratory-based, radiological, and endoscopic evaluation parameters that have been assessed. The Crohn disease activity index (CDAI) is a clinical research score that is used to define clinical activity and response to medical therapy. Although the most widely applied activity score in research studies and publications, the CDAI may not accurately predict postoperative Crohn disease recurrence.[17]

Currently, colonoscopy seems to be the best modality for evaluation of mucosal Crohn disease recurrence at the ileocolic anastomosis and neoterminal ileum. Proactive evaluation for endoscopic recurrence often detects mucosal inflammatory changes that precede clinical recurrence. Effective treatment of endoscopically recurrent Crohn disease in the postoperative setting is an area of great research interest. Early treatment of mucosally evident inflammation may prove effective in altering the natural course of disease, with prevention of clinical recurrence and of need for future surgery. It is currently not known whether prophylactic treatment immediately after surgery is more effective than treatment that is based on subsequent endoscopic findings.

MEDICAL TREATMENT TRIALS FOR POSTOPERATIVE CROHN DISEASE

In the following sections, the authors review the data from prospective randomized trials on postoperative prevention of Crohn disease.

Table 1
Endoscopic recurrence score[6]

Endoscopic Score	Definition
i0	No lesions
i1	≤5 aphthous lesions
i2	>5 aphthous lesions with normal mucosa between the lesions, or skip areas of larger lesions, or lesions confined to the ileocolic anastomosis
i3	Diffuse aphthous ileitis with diffusely inflamed mucosa
i4	Diffuse inflammation with already larger ulcers, nodules, and/or narrowing

Remission: endoscopic score of i0 or i1; Recurrence: endoscopic score of i2–i4.
From Rutgeerts P, Geboes K, Vantrappen G, et al. Predictability of the postoperative course of Crohn's disease. Gastroenterology 1990;99:956–83; with permission.

I1   I3   I4

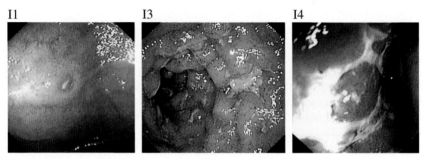

Fig. 1. Endoscopic view of recurrence score (example of I1, I3, and I4 findings).

5-Aminosalicylic Acid Medications

5-Aminosalicylic acid (5-ASA) medications have been most extensively studied in postoperative treatment of Crohn disease. Despite several randomized trials evaluating the efficacy of 5-ASAs in the prevention of postoperative recurrence, the benefit of these agents has not been uniformly established. This is probably due to the heterogeneity of trial designs and the drug preparations and doses that are administered in the studies.

Early randomized trials on the use of sulfasalazine (salazosulfapyridine) did not show benefit of its use in the postoperative setting.[18,19] In the largest study of 5-ASAs in the postoperative setting by Lochs and colleagues,[20] patients either received 5-ASA (mesalamine 4 g/d) or placebo over 18 months after initial surgery for Crohn disease. The clinical recurrence rates were lower in the 5-ASA–treated group than in the control group (24.5% vs 31.4%; $P = .10$), but they did not reach statistical significance. In another randomized trial, 5-ASA (mesalamine 2.4 g/d) did reduce symptomatic recurrence rates at 24 months of follow-up (18% vs 41% among those receiving mesalamine vs placebo; $P = .006$).[21] Regarding endoscopic recurrence, Florent and colleagues[22] found that mesalazine (1 g, 3 times a day) did not significantly reduce endoscopic recurrence rates at 12 weeks (50% vs 63%; $P = .16$).

Ewe and colleagues[23] found that sulfasalazine (3 g/d) significantly reduced clinical recurrence rates at 1 year (16% vs 28%; $P<.01$), and this effect was sustained at 2 years of follow-up. In another large multicenter randomized trial, Brignola and colleagues[24] found that 12 months of mesalazine (3 g/d) was associated with lower rates of endoscopic recurrence and severity score. However, clinical recurrence rates were similar in the 2 groups. In another study, 5-ASA (mesalamine 3 g/d) was found to significantly reduce symptomatic recurrence rates (31% vs 41%; $P = .031$) and endoscopic and radiological recurrence rates.[25] In this study, 5-ASA was generally safe, with only 1 case of serious side effects (pancreatitis).

Recently, a double-blind, randomized, multicenter trial was performed to evaluate efficacy of different doses of mesalazine in preventing postoperative endoscopic and clinical recurrence.[26] Two hundred six patients, who had undergone surgery for terminal ileum involvement, were randomized to receive 4.0 g/d or 2.4 g/d of mesalazine, 2 weeks after surgery. At 12 months after surgery, endoscopic recurrence was more frequent in the 2.4 g/d group than in the 4.0 g/d group, but clinical recurrence rates were similar in the 2 groups.

A meta-analysis of available trials suggests that 5-ASA reduces overall postoperative recurrence rates by only 13%.[27] Therefore, the current evidence indicates that the 5-ASAs are generally safe for postoperative Crohn disease prophylaxis, but they may only slightly reduce clinical and endoscopic recurrence.

Nitroimidazole Antibiotics

Rutgeerts and colleagues[28] studied the efficacy of metronidazole after ileocecal resection for Crohn disease, in a placebo-controlled randomized fashion. Metronidazole (20 mg/kg/d) was started within 1 week of surgery and was administered for 3 months. Endoscopic recurrence rates and severity at 3 months were evaluated. The metronidazole group had lower incidence of early endoscopic recurrence of Crohn disease in the neoterminal ileum, compared with placebo group (75% vs 52%; $P = .09$). Compared with the placebo group, metronidazole significantly reduced the clinical recurrence rates at 1 year (4% vs 25%).[28] However, patients in the metronidazole arm experienced more frequent side effects (23.3% vs 6.7%). In another study using ornidazole (1 g/d), the same group found significantly lower clinical recurrence rates in the treatment group, compared with the placebo group, at 12 months (7.9% vs 37.5%; $P = .0046$).[29] Ornidazole also significantly reduced endoscopic recurrence rates at 12 months (53.6% vs 79%; $P = .037$), and endoscopic findings at 3 and 12 months predicted clinical course. In terms of side effects, however, the ornidazole group was associated with a higher rate of discontinuation of therapy, compared with the placebo group (31.6% vs 12.5%). Unlike the 5-ASAs, the nitroimidazole antibiotics may have a role in preventing postoperative Crohn disease recurrence, but long-term tolerance of these agents is limited.

Budesonide

In 2 large randomized trials, oral budesonide was found to be ineffective in reducing recurrence rates. In both studies, the frequency of clinical recurrences was similar in the budesonide group and the placebo group at 3 and 12 months.[30,31] Ewe and colleagues[31] found that the endoscopic and clinical recurrence rates after 1 year were not significantly different in the treatment group, compared with the placebo group. Hellers and colleagues[30] found that the endoscopic recurrence rates did not differ between the groups at 3 and 12 months. However, they found significantly lower endoscopic recurrence rates in the subgroup of patients who underwent surgery for inflammatory Crohn disease, but not in the subgroup whose surgical indication was a fibrostenotic stricture. Overall, data are lacking in support of budesonide use for prevention of Crohn disease in the postoperative setting.

6-Mercaptopurine/Azathioprine

Immunomodulators, such as 6-mercaptopurine (6MP) and azathioprine (AZA) are commonly used to maintain medically induced remission in Crohn disease. In a randomized open-label study, AZA (2 mg/kg/d) was compared with mesalamine (3 g/d) as a secondary preventive treatment after bowel resection for Crohn disease.[32] The clinical relapse rates were similar in the 2 groups at 24 months. In a subgroup analysis, patients with a prior history of bowel resections benefited more from AZA than from mesalamine in the prevention of clinical relapse, with an odds ratio of 4.83. However, significantly more patients receiving AZA experienced side effects than those receiving mesalamine (22% vs 8%). In another study, Hanauer and colleagues[33] randomized 131 patients after bowel resection and ileocolic anastomosis to placebo, mesalamine (3 g/d), or 6MP (50 mg/d). They found that clinical recurrence at 2 years was 50% in the 6MP group, 58% in mesalamine group, and 77% in the placebo group. However, this study also demonstrated the limitation of 6MP as a prophylactic therapy; only 69% of patients were able to complete the treatment course and were evaluable at the end of the study, because of the significant side effects of 6MP. These 2 studies show that immunomodulators are more effective than mesalamine in the prevention of postoperative recurrence, albeit with a higher side-effect profile.

A regimen that combined an immunosuppressive drug with an antibiotic was studied in a double-blind randomized trial. Eighty-one patients were given metronidazole (250 mg, 3 times a day) for 3 months. The patients were then randomized to receive either AZA (100 mg/d for body weight<60 kg or 150 mg/d for body weight>60 kg) or placebo for 12 months. The endoscopic recurrence rates were significantly lower at 12 months in the group which was given AZA and metronidazole, compared with the metronidazole-alone group (69% vs 44%; P = .048).[34]

Biologic Therapy

The use of infliximab in Crohn disease has been a major therapeutic advance and is effective for fistulizing disease and for the induction and maintenance of remission in patients with moderately to severely active Crohn disease. In a double-blind placebo-controlled trial to assess efficacy of infliximab in the postoperative setting, infliximab significantly reduced recurrence rates after ileocolic resection.[35] In this study, patients who underwent surgery for Crohn disease were randomized to either infliximab (5 mg/kg administered as a standard 3-dose induction, with a maintenance dose every 8 weeks) or placebo for 1 year. Infliximab or placebo was started within 4 weeks of surgery. Corticosteroids and antibiotics were discontinued within 12 weeks of surgery. AZA, 6MP, or 5-ASA products were continued as long as the patients were maintained on stable doses for at least 12 weeks before starting the study. The study found that 9.1% in the infliximab group developed endoscopic recurrence, compared with 84.6% in the placebo group (P = .0006). Furthermore, the infliximab patients had a lower risk of endoscopic, histologic, and clinical recurrence at 1 year. Further study is needed to confirm the results from this small study and determine the length of infliximab treatment that is required beyond 1 year.

SUMMARY OF MEDICAL TREATMENT TRIALS FOR POSTOPERATIVE CROHN DISEASE

There is a wide range of efficacy response between medications and within treatment groups (**Table 2**). Much of this disparity probably results from the wide variation in study design and definition of outcomes. Most postoperative studies define recurrence by endoscopic and clinical recurrence, but the time to recurrence and duration of trials vary widely. Thus, there may be large ranges of therapeutic efficacy for any given agent, which may not be dissimilar to placebo ranges. Weighing the risk and

Table 2		
Clinical and endoscopic 1-year recurrence rates from randomized treatment trials		
Medication Class	Clinical Recurrence (%)	Endoscopic Recurrence (%)
Placebo	25–77	53–79
5-ASA	24–58	63–66
Budesonide	19–32	52–57
Nitroimidazole	7–8	52–54
AZA/6MP	34–50	42–44
Infliximab	0	9

Data from Regueiro M. Management and prevention of postoperative Crohn's disease. Inflamm Bowel Dis 2009;15:1583–90.

benefit of any given medication and the associated costs are important factors in deciding which postoperative treatment is most appropriate.

MANAGEMENT OF POSTOPERATIVE CROHN DISEASE

Management of postoperative Crohn disease presents a difficult treatment dilemma. Although it is common for Crohn disease to recur postoperatively, not all patients have recurrence and some may not require treatment. The authors recommend stratifying patients' risk to determine which medication is most appropriate. Additionally, colonoscopic inspection of the ileocolic anastomosis within 1 year of surgery is suggested. In any postoperative management strategy, cigarette-smoking cessation is imperative and is currently the only known modifiable risk factor.

The authors recommend selecting treatment that is based on the individual patient's risk of recurrence and stratifying patients into high, moderate, and low risk of recurrence. The authors propose the treatment algorithm shown in **Fig. 2**.[36] For those at very low risk of recurrence, that is, those with a longstanding history of Crohn disease who come to their first surgery for a short stricture, no maintenance medication may be necessary. The authors typically perform a colonoscopy 6 to 12 months postoperatively, and if there is significant endoscopic recurrence, they would start immunomodulators or anti-TNF (tumor necrosis factor) therapy; if there is no recurrence, then the authors repeat a colonoscopy 1 to 3 years later.

For those at low-to-moderate risk of disease recurrence, that is, those with less than 10 years of disease duration, a long stricture (>10 cm), or significant inflammation, the authors suggest 6MP/AZA, with or without a 3-month course of metronidazole. If there

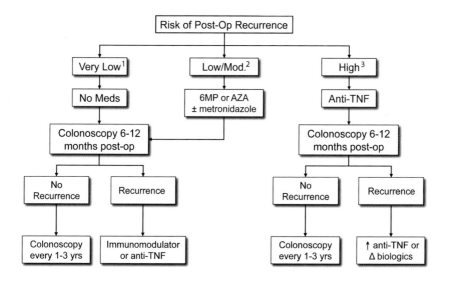

1. Long-standing CD, 1st surgery, short stricture
2. <10yrs CD, long stricture or inflammatory CD
3. Penetrating disease, > 2 surgeries

Fig. 2. Assessment and management of postoperative Crohn disease. (*Data from* Regueiro M. Management and prevention of postoperative Crohn's disease. Inflamm Bowel Dis 2009;15:1583–90.)

is evidence of endoscopic recurrence within 12 months after surgery, then anti-TNF therapy is recommended.

For those at high risk of recurrence, that is, those with penetrating disease and more than 2 intestinal resections, postoperative anti-TNF therapy is recommended. The authors typically initiate anti-TNF treatment after the postoperative visit with the surgeon; this is usually 2 to 4 weeks after surgery. If endoscopic surveillance reveals disease recurrence, then the authors either intensify the dose of anti-TNF therapy or change to another agent.

SUMMARY

Postoperative Crohn disease recurrence is common. Several factors, such as smoking status, disease phenotype, type of surgical anastomosis, and endoscopic disease activity have been associated with risk of recurrence. In the authors' opinion, patients with a high probability of recurrence should receive anti-TNF therapy; those with less severe disease, 6MP/AZA with or without metronidazole; and those at low risk, no treatment. Regardless of postoperative treatment, a colonoscopy within 1 year of surgery is the only definitive way to detect early Crohn disease recurrence.

REFERENCES

1. Bennell O, Lapidus A, Hellers G. Risk factors for surgery and postoperative recurrence in Crohn's disease. Ann Surg 2000;231:38–45.
2. Fazio VW, Marchetti F, Church M, et al. Effect of resection margins on the recurrence of Crohn's disease in the small bowel: a randomized controlled trial. Ann Surg 1996;224:563–71.
3. Sachar DB. The Problem of post operative recurrence of Crohn's disease. Med Clin North Am 1990;74:183–8.
4. Renna S, Camma C, Modesto I, et al. Meta-analysis of the placebo rates of clinical relapse and severe endoscopic recurrence in postoperative Crohn's disease. Gastroenterology 2008;135:1500–9.
5. Olaison G, Smedh K, Sjodahl R. Natural course of Crohn's disease after ileocolic resection: endoscopically visualized ileal ulcers preceding symptoms. Gut 1992; 33:331–5.
6. Rutgeerts P, Geboes K, Vantrappen G, et al. Predictability of the postoperative course of Crohn's disease. Gastroenterology 1990;99:956–83.
7. Cameron JL, Hamilton SR, Coleman J, et al. Patterns of ileal recurrence in Crohn's disease: A prospective randomized study. Ann Surg 1992;546–52.
8. Yamamoto T. Factors affecting recurrence after surgery for Crohn's disease. World J Gastroenterol 2005;11:3971–9.
9. Cosnes J, Carbonnel F, Beaugerie L, et al. Effects of cigarette smoking on the long-term course of Crohn's disease. Gastroenterology 1996;110:424–31.
10. Avidan B, Sakhnini E, Lahat A, et al. Risk factors regarding the need for a second operation in patients with Crohn's disease. Digestion 2005;72:563–71.
11. Greenstein AJ, Lachman P, Sachar DB, et al. Perforating and non-perforating indications for repeated operations in Crohn's disease: evidence for two clinical forms. Gut 1988;29:588–92.
12. Lautenbach E, Berlin JA, Lichtenstein GR. Risk factors for early postoperative recurrence of Crohn's disease. Gastroenterology 1998;115:259–67.
13. Post S, Herfarth C, Bohm E, et al. The impact of disease pattern, surgical management, and individual surgeons on the risk for relaparotomy for recurrent Crohn's disease. Ann Surg 1996;223(3):253–60.

14. Munoz-Juarez M, Yamamoto T, Wolff BG, et al. Wide-lumen stapled anastomosis vs. conventional end-to end anastomosis in the treatment of Crohn's disease. Dis Colon Rectum 2001;44:20–5.
15. Caprilli R, Corrao G, Taddei G, et al. Prognostic factors for postoperative recurrence of Crohn's disease. Gruppo Italiano per lo Studio del Colon e del Retto (GISC). Dis Colon Rectum 1996;39:335–41.
16. Scarpa M, Ruffolo C, Bertin E, et al. Surgical predictors of recurrence of Crohn's disease after ileocolonic resection. Int J Colorectal Dis 2007;22:1061–9.
17. Viscido A, Corrao G, Taddei G, et al. Crohn's disease activity index is inaccurate to detect the post-operative recurrence in Crohn's disease. A GISC study. Ital J Gastroenterol Hepatol 1999;31:274–9.
18. Wenckert A, Kristensen M, Eklund AE, et al. The long-term prophylactic effect of salazosulphapyridine (Salazopyrin) in primarily resected patients with Crohn's disease. A controlled double-blind trial. Scand J Gastroenterol 1978;13:161–7.
19. Summers RW, Switz DM, Sessions JT Jr, et al. National Cooperative Crohn's Disease Study: results of drug treatment. Gastroenterology 1979;77(4 Pt 2):847–69.
20. Lochs H, Mayer M, Fleig WE, et al. Prophylaxis of postoperative relapse in Crohn's disease with mesalamine: European Cooperative Crohn's Disease Study VI. Gastroenterology 2000;118:264–73.
21. Caprilli R, Andreoli A, Capurso L, et al. Oral mesalazine (5-aminosalicylic acid; Asacol) for the prevention of post-operative recurrence of Crohn's disease. Gruppo Italiano per lo Studio del Colon e del Retto (GISC). Aliment Pharmacol Ther 1994;8:35–43.
22. Florent C, Cortot A, Quandale P, et al. Placebo-controlled clinical trial of mesalazine in the prevention of early endoscopic recurrences after resection for Crohn's disease. Groupe d'Etudes Thérapeutiques des Affections Inflammatoires Digestives (GETAID). Eur J Gastroenterol Hepatol 1996;8:229–33.
23. Ewe K, Herfarth C, Malchow H, et al. Postoperative recurrence of Crohn's disease in relation to radicality of operation and sulfasalazine prophylaxis: a multicenter trial. Digestion 1989;42:224–32.
24. Brignola C, Cottone M, Pera A, et al. Mesalamine in the prevention of endoscopic recurrence after intestinal resection for Crohn's disease. Italian Cooperative Study Group. Gastroenterology 1995;108:345–9.
25. Mcleod RS, Wolff BG, Steinhart AH, et al. Prophylactic mesalamine treatment decreases postoperative recurrence of Crohn's disease. Gastroenterology 1995;109:404–13.
26. Caprilli R, Cottone M, Tonelli F, et al. Two mesalazine regimens in the prevention of the post-operative recurrence of Crohn's disease: a pragmatic, double-blind, randomized controlled trial. Aliment Pharmacol Ther 2003;17:517–23.
27. Camma C, Giunta M, Rosselli M, et al. Mesalamine in the maintenance treatment of Crohn's disease: a metaanalysis adjusted for confounding variables. Gastroenterology 1997;113:1465–73.
28. Rutgeerts P, Hiele M, Geboes K, et al. Controlled trial of metronidazole treatment for prevention of Crohn's recurrence after ileal resection. Gastroenterology 1995; 108:1617–21.
29. Rutgeerts P, Van Assache G, Vermeire S, et al. Ornidazole for prophylaxis of post-operative Crohn's disease recurrence: a randomized, double blind, placebo-controlled trial. Gastroenterology 2005;128:856–61.
30. Hellers G, Cortot A, Jewell D, et al. Oral budesonide for prevention of postsurgical recurrence in Crohn's disease. The IOIBD Budesonide Study Group. Gastroenterology 1999;116:294–300.

31. Ewe K, Bottger T, Buhr HJ, et al. Low-dose budesonide treatment for prevention of postoperative recurrence of Crohn's disease: a multicentre randomized placebo-controlled trial. German Budesonide Study Group. Eur J Gastroenterol Hepatol 1999;11:277–82.

32. Ardizzone S, Maconi G, Sampietro GM, et al. Azathioprine and mesalamine for prevention of relapse after conservative surgery for Crohn's disease. Gastroenterology 2004;127:730–40.

33. Hanauer SB, Korelitz BI, Rutgeerts P, et al. Postoperative maintenance of Crohn's disease remission with 6-mercaptopurine, mesalamine, or placebo: a 2-year trial. Gastroenterology 2004;127:723–9.

34. D'Haens G, Vermeire S, Van Assche G, et al. Therapy of metronidazole with azathioprine to prevent postoperative recurrence of Crohn's disease: a controlled randomized trial. Gastroenterology 2008;135(4):1123–9.

35. Regueiro M, Schraut W, Baidoo L, et al. Infliximab prevents Crohn's disease recurrence after ileal resection. Gastroenterology 2009;136:441–50.

36. Regueiro M. Management and prevention of postoperative Crohn's disease. Inflamm Bowel Dis 2009 [Epub ahead of print].

Index

Note: Page numbers of article titles are in **boldface** type.

A

Med Clin N Am 94 (2010) 189–199
doi:10.1016/S0025-7125(09)00147-3
0025-7125/09/$ – see front matter © 2010 Elsevier Inc. All rights reserved.

medical.theclinics.com